Gynecological Oncology: A Comprehensive Outlook

Gynecological Oncology: A Comprehensive Outlook

Editor: Aurora Moran

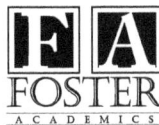

FA
FOSTER
ACADEMICS

www.fosteracademics.com

www.fosteracademics.com

FA
FOSTER
ACADEMICS

Cataloging-in-Publication Data

Gynecological oncology : a comprehensive outlook / edited by Aurora Moran.
    p. cm.
Includes bibliographical references and index.
ISBN 978-1-63242-746-5
1. Generative organs, Female--Cancer. 2. Generative organs, Female--Cancer--Diagnosis.
3. Generative organs, Female--Cancer--Treatment. 4. Oncology. I. Moran, Aurora.
RC280.G5 G85 2019
616.994 65--dc23

Foster Academics,
118-35 Queens Blvd., Suite 400,
Forest Hills, NY 11375, USA

ISBN 978-1-63242-746-5 (Hardback)

Contents

Preface

I am honored to present to you this unique book which encompasses the most up-to-date data in the field. I was extremely pleased to get this opportunity of editing the work of experts from across the globe. I have also written papers in this field and researched the various aspects revolving around the progress of the discipline. I have tried to unify my knowledge along with that of stalwarts from every corner of the world, to produce a text which not only benefits the readers but also facilitates the growth of the field.

Gynecological oncology is a specialized field of medicine, which is concerned with the study, diagnosis and management of cancers of the female reproductive system. Some gynecological cancers are ovarian cancer, uterine cancer, cervical cancer, vaginal cancer and vulvar cancer. Gynecologic ultrasonography, gynoroentgenology and speculoscopy are certain imaging techniques used for detecting gynecological malignancies. Many gynecological malignancies are treated surgically, such as cervical, uterine, ovarian or endometrium tumors and uterine fibroids. Oophorectomy or the surgical removal of the ovaries is frequently combined with hysterectomy to decrease the risk of ovarian cancer or as a therapeutic strategy to treat cancer. In gynecological oncology, the surgical removal of the uterine cervix or cervicectomy is performed as a surgical alternative to radical hysterectomy to treat younger women with cervical cancer. To manage necrosis of the clitoris or remove malignancy of the clitoris, a clitoridectomy is performed. This book is a valuable compilation of topics, ranging from the basic to the most complex advancements in gynecological oncology. It presents researches and studies performed by experts across the globe. Those with an interest in gynecological cancers would find this book helpful.

Finally, I would like to thank all the contributing authors for their valuable time and contributions. This book would not have been possible without their efforts. I would also like to thank my friends and family for their constant support.

Editor

1

The Role of Lymphadenectomy in Ovarian Epithelial Cancer

Hans Nagar

Abstract

High-grade serous ovarian/tubal cancer commonly spreads via the peritoneal and lymphatic routes. This chapter discusses the anatomical lymphatic drainage of the ovary and tube with reference to spread from different epithelial ovarian cancer types. The role of lymph node surgery in apparent early stage curative disease will be discussed with reference to staging and directing the need for adjuvant chemotherapy. In advanced disease, the role of lymph node sampling versus systematic dissection surgery as part of cytoreduction is assessed. The result of two randomised controlled trials (RCTs) published on the subject will be analysed along with the ongoing Lymphadenectomy in Ovarian Neoplasia (LION) study. The chapter adopts an evidence-based approach to the role of lymph node surgery in women with epithelial ovarian/tubal cancer.

Keywords: epithelial ovarian/tubal cancer, high-grade serous, para aortic lymph node, pelvic lymph node, systematic dissection sampling, FIGO staging

1. Introduction

The modern of management of women with ovarian involves complete surgical cytoreduction of all visible disease [1]. It is therefore important to understand that approximately 70% of the women will also have lymphatic spread. Even in disease, apparently confined to one or both ovaries, there is evidence of nodal metastatic spread in up to 24% of women [2].

2. The lymphatic drainage of the ovaries

An understanding of the lymphatic drainage of the ovary and fallopian tube is important in the management of women with ovarian cancer. There are three main lymphatic pathways. The principal pathway is along the ovarian vessels through the infundibulopelvic ligament to the para aortic and para caval nodes surrounding the aorta and inferior vena cava (IVC). The second pathway occurs through the broad ligaments into the pelvic nodal region. Of note, spread to contralateral pelvic nodes in women with a unilateral cancer is reported in up to 30% of women [3]. Therefore, a bilateral pelvic node dissection (PND) is recommended even with unilateral apparent stage 1 tumours.

A third lesser route is through the uterine round ligament to the inguinal nodes. In addition, women with disease involving the rectum or sigmoid colon may have tumour spread to the mesocolic lymph nodes within the sigmoid mesentery.

3. Is histopathological type important?

Over the last decade, the understanding of the pathogenesis of epithelial ovarian cancer has changed. The most common histopathological subtype, high-grade serous cancer (approximately 70–80% of cases) appears to arise in the distal fallopian tube [4]. Most of these women present with disease spread to the transperitoneal surfaces and to the lymph system. The majority of this chapter will be concerned with the role of lymphadenectomy in this group of women.

Less common types of ovarian cancer include endometrioid, clear cell, low grade serous and mucinous tumours. These appear to have separate aetiologies with a different risk of lymphatic spread. The risk of nodal metastases appears to be lower in endometrioid and mucinous cancers. For example, a meta-analysis of 278 women with apparent early mucinous cancer of the ovary who underwent a full pelvic and para aortic nodal dissection reported an incidence of involved nodes of only 1.2% [5]. Most authors no longer recommend a lymphadenectomy in early mucinous cancers.

4. What are the methods of surgical assessment?

A definition of a pelvic node dissection (PND) is widely accepted in the gynaecological oncology literature [6]. PND includes bilateral removal of nodal tissue from the distal one-half of each common iliac artery, the anterior and medial aspect of the external iliac artery and vein to the level of the deep circumflex artery, and obturator fat pad anterior to the obturator nerve. The medial aspect of the dissection is the hypogastric artery. Enlarged nodes below the obturator nerve should also be removed. The obturator nerve should be identified and guarded prior to any sharp dissection. The nodes should be swept away from the nerve with careful attention paid to the area below the nerve to avoid damage to the numerous vessels present in this area. The ideal scenario is to remove the node in a single nodal unit to reduce the risk of nodal fracture leading to possible tumour dissemination and port site metastases. A PND may be performed either as an open procedure or as part of a laparoscopic procedure. Laparoscopic surgery lends itself to PND due to the increased magnification and illumination of the surgical field and dissected nodes can be removed through an 11/12 mm suprapubic port or removed via the vagina if a hysterectomy is performed.

Para aortic assessment/dissection has in contrast to pelvic nodes not been well quantified. Pomel et al. [7] have published a proposed classification of para aortic node assessment which ranges from radiological assessment and palpation to a full systematic dissection of all nodal tissue including the dorsal surfaces of the vessel (**Table 1**).

Open para aortic dissection (type A1 to B1) requires a generous midline abdominal incision to the xiphisternum and a self-retaining retractor to allow access to the great vessels. The right side of the colon and small bowel are mobilised by incising the peritoneum at the level of the right common iliac artery extending medially and caudally to the fourth part of the duodenum and then incising the peritoneum along the right paracolic gutter to the hepatic flexure. This allows the surgeon to perform called 'Kocher manoeuvre' mobilising the bowel off both the right renal fascia and ureter and to be retracted out of the abdomen. Following this, the surgeon should identify the left ureter lying medially underneath the inferior mesenteric vein. The node dissection should not start until all the important anatomical structures have been identified including the inferior mesenteric artery (IMA).

Laparoscopic PA node dissection is well described in the literature and can be performed either via the conventional transperitoneal route or via an extra peritoneal route. Both routes require a high degree of laparoscopic training and is considered unlikely to replicate a systematic node dissection (Pommel type A) but rather an extensive node sampling (Pommel type B1–2).

Type	
A	**Systematic para aortic node dissection**
A1	Complete (includes infrarenal and suprarenal up to coeliac trunk to midpoint of common iliac vessels)
A2	Infrarenal (as above, but does not include suprarenal dissection)
A3	Infra inferior mesenteric artery (IMA) (as above but does not include dissection above IMA)
B	**Para aortic sampling**
B1	Extensive (incudes para aortic areas, but does not allow full visualisation of structures—adventicia of vessels. Renal vessels, anterior common vertebral ligament, psoas muscle and sacrum
B2	Minimal (includes limited para aortic areas, and does not allow visualisation of structures above)
C	**Non-excisional assessment**
C1	Palpation (direct) following full exposure of PA area
C2	Palpation (indirect), transperitoneal without any exposure
C3	Radiological assessment by PET/CT or MRI

Table 1. Proposed classification of para aortic node assessment (Pomel et al. [7]).

5. What is the role of lymphadenectomy in apparent early stage ovarian cancer?

A number of women will undergo surgery for an apparently benign ovarian cyst. Postoperatively, those women with confirmed malignancy can be offered staging including lymphadenectomy. Approximately, 30% of women with ovarian cancers apparently confined to the ovaries will be upstaged following further surgery including a pelvic/para aortic node dissection/sampling (Pommel type B1) with a gynaecological oncologist [8].

It is important to understand that lymph node status is not the only factor that determines the need for adjuvant chemotherapy. Many centres offer chemotherapy to women with stage Ic or above cancers, high-grade lesions and all clear cell cancers of the ovary [9].

However, node status is important for a number of reasons: it may influence whether or not chemotherapy is given, the number of cycles or types of chemotherapy and it may result in complete cytoreduction of the cancer. Node status also partially determines the true FIGO stage and prognosis.

The ACTION trial was a randomised controlled trial (RCT) of 448 women with stage IA, IB grades 2–3, all IC, IIA and all clear cell cancer stage I–IIA and compared the administration of adjuvant chemotherapy with a control arm. The main finding showed overall survival was significantly better with the administration of chemotherapy. A subset analysis revealed that stage I patients with complete surgical staging did not benefit from chemotherapy contrast to patients that underwent incomplete staging [10]. Long-term follow-up of this study has confirmed these results [11]. It has been surmised that patients that have not being staged harbour more advanced disease, and therefore have a poorer prognosis and chemotherapy does not compensate for incomplete staging.

In older women with complex masses or those felt to have a high risk of cancer, an intraoperative frozen section histopathological analysis may be performed. A study from the Gateshead Gynaecological Oncology Centre reported a with a sensitivity of 92%, specificity of 88%, positive predictive value of 82% and negative predictive value of 95% for frozen section analysis [12]. This is equally important in determining which women should not be exposed to unnecessary surgery such as a para aortic node dissection.

Laparoscopic staging is possible, though requires a high degree of specialist training. Several centres have reported on full laparoscopic staging and have found it feasible [13, 14]. Chi et al. performed a case control study comparing staging via laparoscopy or laparotomy in 80 women [13]. They found no difference in specimen sizes and lymph nodal counts. The laparoscopic group had levels of reduced blood loss and a reduced hospital stay. A laparoscopic nodal dissection/sampling should include both the pelvic and para aortic basins to the level of the renal vessels. A case series by Nezhat et al. [15] concluded that laparoscopic staging when performed by a gynaecological oncologist did not compromise survival.

Robotically assisted laparoscopic surgery is an evolution of minimal access surgery rather than a revolution. Perceived benefits include three-dimensional vision, control of the laparoscope by the operating surgeon, more precise instrument movement and a shortened learning curve. Perhaps, the biggest advantage is the use of instruments that fully articulate at the end in the manner of a human wrist allowing fine delicate movements. This is particularly important in the obese patient, where the increased thickness of the anterior abdominal wall produces an increased torque effect leading to decrease manoeuvrability of standard laparoscopic instruments. Robotic platforms have been used in staging apparent ovarian cancer and appear comparable to laparoscopic surgery [16–19].

Maggioni et al. [20] reported a randomised controlled trial of 268 women with apparent stage 1 or 2 ovarian epithelial cancer. The women were randomised to either a random sampling of pelvic and PA nodal basin or systematic dissection (pommel type A) of the same areas. Positive nodes were found in 9% of the control group and in 22% of the SLD group. No significant difference was recorded in 5 years year overall survival (84.2 vs. 81.3%) or progression free survival (PFS) (78.3 vs. 71.3). The SLD group had a significantly longer operating time, blood loss and blood transfusion.

In view of the results of this study, SLD should not be offered over more limited dissection/ sampling (pommel B) in women with apparent early ovarian cancer.

6. What is the role of lymphadenectomy in advanced ovarian cancer?

The goal of surgery in advanced ovarian cancer is to remove all visible disease including a removal of all enlarged lymph nodes. This requires intraoperative assessment of the bilateral pelvic nodes and the para aortic region (pommel type C1–B1).

Given that the nodal basin is considered by some to be relatively chemotherapy insensitive, this to the question whether removal of all involved microscopically and macroscopically involved nodes has a therapeutic benefit.

Panici et al. [21] reported a randomised controlled trial of 268 women with apparent stage IIIB, IIIC/IV cancer. The women were randomised to either resection bulky of pelvic and PA nodes or systematic dissection of the same areas. Positive nodes were found in 42% of the control group and in 42% of the SLD group. No significant difference was recorded in 5 years year overall survival (47 vs. 48.4%). A significant 7-month extension in progression free survival (PFS) was demonstrated (29.4 vs. 22.4 months). The SLD group had a significantly longer operating time, blood loss and blood transfusion. Subsequently, the authors have suggested that the study may be underpowered to detect an overall survival difference.

7. Common complications

7.1. Vascular injury

Working in close proximity to the large blood vessels poses a risk of major haemorrhage. Reducing this risk involves an appropriate surgical incision with a good operative exposure involving dissection/identification of anatomical structures. This allows easier identification of vascular anomalies and reduces the risk of collateral damage to structures such as the kidney and ureter. Initial management includes pressure to the area and appropriate communication with the rest of the team including the anaesthetist. Small vascular injuries may be oversewn using a vascular needle and small monofilament suture, ideally avoiding constricting the vessel's diameter. Larger defects require the vascular clamp and the expertise of a vascular surgeon.

7.2. Lymphocyst formation

The incidence of lymphocyst after the para aortic/pelvic dissection maybe as high as 43% [22]. The vast majority of these will resolve spontaneously and do not require any intervention. Occasionally, a larger lymphocyst may require aspiration typically by interventional radiological drainage. Occasionally, chylous ascites develop in association with an aortic node dissection especially at the level of the renal vessels. This illustrates the importance clipping large lymphatic channels especially in this region. Management of how chylous ascites includes the low-fat diet, the administration of somatosatin and occasionally total parenteral nutrition.

7.3. Other complications

Other complications associated with lymph node dissection include postoperative ileus, damage to the duodenum, damage to relevant nerves and long-term lymphoedema.

8. Ongoing research into lymphadenectomy

8.1. Early stage ovarian/tubal cancer

Serous tubal intraepithelial carcinoma (STIC) is now considered the precursor lesion for high-grade serous cancer [4]. STIC may be an incidental finding in women undergoing a salpingectomy for benign reasons and the incidence is expected to rise in women undergoing risk reducing surgery for ovarian/tubal cancer. The management of women with STIC as an incidental finding it is unclear. It is apparent, the percentage of these women will have disseminated spread of high-grade serious cancer. Based on small series, authors have suggested comprehensive surgical staging including lymphadenectomy [23, 24]. This is relatively a new condition with larger case series publication expected over the next few years.

8.2. Advanced stage cancer

Following the Panici study reporting a significant difference in PFS, the role of a full systematic node dissection is the subject of two randomised controlled trials, the Lymphadenectomy in Ovarian Neoplasia (LION) and CURACO trials [21].

The Lymphadenectomy in Ovarian Neoplasia (LION) study is an AGO randomised controlled trial including women with FIGO stage IIB–IV ovarian epithelial cancer and complete macroscopic resection of all disease. Around 640 women were randomised to either a full systematic lymph node (SLN) or no lymph node dissection and the study results are due in late 2017. The primary end point is overall survival (OS) and secondary endpoints include progression free survival (PFS) and quality of life (QOL).

The French CURACO trial is a randomised controlled trial including women with stage III–IV epithelial ovarian cancer with complete macroscopic resection. The women are being randomised to SLN versus no node dissection. The primary end point is progression free survival.

9. Conclusion

Spread to the lymphatic system is common in epithelial ovarian cancer is common and is an early event. Para aortic and bilateral pelvic node dissection sampling (Pommel type B1) should be included in surgical staging to determine chemotherapy use and to improve prognosis in ovarian cancer apparently confined to the ovary based on the results of the ACTION trial.

In women with advanced ovarian, the retroperitoneal lymph nodes should be assessed and bulky lymph nodes removed in an attempt to achieve complete cytoreduction. Systematic lymph node (SLN) of the para aortic nodes should not be routinely performed pending the results of the LION and CURACO studies.

Author details

Hans Nagar

Address all correspondence to: hans.nagar@mac.com

Northern Ireland Cancer Centre, Belfast Trust, UK

References

[1] Elattar A, Bryant A, Winter-Roach BA, et al. Optimal primary surgical treatment for advanced epithelial ovarian cancer. The Cochrane Database of Systematic Reviews. 2011; 8:CD007565. DOI: 10.1002/14651858.CD007565.pub2

[2] Burghardt E, Girardi F, Lahousen M, et al. Patterns of pelvic and paraaortic lymph node involvement in ovarian cancer. Gynecologic Oncology. 1991;**40**(2):103-106

[3] Cass I, Li AJ, Runowicz CD, et al. Pattern of lymph node metastases in clinically unilateral stage I invasive epithelial ovarian carcinomas. Gynecologic Oncology. 2001;**80**(1):56-61. DOI: 10.1006/gyno.2000.6027

[4] Carlson JW, Miron A, Jarboe EA, et al. Serous tubal intraepithelial carcinoma: Its potential role in primary peritoneal serous carcinoma and serous cancer prevention. Journal of Clinical Oncology. 2008;**26**(25):4160-4165. DOI: 10.1200/JCO.2008.16.4814

[5] Hoogendam JP, Vlek CA, Witteveen PO, Verheijen R, Zweemer RP. Surgical lymph node assessment in mucinous ovarian carcinoma staging: a systematic review and meta-analysis. BJOG. 2017;**124**(3):370-8

[6] CW Whitney, N Spirtos. Gynecologic Oncology Group Surgical Procedures Manual. Philadelphia: Gynecologic Oncology Group; 2010

[7] Pomel C, Naik R, Martinez A, et al. Systematic (complete) para-aortic lymphadenectomy: Description of a novel surgical classification with technical and anatomical considerations. BJOG. 2012;**119**(2):249-253. DOI: 10.1111/j.1471-0528.2011.03171.x

[8] Young RC, Decker DG, Wharton JT, et al. Staging laparotomy in early ovarian cancer. JAMA. 1983;**250**(22):3072-3076

[9] Chan JK, Tian C, Teoh D, et al. Survival after recurrence in early-stage high-risk epithelial ovarian cancer: A Gynecologic Oncology Group study. Gynecologic Oncology. 2010;**116**(3):307-311. DOI: 10.1016/j.ygyno.2009.10.074

[10] Trimbos JB, Parmar M, Vergote I, et al. International collaborative ovarian neoplasm trial 1 and adjuvant ChemoTherapy in ovarian neoplasm trial: Two parallel randomized phase III trials of adjuvant chemotherapy in patients with early-stage ovarian carcinoma. Journal of the National Cancer Institute. 2003;**95**(2):105-112

[11] Trimbos B, Timmers P, Pecorelli S, et al. Surgical staging and treatment of early ovarian cancer: Long-term analysis from a randomized trial. Journal of the National Cancer Institute. 2010;**102**(13):982-987. DOI: 10.1093/jnci/djq149

[12] Naik R, Cross P, Lopes A, et al. "True" versus "apparent" stage I epithelial ovarian cancer: Value of frozen section analysis. International Journal of Gynecological Cancer. 2006;**16**(Suppl 1):41-46. DOI: IJG312 [pii] 10.1111/j.1525-1438.2006.00312.x [published Online First: 2006/03/07]

[13] Chi DS, Abu-Rustum NR, Sonoda Y, et al. The safety and efficacy of laparoscopic surgical staging of apparent stage I ovarian and fallopian tube cancers. American Journal of Obstetrics and Gynecology. 2005;**192**(5):1614-1619. DOI: 10.1016/j.ajog.2004.11.018

[14] Spirtos NM, Eisekop SM, Boike G, et al. Laparoscopic staging in patients with incompletely staged cancers of the uterus, ovary, fallopian tube, and primary peritoneum: A gynecologic oncology group (GOG) study. American Journal of Obstetrics and Gynecology. 2005;**193**(5):1645-1649. DOI: 10.1016/j.ajog.2005.05.004

[15] Nezhat FR, Ezzati M, Chuang L, et al. Laparoscopic management of early ovarian and fallopian tube cancers: Surgical and survival outcome. American Journal of Obstetrics and Gynecology. 2009;**200**(1):83 e1-83 e6. DOI: 10.1016/j.ajog.2008.08.013

[16] Brown JV 3rd, Mendivil AA, Abaid LN, et al. The safety and feasibility of robotic-assisted lymph node staging in early-stage ovarian cancer. International Journal of Gynecological Cancer. 2014;24(8):1493-1498. DOI: 10.1097/IGC.0000000000000224

[17] Chen CH, Chiu LH, Chen HH, et al. Comparison of robotic approach, laparoscopic approach and laparotomy in treating epithelial ovarian cancer. The International Journal of Medical Robotics. 2016;12(2):268-275. DOI: 10.1002/rcs.1655

[18] Gallotta V, Cicero C, Conte C, et al. Robotic versus laparoscopic staging for early ovarian cancer: A case-matched control study. Journal of Minimally Invasive Gynecology. 2017;24(2):293-298. DOI: 10.1016/j.jmig.2016.11.004

[19] Magrina JF, Zanagnolo V, Noble BN, et al. Robotic approach for ovarian cancer: Perioperative and survival results and comparison with laparoscopy and laparotomy. Gynecologic Oncology. 2011;121(1):100-105. DOI: 10.1016/j.ygyno.2010.11.045

[20] Maggioni A, Benedetti Panici P, Dell'Anna T, et al. Randomised study of systematic lymphadenectomy in patients with epithelial ovarian cancer macroscopically confined to the pelvis. British Journal of Cancer. 2006;95(6):699-704. DOI: 10.1038/sj.bjc.6603323

[21] Panici PB, Maggioni A, Hacker N, et al. Systematic aortic and pelvic lymphadenectomy versus resection of bulky nodes only in optimally debulked advanced ovarian cancer: A randomized clinical trial. Journal of the National Cancer Institute. 2005;97(8):560-566. DOI: 10.1093/jnci/dji102

[22] Tam KF, Lam KW, Chan KK, et al. Natural history of pelvic lymphocysts as observed by ultrasonography after bilateral pelvic lymphadenectomy. Ultrasound in Obstetrics & Gynecology. 2008;32(1):87-90. DOI: 10.1002/uog.5345

[23] Schneider S, Heikaus S, Harter P, et al. Serous tubal intraepithelial carcinoma associated with extraovarian metastases. International Journal of Gynecological Cancer. 2017;27(3):444-451. DOI: 10.1097/IGC.0000000000000920

[24] Chay WY, McCluggage WG, Lee CH, et al. Outcomes of incidental fallopian tube high-grade serous carcinoma and serous tubal intraepithelial carcinoma in women at low risk of hereditary breast and ovarian cancer. International Journal of Gynecological Cancer. 2016;26(3):431-436. DOI: 10.1097/IGC.0000000000000639

2

Secondary Prevention of Uterine Cervical Cancer

Seiya Sato and Hiroaki Itamochi

Abstract

Secondary prevention by cervical cytology has clearly improved the mortality rate of uterine cervical cancer (CC) by enabling early detection and treatment of high-grade squamous intraepithelial lesion (HSIL) or cervical intraepithelial neoplasia (CIN), which is a precancerous lesion. In the past two decades, HPV-DNA testing, including HPV typing, has clearly brought about positive effects on secondary prevention of CC. However, in practice, CC remains a fatal disease and is the second leading cause of cancer deaths in women aged 20–39 years. Although elucidation of the mechanisms of HPV carcinogenesis and development of a prophylactic vaccine have made CC a preventable disease, eradication of CC is expected to take several decades. Therefore, primary screening to decrease the mortality rate of CC will remain important for a while. In addition, the clinical application of simple biomarkers to stratify HPV-positive women is important for maintenance of medical economy and avoidance of overtreatment in women in the reproductive age. Therefore, the development of an inexpensive therapy or vaccine that can be used worldwide is necessary to overcome cancer deaths due to CC.

Keywords: uterine cervical cancer, cervical intraepithelial neoplasia, secondary prevention, human papillomavirus, carcinogenesis, biomarker, therapeutic vaccine

1. Introduction

Secondary prevention with the use of cervical cytology has clearly improved the mortality rate and early treatment of uterine cervical cancer (CC) by enabling early detection of high-grade squamous intraepithelial lesion (HSIL) or cervical intraepithelial neoplasia (CIN), which is a precancerous lesion [1]. In practice, however, CC was estimated to have 12,820 newly diagnosed cases and 4210 women dying of the disease in 2017 [2]. Moreover, according to the United States data in 2014, CC is the second leading cause of cancer deaths in women aged 20–39 years [2]. Therefore, improvement of screening efficiency remains an important issue.

The etiology of CC is persistent uterine cervical infection with the high-risk human papillomavirus (hrHPV). Therefore, HPV-DNA testing or HPV testing, has become widely used for primary screening of CC. Compared with conventional cytology, HPV testing has higher sensitivity and reproducibility in detecting lesions [3]. However, the specificity of HPV testing is low, with an increase in the number of false-positives, especially in women in their twenties who are highly sexually active [3, 4]. Therefore, HPV testing has been adopted in cancer screening for women over 30 years old. In fact, in the United States (US), the guidelines created by the American Cancer Society, American Society for Clinical Pathology, and American Society for Colposcopy and Cervical Pathology suggested CC screening by cytology starting at the age of 21 and every 3 years until 30 years old; beyond the age of 30, combined HPV testing and cytology for every 5 years was recommended [5]. Based on data from large-scale, longitudinal, randomized-controlled trials in European countries, HPV testing has been adopted as the primary screening tool for CC in women aged 30 years or older [6–9]; in those who are tested positive for HPV, cytology is used as the triage test. In ASC-US cases, HPV testing is performed for triage in the management of CIN, based on the results of available large-scale clinical studies [10–13]. Furthermore, HPV typing has already been used as a biomarker for decisions on therapeutic interventions and subsequent follow-up of CIN [14–19]. Both the US and European guidelines recommended HPV testing to confirm the completion of treatment of CIN.

HPVs are classified according to carcinogenic potential. In general, the frequently reported high-risk types are HPV 16, 18, 31, 33, 35, 39, 45, 51, 52, 56, 58, 59, 66, and 68 [20]. Among these, HPV 16 and 18 are the most common types that are related to carcinogenesis worldwide; both HPV types are controllable by prophylactic vaccines that contain virus-like particles with antigenicity [21, 22]. Bivalent vaccines for HPV 16 and 18 are commercially available, but quadrivalent vaccines are also available for HPV 6, 11, 16, and 18. Although these vaccines have some cross-protective effects [23, 24], these are basically ineffective for infection by all HPV types. To overcome these limitations, a nonavalent vaccine containing HPV 6, 11, 16, 18, 31, 33, 45, 52, and 58 has been launched [25, 26].

As mentioned above, hrHPV testing has clearly brought about positive effects on early detection of CIN and prevention of CC in the past two decades [27–30]. Several researchers all over the world continue to pursue efforts to eradicate CC. **Figure 1** shows the schema of the natural

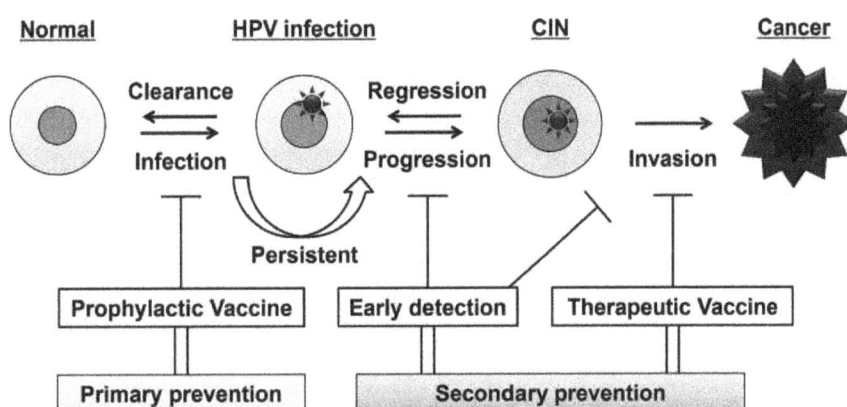

HPV: Human papillomavirus, CIN: Cervical intraepithelial neoplasia

Figure 1. Natural history of HPV and prevention of cervical cancer. Persistent infection of the cervix with high-risk HPV causes cervical cancer (CC), which begins as cervical intraepithelial neoplasia (CIN). Primary prevention of CC can be achieved by prophylactic HPV vaccination. Secondary prevention consists of early detection of CIN and therapeutic vaccination to inhibit progression from CIN to CC.

history of HPV and CC prevention. In this chapter, we will describe the recent developments in secondary prevention of CC.

2. Biology and carcinogenesis of HPV

HPV is a virus with a double-stranded circular DNA in the icosahedral capsid. The genome size is about 8000 bases and contains eight protein-coding genes and a noncoding, regulatory long control region [31]. The early genes (E1, E2, E4, E5, E6, and E7) encode nonstructural proteins involved in replication, transcription, and transformation; whereas the late genes (L1 and L2) encode viral capsid proteins. Among these genes, E6 and E7 play a central role, particularly in carcinogenesis. Notably, a recent whole-genome sequencing study that assessed the risk of viral genetic variation showed that strict preservation of the 98 amino acids of E7, which destroys the function of the retinoblastoma protein (pRB), was critical for HPV 16 carcinogenesis and development of CIN and CC [32].

HPV can infect the epithelial cells of the human mucosa and skin at least once in most women's lives. In other words, HPV infection is a common sexually transmitted disease. Because prophylactic vaccines prevent only initial infection, its value in women is most effective before the first sexual contact [33]. In the early stages of HPV infection, the host is asymptomatic, and in most cases, the virus is eliminated by the immune system within a few years [34]. However, HPV infection can persist in some patients. The reported risk factors for progression of cervical HPV infection to CIN or CC include persistent hrHPV infection, immunosuppression, age over 30 years, and smoking [35].

Persistent hrHPV infection of the cervix is divided into three stages: latent, permissive, and transforming [36–38]. First, HPV invades the epithelial basal cells via minor breaches of the epithelium [39] and become latent as a nuclear episome; the infected cells usually die after virus multiplication. The E6 and E7 genes are rarely integrated into cellular DNA and cause HPV growth in the cells; however, this property also allows continued expression of E6 and E7 proteins at high levels. The expression of E6 and E7 oncogenes in basal cells is tightly controlled; therefore, HPV-infected cells can escape a host's immune defense. In fact, in a small percentage of HPV-infected women, HPV-specific antibodies and T cells are detected at low levels [40, 41]. Recently, it was suggested that the programmed death 1/programmed death 1 ligand (PD-1/PD-L1) pathway might be involved in the mechanism of this immune evasion [42–44].

When infected cells begin to differentiate in the epidermis, the E6 proteins degrade the tumor suppressor protein p53, while the E7 proteins inhibit the function of the pRB; these processes reactivate DNA synthesis and replication of the HPV genome. The cells with integrated E6 and E7 genes will have uncontrolled cell cycles because p53 and pRB are major cell cycle regulators. Furthermore, apoptosis and the tumor suppressor pathway are repressed. During this process, accumulation of genetic mutations and genomic instability ensue [45–50]. As a result, a large number of clones with intratumor heterogeneity are produced, some of which might be able to avoid the host antitumor response [51–54]. Ultimately, with the addition of external factors, these cells will be immortalized and can become cancerous [55].

3. Biomarker for early detection and triage

HPV testing has been introduced for primary screening for CC; it is highly sensitive, but its false-positive rate is high due to the low specificity. Therefore, the need to stratify HPV-positive women with or without abnormal cytology has become a very important issue [56]. At present, HPV-positive women undergo cytology tests and HPV retesting, with colposcopy and tissue biopsy correlations at frequent intervals; however, the precision of this process remains unclear. More objective indicators are required to prevent unnecessary procedures and treatment. As the understanding of the molecular mechanisms of cervical carcinogenesis by HPV has progressed, various biomarkers that predict patient outcomes have been developed not only for early detection but also for triage.

As mentioned earlier, persistent HPV infection of cervical cells leads to tumor formation through several stages. Since HPV infection is often transient, detection of the stage when HPV infection shifts from permissive to transforming is clinically important for cancer screening. Similarly, the histopathologic and molecular diagnostic processes for CIN focus on detection of malignant transformation in HPV-infected cells [57, 58]. The function of HPV-transformed cells is critically dependent on E6 and E7 oncogenes and related molecules such as $p16^{INK4a}$ [59, 60]. Therefore, E6/E7 mRNA and $p16^{INK4a}$ are important targets for early detection and triage. In addition, genetic or epigenetic changes in HPV-transformed cells have been attracting attention as biomarkers for screening of CC, in the triage of HPV-positive women, and as targets of treatment. Because, such new biomarkers can be analyzed from preserved liquid-based cytology (LBC) specimens, their use may be further expanded [61].

3.1. HPV typing

HPV 16 and 18 account for 70% of the causes of CC. The other reported HPV types related to CC are 31, 33, 35, 45, 52, and 58 [62]. Furthermore, the risk of developing CC has been reported to differ according to the type of hrHPV [63]. A cohort study to estimate the risk of disease progression among the HPV genotypes in 570 Japanese women with cytologic low-grade squamous intraepithelial lesion (LSIL) and histologic CIN1/2 showed that the cumulative probability of CIN3 within 5 years was higher in HPV 16, 18, 31, 33, 35, 52, and 58 than in the other hrHPV types [64]. Another Japanese cohort study on cytologic abnormalities, including ASC-US, LSIL, and HSIL (≤CIN2), reported that infection with HPV types 16, 18, and 33 posed a high risk of developing CIN3 [65]. The Japanese gynecologic guideline 2017 recommended HPV typing to evaluate the risk of disease progression for patients with histologically proven CIN1/2 (**Figure 2**). Taken altogether, HPV typing in CIN patients is useful for risk assessment of disease progression [66].

3.2. $p16^{INK4a}$

The $p16^{INK4a}$ is a cyclin-dependent kinase inhibitor that blocks the phosphorylation of various cyclins that control the cell cycle. In many human cancers, including colon and breast, the function of the $p16^{INK4a}$ gene is lost by gene deletions, mutations, or epigenetic silencing. In CC,

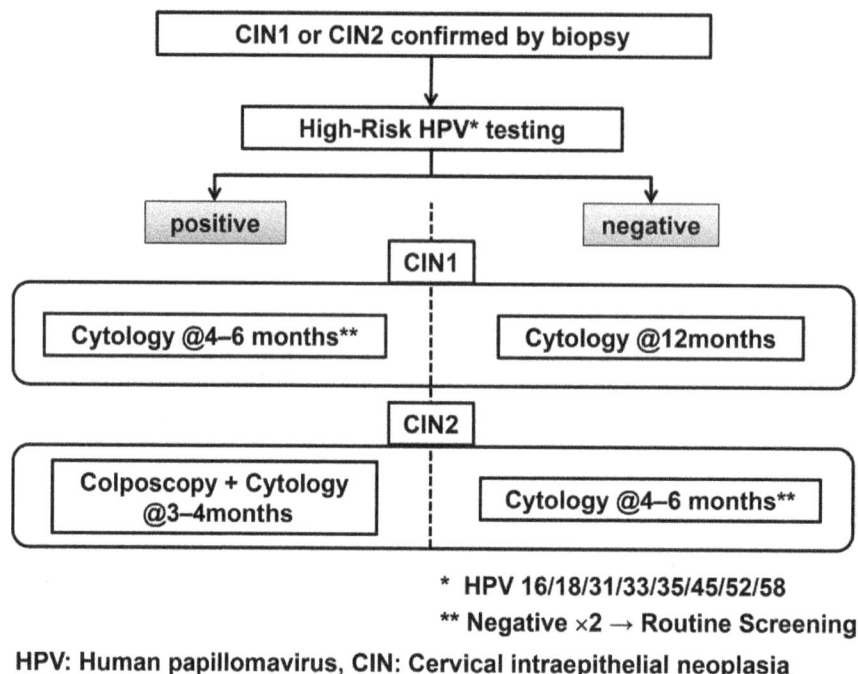

Figure 2. HPV typing for CIN1 and CIN2 in Japan. The Japanese gynecologic guidelines in 2017 recommend HPV typing to evaluate the risk of disease progression in patients with histologically proven CIN1/2. Patients who are positive for high-risk HPV receive more intensive management compared with negative patients.

however, a high level of intracellular E7 expression eliminates the inhibitory methylation mark encoding the CDKN2A gene promoter from p16^{INK4a}, resulting in overexpression of the p16^{INK4a} protein [67]. In addition, since E7 inactivates pRB, there is proliferation of cells that highly express p16^{INK4a}. In other words, high expression of p16^{INK4a} reflects the high expression of E7, which is a good indicator of CIN3 and CC. For this reason, p16^{INK4a} is widely accepted as a valuable surrogate biomarker for the transforming properties of HPV infection [68]. Based on this fact, a therapeutic peptide vaccine using p16^{INK4a} as the antigen has been developed [69]. Moreover, p16^{INK4a} has been used for dual-staining with p16/Ki-67 cytology (p16/Ki-67); this would complement the low sensitivity of cytology and the low specificity of the HPV test for secondary prevention of CC [70–72].

In Europe, p16/Ki-67 was compared with Papanicolaou (Pap) cytology and HPV testing for screening high-grade CIN (CIN2+) in 27,349 women aged 18 years or older; the p16/Ki-67 had high sensitivity and comparable specificity for CIN2 detection, compared with the other tests [73]. This suggested the utility of p16/Ki-67 as a screening method in young women with high HPV infection rates. Other studies showed the effectiveness of p16/Ki-67 as a triage test for CIN2+ detection in Pap-negative and HPV-positive women ≥30 years old [74]. In addition, the usefulness of p16/Ki-67 for follow-up of patients after CIN treatment was suggested [75]. In Germany, a recent study revealed that combined HPV 16/18 testing and p16/Ki-67 resulted in lower cost and clinically efficient CC screening, compared with conventional annual Pap cytology [76]. As described earlier, several evidences on the utility of p16/Ki-67 have accumulated; therefore, p16/Ki-67 will definitely play an important role in the secondary prevention of CC.

3.3. HPV E6/E7 mRNA

The usefulness of HPV E6/E7 mRNA testing in secondary prevention of CC has already been established [77, 78]. Combined testing of LBC cytology and APTIMA® HPV (AHPV) has already been used in the US and Europe. HPV E6/E7 mRNA testing is useful because it can detect HPV infection and the transformation properties of cervical cells. In fact, HPV E6/E7 mRNA testing was reported to detect high-grade CIN with high sensitivity and specificity [79–81].

ASC-US and LSIL on cytology are mainly caused by low-grade cervical lesions that often resolve spontaneously [82]. Currently, the HPV test is used for triage of women with ASC-US and LSIL; however, its low specificity has increased the number of unnecessary examinations and treatment [83]. On the other hand, HPV E6/E7 mRNA testing enables stratification of the risk of developing CIN2+ in women with both hrHPV-positive and hrHPV-negative cytology [84]. A recent meta-analysis to confirm usefulness of HPV E6/E7 mRNA testing for triage revealed that a positive HPV E6/E7 mRNA testing in women with mild cytology findings, such as ASC-US and LSIL, necessitates immediate colposcopy and intensive follow-up because the risk of carcinogenesis is high [85].

3.4. Epigenomic alterations

Epigenetic events in the host and in viral genomic regions and genes are necessary during HPV-mediated cellular transformation and carcinogenesis [86]. DNA methylation is a typical epigenetic change and characterizes the molecular, cellular, and clinical features of HPV-associated neoplasia. Because hypermethylation is a stable and reversible process, detection of methylation marks is used for diagnosis. In addition, new targeted therapies with demethylating compounds have been developed [87].

Combined testing with DNA methylation and hrHPV is one of the promising screening options for CC. The Triage and Risk Assessment of Cervical Precancer by Epigenetic Biomarker (TRACE) study was conducted to examine the usefulness of human epigenetic biomarker testing in the primary prevention of CC. In this study, methylation of the POU4F3 promoter, which is a promising marker for CIN3, showed significantly higher sensitivity and similar specificity for detecting CIN3+, compared with LBC [88]. This finding suggested that detection of POU4F3 methylation is useful for early detection of CIN3. Another study assessed the correlation between CpG methylation of the HPV16 L1 gene and CC in 145 HPV 16-infected Uyghur women who were divided into five groups, as follows: transient infection (n = 32), persistent infection (n = 21), CIN1 (n = 21), CIN2–3 (n = 33), and CC (n = 38) [89]. After quantifying each CPG methylation by pyrosequencing, results revealed that methylation increased at 13 CpG sites in advanced lesions and that high methylation levels were associated with the risk of developing CIN2+ [89]. These findings may be applied to CC screening.

4. Therapeutic vaccine for CIN

Currently, the standard therapy for CIN is surgical excision such as conization or LEEP. Although these treatments are very effective from the viewpoint of removing HPV-induced precancerous lesions, these can cause infertility and menstrual disorders secondary to stenosis of the cervix. In addition, the existing CC prophylactic vaccines are ineffective for HPV-infected women and nontargeted HPV types. Therefore, development of a therapeutic vaccine using immunotherapy as a nonsurgical treatment for CIN is an important strategy for the prevention of CC.

The development of therapeutic vaccines has been mainly targeted for HPV E6 and E7 [90], because these proteins are essential for the malignant transformation of HPV-infected cells and are permanently expressed in CIN. In order to induce an E6 or E7 antigen-specific T cell immune response, several kinds of vaccines have been developed; these include adoptive transfer of tumor-specific T cells, chimeric virus-like particle vaccines, dendritic cell, DNA vaccines, peptide vaccines, protein vaccines, and viral or bacterial vector vaccines. Among these, protein vaccines are the most common therapeutic vaccines for HPV 16 because of the simplicity of the method and the lack of HLA restriction [91]. However, there are currently no available therapeutic HPV vaccines against CIN.

Recently, a randomized, double-blind, placebo-controlled phase 2b trial on CIN2/3 patients showed promising results on the efficacy and safety of VGX-3100, which is a synthetic plasmid targeting human HPV 16 and HPV 18 E6 and E7 proteins (ClinicalTrials. gov Identifier: NCT01304524). In the study, the primary endpoint for efficacy was regression to CIN1 or normal pathology at 36 weeks after the first dose. This study enrolled 167 people who were randomized (3:1) to the VGX-3100 group (n = 125) and the placebo group (n = 42); the rate of histopathologic regression was significantly higher by 18.2% [95% CI 1.3–34.4] in the VGX-3100 group, compared with the placebo group (48.2% vs. 30.0%; p = 0.034). The incidence of erythema at the injection site was significantly higher in the VGX-3100 group than in the placebo group (78.4% vs. 57.1%, p = 0.007). On the other hand, there was no significant increase in the number of severe side effects that could interfere with the performance of vaccine therapy [92]. Therefore, this vaccine might be a nonsurgical therapeutic option for CIN2/3, but further research and development are needed in this field. A clinical trial on HPV therapeutic vaccines was detailed in a recent review [93].

5. Discussion

The mathematical model by a German group estimated that the incidence and mortality of CC will drastically decrease in the next 30 years due to the increasing number of screening participants since the 1990s [94]. Furthermore, even at a vaccination rate of only 50%, more than 40% of CC is considered to be preventable in the next 100 years [94]. Nevertheless, more effective primary prevention is necessary to eradicate CC. Currently, an effective vaccine can be used to inhibit a part of the hrHPV infection process that leads to cancer. However, several individuals cannot receive vaccination due to economic or geographical problems. In order to solve this problem, international cooperation and national policy are necessary to construct a CC prevention system. One possible problem in the future would be the changes in the distribution of hrHPV types due to an increase in the number of vaccinated cohorts; this would likely decrease the efficiency of the current screening system. Therefore, it may be necessary to monitor the distribution of hrHPV in each country and region, and to develop screening methods that are suitable for each situation.

Secondary prevention remains important because vaccines only prevent infection with a limited number of HPV types. In order to reduce the mortality rate of CC, the coverage of a screening program needs to be increased and include patients with advanced CC. To address this issue, the usefulness of self-sampling for HPV testing has been studied [95, 96]. The US National Health and Nutrition Examination Survey in 2007–2010 on women aged 18–59 years revealed a 41.9% prevalence of genital HPV infection [97]. Multivariate analysis in this cohort revealed that HPV infection was related to age, number of sexual partners, smoking, educational level, income, and insurance status [97]. Similar results on the risk of persistent HPV infection have been confirmed in other studies [98, 99]. Therefore, populations with these risk factors require more rigorous and continuous monitoring for effective prevention; in these cases, self-sampling may be particularly useful. Importantly, the hrHPV detection rate by continuous self-sampling of vaginal fluid for 28 days was reported to be consistent regardless of the hormonal cycle [100]. In other words, hrHPV detection by self-sampling can be adapted to all women, even those in the nonmenstrual period, including menopause. A recent meta-analysis of 37 studies including 18,516 women revealed that HPV-DNA sampling screening was highly accepted compared with clinician's sampling. In the future, the importance of self-collection method will increase, especially from the viewpoint

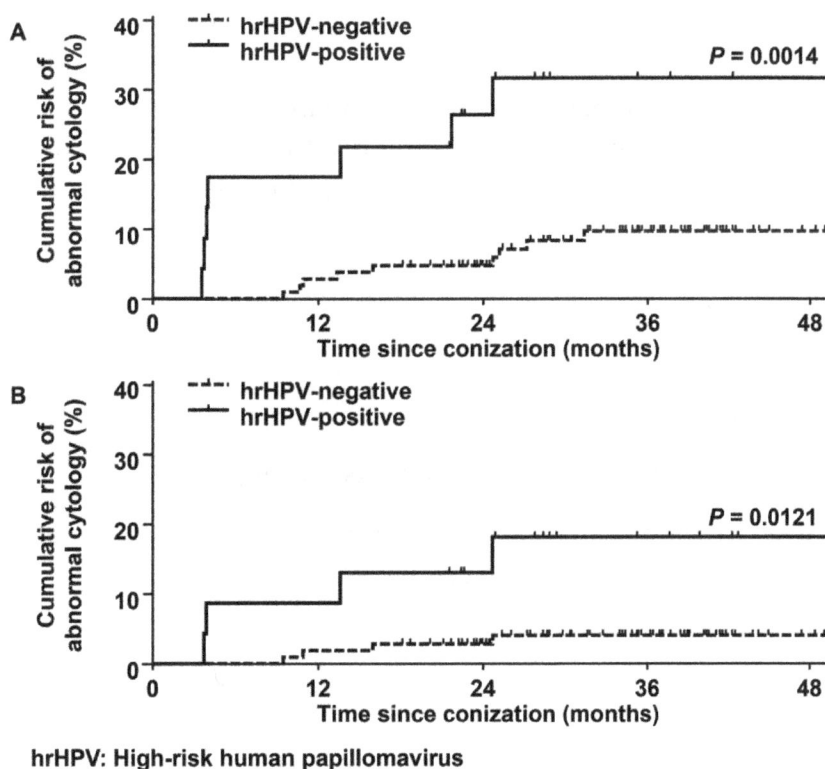

Figure 3. Postoperative infection with high risk (hr) HPV and risk of abnormal cytology. The cumulative risk curves for (a) atypical squamous cells of undetermined significance (ASC-US) or higher and (b) low-grade squamous intraepithelial lesion (LSIL) or higher show that the cumulative risks for recurrence of abnormal cytology and LSIL or higher were significantly increased in postoperative hrHPV-positive patients than in hrHPV-negative patients.

of cost-effectiveness and expansion of screening services [101]. Therefore, HPV-DNA testing by self-sampling has the potential to become the mainstream in cancer prevention.

CIN frequently regresses spontaneously within months or a few years [102, 103]. However, there is no biomarker to predict spontaneous regression of CIN. The standard treatment for CIN is still surgical resection such as conization; for a long time, there had been no other options for treatment. Although surgical excision is successful for CIN treatment most of the time, HPV infection cannot be completely eliminated. We reported that postsurgical hrHPV infection was a positive predictor of the recurrence of abnormal cytology (**Figure 3**). Furthermore, surgical procedure can lead to complications such as pregnancy problems, infertility, incontinence, and sexual dysfunction [104–106]. At the very least, overtreatment of women with fertility must be avoided. With the progression of CC screening, the importance of these problems has increased. In order to overcome this problem, development of a therapeutic vaccine as a new treatment option without surgery is urgently needed. The availability of low-cost therapeutic vaccines for patients with CIN or stage IA CC in the future will lead to a long-term reduction in medical costs [107].

6. Conclusions

Although elucidation of the mechanisms of HPV carcinogenesis and development of a prophylactic vaccine have made CC a preventable disease, eradication of CC is expected to take several decades. To decrease the mortality rate of CC, early detection by screening will remain important for a while. The clinical application of simple biomarkers to stratify HPV-positive women is important for maintenance of medical economy and avoidance of overtreatment of women in the reproductive age. To overcome cancer deaths due to CC, the development of inexpensive treatment options or therapeutic vaccines that can be readily used worldwide is necessary.

Author details

Seiya Sato and Hiroaki Itamochi*

*Address all correspondence to: itamochi@iwate-med.ac.jp

Department of Obstetrics and Gynecology, Iwate Medical University School of Medicine, Iwate, Morioka, Japan

References

[1] Saslow D. American Cancer Society, American Society for Colposcopy and Cervical Pathology, and American Society for Clinical Pathology screening guidelines for the prevention and early detection of cervical cancer. Journal of Lower Genital Tract Disease. 2012; **16**(3):175-204

[2] Siegel RL. Cancer statistics, 2017. CA: A Cancer Journal for Clinicians. 2017;**67**(1):7-30

[3] Wright TC Jr. Interim guidance for the use of human papillomavirus DNA testing as an adjunct to cervical cytology for screening. Obstetrics and Gynecology. 2004;**103**(2): 304-309

[4] Massad LS. 2012 updated consensus guidelines for the management of abnormal cervical cancer screening tests and cancer precursors. Obstetrics and Gynecology. 2013; **121**(4):829-846

[5] Saslow D. American Cancer Society, American Society for Colposcopy and Cervical Pathology, and American Society for Clinical Pathology screening guidelines for the prevention and early detection of cervical cancer. CA: A Cancer Journal for Clinicians. 2012;**62**(3):147-172

[6] Ronco G. Efficacy of human papillomavirus testing for the detection of invasive cervical cancers and cervical intraepithelial neoplasia: A randomised controlled trial. The Lancet Oncology. 2010;**11**(3):249-257

[7] Bulkmans NW. Human papillomavirus DNA testing for the detection of cervical intraepithelial neoplasia grade 3 and cancer: 5-year follow-up of a randomised controlled implementation trial. Lancet. 2007;**370**(9601):1764-1772

[8] Rijkaart DC. Human papillomavirus testing for the detection of high-grade cervical intraepithelial neoplasia and cancer: Final results of the POBASCAM randomised controlled trial. The Lancet Oncology. 2012;**13**(1):78-88

[9] Kitchener HC. HPV testing in combination with liquid-based cytology in primary cervical screening (ARTISTIC): A randomised controlled trial. The Lancet Oncology. 2009; **10**(7):672-682

[10] Results of a randomized trial on the management of cytology interpretations of atypical squamous cells of undetermined significance. American Journal of Obstetrics and Gynecology. 2003;**188**(6):1383-1392

[11] A randomized trial on the management of low-grade squamous intraepithelial lesion cytology interpretations. American Journal of Obstetrics and Gynecology. 2003;**188**(6): 1393-1400

[12] Katki HA. Benchmarking CIN 3+ risk as the basis for incorporating HPV and Pap cotesting into cervical screening and management guidelines. Journal of Lower Genital Tract Disease. 2013;**17**(5 Suppl 1):S28-S35

[13] Wright TC Jr. Evaluation of HPV-16 and HPV-18 genotyping for the triage of women with high-risk HPV+ cytology-negative results. American Journal of Clinical Pathology. 2011;**136**(4):578-586

[14] Hoffman SR. Patterns of persistent HPV infection after treatment for cervical intraepithelial neoplasia (CIN): A systematic review. International Journal of Cancer. 2017; **141**(1):8-23

[15] Kocken M. Risk of recurrent high-grade cervical intraepithelial neoplasia after success-
      ful treatment: A long-term multi-cohort study. The Lancet Oncology. 2011;**12**(5):441-450

[16] van der Heijden E. Follow-up strategies after treatment (large loop excision of the
      transformation zone (LLETZ)) for cervical intraepithelial neoplasia (CIN): Impact of
      human papillomavirus (HPV) test. The Cochrane Database of Systematic Reviews.
      2015;**1**:CD010757

[17] Katki HA. Five-year risk of recurrence after treatment of CIN 2, CIN 3, or AIS: Per-
      formance of HPV and Pap cotesting in posttreatment management. Journal of Lower
      Genital Tract Disease. 2013;**17**(5 Suppl 1):S78-S84

[18] Cubie HA. Evaluation of commercial HPV assays in the context of post-treatment fol-
      low-up: Scottish Test of Cure Study (STOCS-H). Journal of Clinical Pathology. 2014;
      67(6):458-463

[19] Gosvig CF. Long-term follow-up of the risk for cervical intraepithelial neoplasia grade
      2 or worse in HPV-negative women after conization. International Journal of Cancer.
      2015;**137**(12):2927-2933

[20] Brianti P. Review of HPV-related diseases and cancers. The New Microbiologica.
      2017;**40**(2):80-85

[21] Quadrivalent vaccine against human papillomavirus to prevent high-grade cervical
      lesions. The New England journal of medicine. 2007;**356**(19):1915-1927

[22] Lehtinen M. Overall efficacy of HPV-16/18 AS04-adjuvanted vaccine against grade 3
      or greater cervical intraepithelial neoplasia: 4-year end-of-study analysis of the ran-
      domised, double-blind PATRICIA trial. The Lancet Oncology. 2012;**13**(1):89-99

[23] Wheeler CM. Cross-protective efficacy of HPV-16/18 AS04-adjuvanted vaccine against
      cervical infection and precancer caused by non-vaccine oncogenic HPV types: 4-year
      end-of-study analysis of the randomised, double-blind PATRICIA trial. The Lancet
      Oncology. 2012;**13**(1):100-110

[24] Brown DR. The impact of quadrivalent human papillomavirus (HPV; types 6, 11, 16, and 18)
      L1 virus-like particle vaccine on infection and disease due to oncogenic nonvaccine
      HPV types in generally HPV-naive women aged 16-26 years. The Journal of Infectious
      Diseases. 2009;**199**(7):926-935

[25] Herrero R. Present status of human papillomavirus vaccine development and imple-
      mentation. The Lancet Oncology. 2015;**16**(5):e206-e216

[26] Pista A. Potential impact of nonavalent HPV vaccine in the prevention of high-grade
      cervical lesions and cervical cancer in Portugal. International Journal of Gynaecology
      and Obstetrics: the Official Organ of the International Federation of Gynaecology and
      Obstetrics. 2017;**139**(1):90-94

[27] Castle PE. Performance of carcinogenic human papillomavirus (HPV) testing and
      HPV16 or HPV18 genotyping for cervical cancer screening of women aged 25 years and
      older: A subanalysis of the ATHENA study. The Lancet Oncology. 2011;**12**(9):880-890

[28] Rijkaart DC. Evaluation of 14 triage strategies for HPV DNA-positive women in population-based cervical screening. International Journal of Cancer. 2012;**130**(3):602-610

[29] Veldhuijzen NJ. Stratifying HPV-positive women for CIN3+ risk after one and two rounds of HPV-based screening. International Journal of Cancer. 2017;**141**(8):1551-1560

[30] Massad LS. 2012 updated consensus guidelines for the management of abnormal cervical cancer screening tests and cancer precursors. Journal of Lower Genital Tract Disease. 2013;**17**(5 Suppl 1):S1-S27

[31] Bernard HU. Genome variation of human papillomavirus types: Phylogenetic and medical implications. International Journal of Cancer. 2006;**118**(5):1071-1076

[32] Mirabello L. HPV16 E7 genetic conservation is critical to carcinogenesis. Cell. 2017;**170**(6):1164-1174 e1166

[33] Hildesheim A. Human papillomavirus vaccine should be given before sexual debut for maximum benefit. The Journal of Infectious Diseases. 2007;**196**(10):1431-1432

[34] Franco EL. Epidemiology of acquisition and clearance of cervical human papillomavirus infection in women from a high-risk area for cervical cancer. The Journal of Infectious Diseases. 1999;**180**(5):1415-1423

[35] Forcier M. An overview of human papillomavirus infection for the dermatologist: Disease, diagnosis, management, and prevention. Dermatologic Therapy. 2010;**23**(5):458-476

[36] Doeberitz M. Host factors in HPV-related carcinogenesis: Cellular mechanisms controlling HPV infections. Archives of Medical Research. 2009;**40**(6):435-442

[37] Doorbar J. Molecular biology of human papillomavirus infection and cervical cancer. Clinical Science (London, England). 2006;**110**(5):525-541

[38] Doorbar J. The biology and life-cycle of human papillomaviruses. Vaccine. 2012;**30**(Suppl 5):F55-F70

[39] Kines RC. The initial steps leading to papillomavirus infection occur on the basement membrane prior to cell surface binding. Proceedings of the National Academy of Sciences of the United States of America. 2009;**106**(48):20458-20463

[40] Reuschenbach M. Characterization of humoral immune responses against p16, p53, HPV16 E6 and HPV16 E7 in patients with HPV-associated cancers. International Journal of Cancer. 2008;**123**(11):2626-2631

[41] de Jong A. Human papillomavirus type 16-positive cervical cancer is associated with impaired CD4+ T-cell immunity against early antigens E2 and E6. Cancer Research. 2004;**64**(15):5449-5455

[42] Mezache L. Enhanced expression of PD L1 in cervical intraepithelial neoplasia and cervical cancers. Modern Pathology: An Official Journal of the United States and Canadian Academy of Pathology, Inc. 2015;**28**(12):1594-1602

[43] Yang W. Increased expression of programmed death (PD)-1 and its ligand PD-L1 corre- lates with impaired cell-mediated immunity in high-risk human papillomavirus-related cervical intraepithelial neoplasia. Immunology. 2013;**139**(4):513-522

[44] Yang W. Expressions of programmed death (PD)-1 and PD-1 ligand (PD-L1) in cervi- cal intraepithelial neoplasia and cervical squamous cell carcinomas are of prognostic value and associated with human papillomavirus status. The Journal of Obstetrics and Gynaecology Research. 2017;**43**(10):1602-1612

[45] Kuner R. Identification of cellular targets for the human papillomavirus E6 and E7 onco- genes by RNA interference and transcriptome analyses. Journal of Molecular Medicine. 2007;**85**(11):1253-1262

[46] McLaughlin-Drubin ME. Biochemical and functional interactions of human papilloma- virus proteins with polycomb group proteins. Virus. 2013;**5**(5):1231-1249

[47] Munger K. Complex formation of human papillomavirus E7 proteins with the retino- blastoma tumor suppressor gene product. The EMBO Journal. 1989;**8**(13):4099-4105

[48] Scheffner M. The E6 oncoprotein encoded by human papillomavirus types 16 and 18 promotes the degradation of p53. Cell. 1990;**63**(6):1129-1136

[49] Duensing S. The human papillomavirus type 16 E6 and E7 oncoproteins cooperate to induce mitotic defects and genomic instability by uncoupling centrosome duplication from the cell division cycle. Proceedings of the National Academy of Sciences of the United States of America. 2000;**97**(18):10002-10007

[50] White AE. Differential disruption of genomic integrity and cell cycle regulation in normal human fibroblasts by the HPV oncoproteins. Genes & Development. 1994;**8**(6):666-677

[51] Akagi K. Genome-wide analysis of HPV integration in human cancers reveals recurrent, focal genomic instability. Genome Research. 2014;**24**(2):185-199

[52] Heselmeyer K. Gain of chromosome 3q defines the transition from severe dysplasia to invasive carcinoma of the uterine cervix. Proceedings of the National Academy of Sciences of the United States of America. 1996;**93**(1):479-484

[53] Cahill DP. Genetic instability and darwinian selection in tumours. Trends in Cell Biology. 1999;**9**(12):M57-M60

[54] Thomas LK. Chromosomal gains and losses in human papillomavirus-associated neo- plasia of the lower genital tract—A systematic review and meta-analysis. European Journal of Cancer. 2014;**50**(1):85-98

[55] Moody CA. Human papillomavirus oncoproteins: Pathways to transformation. Nature Reviews Cancer. 2010;**10**(8):550-560

[56] Wentzensen N. Triage of HPV positive women in cervical cancer screening. Journal of Clinical Virology: The Official Publication of the Pan American Society for Clinical Virology. 2016;**76**(Suppl 1):S49-S55

[57] Steenbergen RD. Clinical implications of (epi)genetic changes in HPV-induced cervical precancerous lesions. Nature Reviews Cancer. 2014;**14**(6):395-405

[58] Reuschenbach M. Diagnostic tests for the detection of human papillomavirus-associated cervical lesions. Current Pharmaceutical Design. 2013;**19**(8):1358-1370

[59] von Knebel Doeberitz M. Correlation of modified human papilloma virus early gene expression with altered growth properties in C4-1 cervical carcinoma cells. Cancer Research. 1988;**48**(13):3780-3786

[60] Zur Hausen H. Papillomaviruses in anogenital cancer as a model to understand the role of viruses in human cancers. Cancer Research. 1989;**49**(17):4677-4681

[61] Tota JE. Approaches for triaging women who test positive for human papillomavirus in cervical cancer screening. Preventive Medicine. 2017;**98**:15-20

[62] de Sanjose S. Human papillomavirus genotype attribution in invasive cervical cancer: A retrospective cross-sectional worldwide study. The Lancet Oncology. 2010;**11**(11): 1048-1056

[63] Skinner SR. Progression of HPV infection to detectable cervical lesions or clearance in adult women: Analysis of the control arm of the VIVIANE study. International Journal of Cancer. 2016;**138**(10):2428-2438

[64] Matsumoto K. Predicting the progression of cervical precursor lesions by human papillomavirus genotyping: A prospective cohort study. International Journal of Cancer. 2011;**128**(12):2898-2910

[65] Hosaka M. Incidence risk of cervical intraepithelial neoplasia 3 or more severe lesions is a function of human papillomavirus genotypes and severity of cytological and histological abnormalities in adult Japanese women. International Journal of Cancer. 2013;**132**(2):327-334

[66] Kudoh A. Human papillomavirus type-specific persistence and reappearance after successful conization in patients with cervical intraepithelial neoplasia. International Journal of Clinical Oncology. 2016;**21**(3):580-587

[67] McLaughlin-Drubin ME. Human papillomavirus E7 oncoprotein induces KDM6A and KDM6B histone demethylase expression and causes epigenetic reprogramming. Proceedings of the National Academy of Sciences of the United States of America. 2011;**108**(5):2130-2135

[68] Bergeron C. The clinical impact of using p16(INK4a) immunochemistry in cervical histopathology and cytology: An update of recent developments. International Journal of Cancer. 2015;**136**(12):2741-2751

[69] Reuschenbach M. A phase 1/2a study to test the safety and immunogenicity of a p16(INK4a) peptide vaccine in patients with advanced human papillomavirus-associated cancers. Cancer. 2016;**122**(9):1425-1433

[70] Tjalma WAA. Diagnostic performance of dual-staining cytology for cervical cancer screening: A systematic literature review. European Journal of Obstetrics, Gynecology, and Reproductive Biology. 2017;**210**:275-280

[71] Ebisch RM. Evaluation of p16/Ki-67 dual-stained cytology as triage test for high-risk human papillomavirus-positive women. Modern Pathology: An Official Journal of the United States and Canadian Academy of Pathology, Inc. 2017;**30**(7):1021-1031

[72] Wright TC Jr. Triaging HPV-positive women with p16/Ki-67 dual-stained cytology: Results from a sub-study nested into the ATHENA trial. Gynecologic Oncology. 2017;**144**(1):51-56

[73] Ikenberg H. Screening for cervical cancer precursors with p16/Ki-67 dual-stained cytology: Results of the PALMS study. Journal of the National Cancer Institute. 2013;**105**(20):1550-1557

[74] Petry KU. Triaging Pap cytology negative, HPV positive cervical cancer screening results with p16/Ki-67 dual-stained cytology. Gynecologic Oncology. 2011;**121**(3):505-509

[75] Polman NJ. Good performance of p16/ki-67 dual-stained cytology for surveillance of women treated for high-grade CIN. International Journal of Cancer. 2017;**140**(2): 423-430

[76] Petry KU. A model to evaluate the costs and clinical effectiveness of human papilloma virus screening compared with annual papanicolaou cytology in Germany. European Journal of Obstetrics, Gynecology, and Reproductive Biology. 2017;**212**:132-139

[77] Monsonego J. Evaluation of oncogenic human papillomavirus RNA and DNA tests with liquid-based cytology in primary cervical cancer screening: The FASE study. International Journal of Cancer. 2011;**129**(3):691-701

[78] Arbyn M. Evidence regarding human papillomavirus testing in secondary prevention of cervical cancer. Vaccine. 2012;**30**(Suppl 5):F88-F99

[79] Dockter J. Clinical performance of the APTIMA HPV Assay for the detection of high-risk HPV and high-grade cervical lesions. Journal of Clinical Virology: The Official Publication of the Pan American Society for Clinical Virology. 2009;**45**(Suppl 1):S55-S61

[80] Monsonego J. Risk assessment and clinical impact of liquid-based cytology, oncogenic human papillomavirus (HPV) DNA and mRNA testing in primary cervical cancer screening (the FASE study). Gynecologic Oncology. 2012;**125**(1):175-180

[81] Origoni M. E6/E7 mRNA testing for human papilloma virus-induced high-grade cervical intraepithelial disease (CIN2/CIN3): A promising perspective. Ecancermedicalscience. 2015;**9**(533). DOI: 10.3332/ecancer.2015.533

[82] Alanen KW. Assessment of cytologic follow-up as the recommended management for patients with atypical squamous cells of undetermined significance or low grade squamous intraepithelial lesions. Cancer. 1998;**84**(1):5-10

[83] Szarewski A. Comparison of seven tests for high-grade cervical intraepithelial neo-plasia in women with abnormal smears: The predictors 2 study. Journal of Clinical Microbiology. 2012;**50**(6):1867-1873

[84] Rijkaart DC. High-risk human papillomavirus (hrHPV) E6/E7 mRNA testing by PreTect HPV-Proofer for detection of cervical high-grade intraepithelial neoplasia and can-cer among hrHPV DNA-positive women with normal cytology. Journal of Clinical Microbiology. 2012;**50**(7):2390-2396

[85] Yang L. The clinical application of HPV E6/E7 mRNA testing in triaging women with atypical squamous cells of undetermined significance or low-grade squamous intra-epi-thelial lesion Pap smear: A meta-analysis. Journal of Cancer Research and Therapeutics. 2017;**13**(4):613-620

[86] Clarke MA. Human papillomavirus DNA methylation as a potential biomarker for cervical cancer. Cancer Epidemiology, Biomarkers & Prevention: A Publication of the American Association for Cancer Research, cosponsored by the American Society of Preventive Oncology. 2012;**21**(12):2125-2137

[87] Prigge ES. Clinical relevance and implications of HPV-induced neoplasia in different anatomical locations. Mutation Research Reviews in Mutation Research. 2017;**772**:51-66

[88] Kocsis A. Performance of a new HPV and biomarker assay in the management of hrHPV positive women: Subanalysis of the ongoing multicenter TRACE clinical trial (n > 6,000) to evaluate POU4F3 methylation as a potential biomarker of cervical precancer and can-cer. International Journal of Cancer. 2017;**140**(5):1119-1133

[89] Niyazi M. Correlation between methylation of human Papillomavirus-16 L1 gene and cervical carcinoma in Uyghur women. Gynecologic and Obstetric Investigation. 2017;**82**(1):22-29

[90] Rosales R. Immune therapy for human papillomaviruses-related cancers. World Journal of Clinical Oncology. 2014;**5**(5):1002-1019

[91] Li J. A novel therapeutic vaccine composed of a rearranged human papillomavirus type 16 E6/E7 fusion protein and Fms-like tyrosine kinase-3 ligand induces CD8+ T cell responses and antitumor effect. Vaccine. 2017;**35**(47):6459-6467

[92] Trimble CL. Safety, efficacy, and immunogenicity of VGX-3100, a therapeutic synthetic DNA vaccine targeting human papillomavirus 16 and 18 E6 and E7 proteins for cervical intraepithelial neoplasia 2/3: A randomised, double-blind, placebo-controlled phase 2b trial. Lancet. 2015;**386**(10008):2078-2088

[93] Vici P. Targeting immune response with therapeutic vaccines in premalignant lesions and cervical cancer: Hope or reality from clinical studies. Expert Review of Vaccines. 2016;**15**(10):1327-1336

[94] Horn J. Estimating the long-term effects of HPV vaccination in Germany. Vaccine. 2013;**31**(19):2372-2380

[95] Belinson JL. Improved sensitivity of vaginal self-collection and high-risk human papillomavirus testing. International Journal of Cancer. 2012;**130**(8):1855-1860

[96] Castle PE. Comparative community outreach to increase cervical cancer screening in the Mississippi Delta. Preventive Medicine. 2011;**52**(6):452-455

[97] Shi R. Factors associated with genital human papillomavirus infection among adult females in the United States, NHANES 2007-2010. BMC Research Notes. 2014;**7**:544

[98] Moscicki AB. Natural history of anal human papillomavirus infection in heterosexual women and risks associated with persistence. Clinical Infectious Diseases: An Official Publication of the Infectious Diseases Society of America. 2014;**58**(6):804-811

[99] Rositch AF. Patterns of persistent genital human papillomavirus infection among women worldwide: A literature review and meta-analysis. International Journal of Cancer. 2013;**133**(6):1271-1285

[100] Sanner K. Daily self-sampling for high-risk human papillomavirus (HR-HPV) testing. Journal of Clinical Virology: The Official Publication of the Pan American Society for Clinical Virology. 2015;**73**:1-7

[101] Nelson EJ. The acceptability of self-sampled screening for HPV DNA: A systematic review and meta-analysis. Sexually Transmitted Infections. 2017;**93**(1):56-61

[102] Moscicki AB. Rate of and risks for regression of cervical intraepithelial neoplasia 2 in adolescents and young women. Obstetrics and Gynecology. 2010;**116**(6):1373-1380

[103] Trimble CL. Spontaneous regression of high-grade cervical dysplasia: Effects of human papillomavirus type and HLA phenotype. Clinical Cancer Research: An Official Journal of the American Association for Cancer Research. 2005;**11**(13):4717-4723

[104] Kyrgiou M. Obstetric outcomes after conservative treatment for intraepithelial or early invasive cervical lesions: Systematic review and meta-analysis. Lancet. 2006;**367**(9509): 489-498

[105] Vrzackova P. Sexual morbidity following radical hysterectomy for cervical cancer. Expert Review of Anticancer Therapy. 2010;**10**(7):1037-1042

[106] Wit EM. Urological complications after treatment of cervical cancer. Nature Reviews Urology. 2014;**11**(2):110-117

[107] Luttjeboer J. Threshold cost-effectiveness analysis for a therapeutic vaccine against HPV-16/18-positive cervical intraepithelial neoplasia in the Netherlands. Vaccine. 2016;**34**(50):6381-6387

3

Genomic Copy Number Alterations in Serous Ovarian Cancer

Joe R. Delaney and Dwayne G. Stupack

Abstract

Precision medicine in cancer is the idea that the recognition and targeting of key genetic drivers of a patient's tumor can permit more effective and less toxic outcomes. Point mutations that alter protein function have been primary targets. Yet in ovarian cancer, unique genetic mutations have been identified only in adult granulosa cell tumors, with a number of other point mutations present in mucinous, clear cell and endometrioid carcinoma subtypes. By contrast, the serous subtype of ovarian cancer shows many fewer point mutations but cascading defects in DNA damage repair that leads to a network of gains and losses of entire genes called somatic copy number alterations. The shuffling and selection of the thousands of genes in serous ovarian cancer has made it a complex disease to understand, but patterns are beginning to emerge based on our understanding of key cellular protein networks that may provide a better basis for future implementation of precision medicine for this most prevalent subtype of disease.

Keywords: SCNA, aneuploidy, autophagy, beclin-1, p53

1. Introduction

When a patient asks an oncologist what tumor cells are, the frequent explanation is that the "Cancer cells are normal cells that accumulate genetic mutations, which causes them to grow out of control." Yet the idea of what a mutation is, and what it can do, varies. It has essentially become dogma that mutations be grouped into two broad categories. One class has been described as either *drivers*, which are key genetic changes that are known to potentiate tumor development. If a gene is not a driver, then it is typically considered a *passenger*,—a bystander mutation occurring due to the tumor-associated genomic instability. Passenger mutations are generally considered to be 'noise' in the system which do not influence tumor progression [1].

This categorization has now had clinical impact. Genes that are known as *drivers* are prioritized for diagnostic testing, and have become a focus for "molecular tumor boards" that review patient data in hospitals across the United States. These boards focus foremost on reviewing a molecular profiling of the tumor, rather than on histopathological features. Thus, tumors with similar genetic features may call for similar therapy regardless of whether they originate in the colon, breast or lung. The division of mutation into drivers and passengers fosters an environment where new mutations may be missed, because we are focused on the pre-established clinical screening protocols, because we both profile and act upon well characterized genetic problems. Even when they are reported, their impact may not be appreciated if they have not had a role as a driver assigned to them in prior peer-reviewed study.

The *driver* assignment comes from a breadth of work that focuses on a type of mutation called a somatic single-nucleotide variant (SNV). Driver SNVs are noted for their critical roles in tumor formation, frequently occur at precise locations within *oncogenes*, and can now be rapidly identified. Notable examples include K-Ras, where mutation of the glycine residue at position 12 (G12) inhibits GTPase activity, leaving the protein in an active, GTP-bound effector state. A second example is phosphoinositide 3'kinase, where mutation of the histidine residue at 1047 (H1047) similarly alters the ability of the protein to regulate activity. The gold standard for such driver mutations is their capacity to facilitate neoplastic disease in murine genetic models, most frequently by providing a dysregulated positive stimulus that drives mitosis and cell survival. Transcription factor mutations, such as the FOXL2 C243W mutation found in all adult type granulosa cell tumors, provide a good example of a key genetic driver.

A second class of drivers involve SNV-mediated inactivation of *tumor suppressor* genes, which act to ameliorate the effects of oncogenes, shunt tumors towards programmed cell death, and maintain the fidelity of DNA replication and repair. Tumor formation requires both oncogenic activation and the disruption of tumor suppressors. Mutation in TS genes do not require the same precision as those in oncogenes; SNV's occur across a swath of locations, any of which may be sufficient to disrupt tumor suppressor function. This chapter will focus on serous

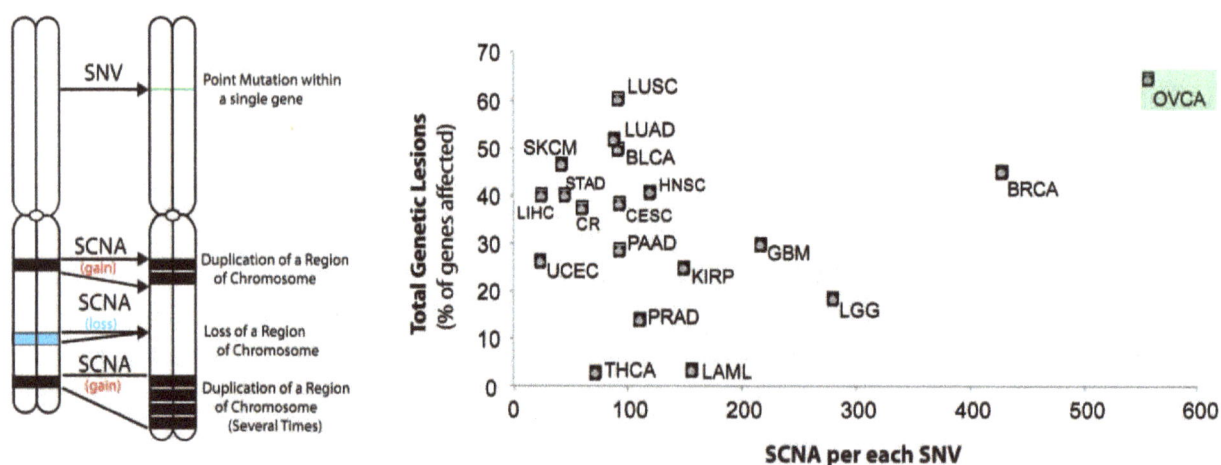

Figure 1. (Left) Possible changes in a single chromosome's architecture. One chromosome is shown; each copy of a chromosome can have different SCNA or SNV. (Right) A plot of the major cancers in the TCGA database, showing total genetic lesions (as percentage of genes) vs. the number of SCNA for each SNV. In each case SCNA are more abundant, with serous ovarian cancer (SOC, denoted as OVCA in the green box) bearing the greatest number.

ovarian cancer (SOC), a lethal tumor whose '*drivers*' are only beginning to be understood. The tumor suppressor gene *TP53* is mutated in more than 85% of serous ovarian cancer (SOC) cases [2], and disruption of DNA repair proteins is commonly identified. Yet most patients bear no SNV that results in oncogene activation.

However, SOC has a further characteristic related to its poor capacity to repair DNA. SOC has the highest ratio of somatic copy number alterations (SCNAs) to SNVs for any major cancer. SCNAs are a broad group of genetic changes that encompass a myriad of short insertions, short deletions, translocations and inversions (**Figure 1**, left panel). SCNAs contribute to the mutational landscape of cancer, expanding the scope of changes beyond the more 'simple' SNVs. The impact of this on SOC malignancy will be the focus of this chapter.

2. SCNA overview and incidence

A gene normally occurs in the human nucleus twice. This normal 2N "dosage" of copy number, which originates from zygote formation, consists of one paternal gene and one maternal gene. SCNAs, which alter this occur in two types: amplifications and deletions. An amplification occurs when a chromosomal region containing a gene is copied. That gene will no longer have the normal 2N copy number, but, depending upon the number of times it is copied, could be 3N, 4N, or in cases of massive amplification, up to 200 N and more. Contrasting with this expansive range, SCNAs that result from deletions most frequently reduce the copy number to 1N. Total gene loss (0N) can occur in rare cases, and is associated with a very small fraction of the overall number of deletions. Nonetheless, these rarer SCNA-derived genotypes will obviously impact function most, since the lack of any gene copy means that the encoded protein cannot be produced. SCNAs are the most common lesions in cancer, occurring much more commonly than SNVs (**Figure 1**, right panel).

SCNAs occur via a variety of mechanisms in cancer [3]. Entire chromosomes may be gained/lost during cell division, generating 3N or 1N copy number status for all genes on the chromosome. This occurs due to failed cell-division checkpoints resulting in chromosome missegregation. In contrast to such gains at the total chromosome level, tiny "focal" SCNAs may alter a single gene (or even part of a gene). The most common example of this is *CDKN2A*, a checkpoint protein which is fully deleted (0N) in 3% of SOC tumors. These focal deletions typically occur during repair of double-stranded DNA (dsDNA) breaks. During the attempted repair, short regions of homology can result in accidental deletion of DNA in between [4]. Focal amplifications occur through unknown mechanisms [5] and can form "double minute" chromosomes containing hundreds of copies of a gene, such as *ERBB2* or *EGFR* [6]. Finally, between the focal alterations and the whole chromosome losses, SCNAs can also encompass large regions of DNA through similar defects in dsDNA break repair. These intermediate sized SCNAs can contain many genes. However, they rarely contribute to a 0N copy numbers (loss on both chromosomes) since the regions affected frequently contain essential genes [7].

Within the Cancer Genome Atlas (TCGA) data sets, the presence of 3N and 1N gene copies dominate the SCNA genomic landscape. This is true across all tumors, including those tumors where SCNAs are highly prevalent, such as SOC [8]. SCNAs are prevalent in SOC. In fact, only about one third of all genes in primary tumors have a normal 2N gene dosage. Roughly a quarter of the total genes in the tumors show an extra gene copy (to 3N) and just over a third lose a gene copy (to 1N). By contrast, only 0.7% loses both gene copies (0N), while 4.2% are amplified to 4N or greater. In practice, the focus on understanding tumor biology has been only on these last two cases (total deletion and gross amplification, respectively). This has a reasonable basis; the effects of total loss or gross amplification are easiest to study.

The common gene changes (i.e., 1N and 3N) have not been the subject of focused study. Many scientists assume that the deletion, or addition, of a single gene copy has limited effect. Recessive genetic alleles are not uncommon in nature, supporting the idea that the loss of a single gene copy can be compensated for. However, the loss of a single gene may not reflect the situation in ovarian cancer, where massive genetic alteration occurs, and compensation may not be possible if the same cellular pathway is repeatedly targeted by SCNAs (**Figure 2**).

More than 80% of genes affected by SCNAs show concordant alteration of mRNA levels [9, 10]. For ~70% of genes, this correlates with steady-state protein levels [11]. Thus, SCNAs offer a predictable, but not absolute, indication of protein expression. This is relevant to ovarian cancer, as SCNAs modify on average 67% of the SOC genome, whereas SNVs modify only

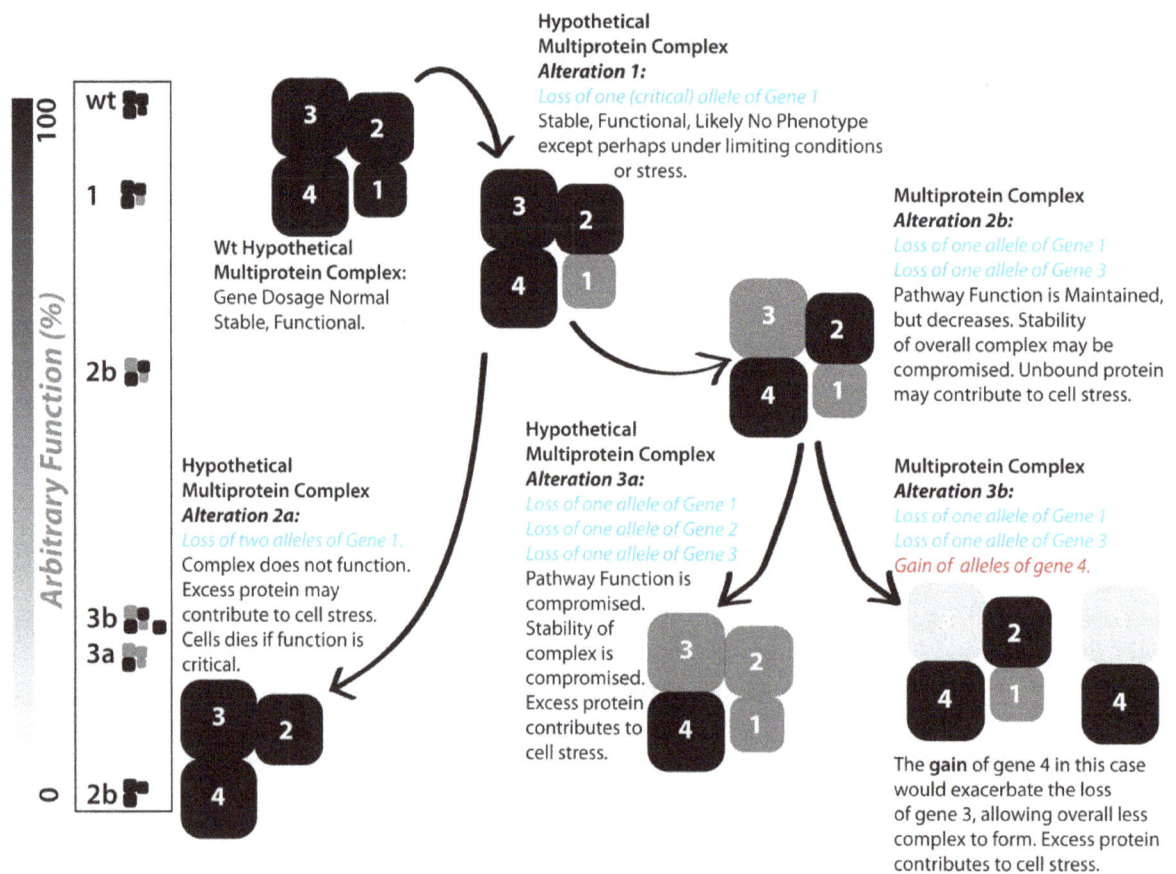

MODEL: *Additive Biological Impact of Multiple SCNA in a Single Protein Complex*

Figure 2. Model showing how SCNA changes resulting in differences in protein expression might impact overall function within a single multiprotein complex. The relative function of the complex as a % is shown at left. The right side shows how a sequence of SCNA changes within a pathway could cumulatively impact its function.

0.12% of the average SOC genome [12]. Less than 10% of SOC patients are mutated in a targetable driver gene [12, 13].

3. Ovarian cancer and copy number alterations

It seems self-evident that an understanding of "driver SCNAs" is absolutely essential to our capacity to target the biology of the disease. Genetic disorders such as Down's syndrome (trisomy 21) and Cri du Chat (5p monosomy) and DiGeorge Syndrome (loss of only 30–40 alleles on 22q11) clearly indicate the penetrative biology of multiple SCNA. More importantly, such lesions affect only ~2% of the genome, while SCNA in SOC affect 67% of genes. Other subtypes of ovarian cancer vary widely in their SCNA burden, but are typically much lower, and are associated with SNVs.

As most SCNA are "monoallelic" changes resulting in a 1N or 3N genotype, is there any reason to expect a phenotype, given our understanding of recessive alleles? Recurrent patterns in serous ovarian cancer suggest that frequently affected regions may be selected for as the tumor evolves. In high grade SOC, the most prevalent SNVs could have been predicted from literature preceding the genomics era. For decades, the mutation of *TP53*, the "guardian of the genome" has been appreciated due to its master control of multiple DNA repair pathways, cell cycle control, and metabolism. Interestingly, there is selection for SCNA deletion of the chromosome with the wild-type copy of p53, suggesting further suppression or misdirection of p53 furthers SOC development [14]. Inheritance studies have associated the *BRCA1/2* mutation with an increased risk of ovarian cancer, and not surprisingly these mutants contain opposite-chromosome deletions just like p53. *BRCA* genes are necessary to maintain the genome. Like p53, they play a coordinating role in facilitating homology-directed repair of DNA. However, single nucleotide variant mutation is not the most common mechanism of BRCA gene disruption. Only ~6% of patients display non-germline SNVs, while copy number deletions (to 1N) occur in more than 70% of tumors. PTEN, a tumor suppressor commonly mutated in many tumor types but not ovarian, was found as early as 2001 to have reduced expression due to shallow deletions across ~40% of samples [15].

Aside from very infrequent gene losses paired with mutations, there are also a few SCNAs which drive cancer through amplification of oncogenes. The stem-cell transcription factor *MYC* is the most amplified gene in the TCGA cohort (42% with at least a 4N copy number, and an additional 37% with 3N). Myc has been appreciated as a common SOC driver oncogene since 1990 [16]. Homozygous deletions in Rb were discovered around the same time [17, 18], and occur in 9% of tumors. *KRAS* amplifications and gene overexpression were discovered around the same time, but in a smaller minority (13%) of patients [19]. Her2, encoded by *ERBB2*, can be overexpressed but this appears to be a case unrelated to SCNA amplification, which occurs in only 3% of cases [20, 21]. Drug resistance can occur following increases in drug efflux genes, and one of the first identified was *MDR1* (*ABCB1*) [22]. Again, this is only found in a small minority of patients (4%). Comparative genomic hybridization in 2006 identified significantly amplified CCNE1 (cyclin E1) and MDM2 (a negative regulator of p53 from its E3 ubiquitin ligase activity) [23, 24]. The year these studies were published provides a historical context to our knowledge. Were we missing a key driver for SOC? Despite the hundreds of genomes sequenced, few additional single-gene drivers were discovered in the recent "brute-force" landmark studies on SOC from either the TCGA [12] or the AOC [13].

There are plausible reasons for this. It may be that every SOC tumor is truly unique from a mutational standpoint: that those SNVs found in only one tumor nonetheless are driver genes, collaborating in ways that we understand poorly [25]. It is thus possible that drivers have already been sequenced and annotated by SCNA studies, but due to high "background" or "passenger" SCNAs it remains unclear which SCNAs are critical to the tumor's biology [8]. The implications of this are enormous, and would necessitate an unparalleled level of personalized therapies targeting such extremely rare mutations. A second reason that SNVs have not yielded common drivers may be that further sequencing of whole genomes and epigenomes will reveal additional drivers prevalent across patients which have remained undetected by exome sequencing.

The problem investigators consistently encounter is the ubiquitous heterogeneity in SOC. Heterogeneity exists at all levels of genetics, manifesting as *between-patient* heterogeneity, *between-tumor* (intra-patient) heterogeneity [14], heterogeneity in SNVs within a single tumor [12], heterogeneity in SCNAs [26], and heterogeneity in mRNA expression (correlating with protein expression) [11] or flux in SCNA status [10]. While such problems are not unique to SOC, they are magnified compared to many other tumor types because of the gross incidence of SCNA. Genetic and phenotypic heterogeneity remains the hardest issue to tackle [27, 28], and our own opinion mirrors that of several other groups working in this area: the analysis of affected pathways will offer new approaches to find hidden patterns of tumor suppressors and oncogenes within these heterogeneous data [8, 9, 29].

Fewer genomic studies have been performed on other types of ovarian cancer. Some limited data are available on SCNAs for Clear cell and endometrioid subtypes, which share the amplification of PIK3CA and the MYC-containing 8q24 region with SOC [30–32]. Larger SCNAs encompassing whole chromosome arms rather than smaller changes dominate the clear cell ovarian cancer SCNA landscape [32]. With the exception of 17p loss (containing *TP53*), focal *TPM3* amplification, and focal *ERBB2* amplification, SCNAs are infrequent in mucinous ovarian cancer, suggesting this histotype is SNV or epigenetic driven [30]. Generally, clear cell and endometrioid are intermediate in SCNA quantity between SOC and mucinous subtypes of ovarian cancer.

Despite the limited data on these non-serous subtypes, there is good reason to expect much more data is coming soon. The copy-number arrays employed in the Cancer Genome Atlas studies sell for less than $100USD per sample, which bests the current, but constantly decreasing, cost of whole-genome sequencing. Eight oncology treatment and research centers are participating in project GENIE, which has just released 19,000 new tumor datasets to the public and will continue to grow [33]. As sequencing becomes a normal part of the treatment strategy for patients, the number of samples will likely outpace scientists' ability to fully analyze and comprehend the complex data. Nonetheless, gathering these data is essential to progressing our understanding of the differences between cancer subtypes, which will facilitate the matching of pharmaceuticals to genotype. For now, the largest datasets exist in SOC, and will be the focus of the remainder of discussion.

4. The interplay of p53 mutation with copy number instability

Mutation in p53 has a long research history in many cancer types, and ovarian cancer is no exception. Ovarian cancer mutations within *TP53* have been observed since 1991 [34], and have been confirmed in every genetic study since. *TP53* has often been referred to as "the" primary tumor suppressor for its central role in responding to stresses: it can halt the cell cycle, divert metabolism, induce transcription of DNA damage response genes, or if the damage cannot be repaired, induce apoptosis or senescence [35–37]. For serous ovarian cancer, it has been used as a marker for false diagnosis as some studies presume that genuine serous ovarian cancers must contain mutant p53. Similarly, since the beginning of genomic copy number studies using comparative genomic hybridization, SCNAs have been labeled as a ubiquitous event in all types of epithelial ovarian cancer [31]. Not all p53 mutant tumors are high in SCNAs [38]. Nonetheless, tumors with higher than average SCNAs are much more likely to have a facilitating mutation in p53 [26, 39, 40]. This implies a basic premise: ovarian cancer tumors utilize the mutation in *TP53* to enable the proliferation of SCNAs. SCNAs can subsequently occur in additional tumor suppressors and oncogenes, which leads to SOC as we know it.

Mechanistically this could occur via the deletion or duplication of entire chromosomes or genomes, followed by many subsequent changes enabled by the extra copies of genes, or via chromosome missegregation event, leading one or more chromosomes to acquire massive damage [41]. Either possibility can explain the high frequency of chromothripsis, a highly-disorganized form of hundreds or thousands of SCNAS, in SOC. Mutant p53 enables such mechanisms of SCNA formation by preventing the death of the cell that bears them, as missegregation directly induces p53-dependent cell-cycle arrest followed by apoptosis [42]. In one well-controlled study, 'dominant negative' p53 reduced the cell cycle delay associated with trisomy in mammalian cells, yet it was rare that gain of any single chromosome in those cells resulted in any proliferative advantage [43]. Thus, partial or gained p53 function may contribute. Many p53 mutations maintain partial function, while mutations such as R273H (the most common variant of TP53 found in SOC) provide a gain of function by directly impairing Mre11/ATM-dependent DNA damage responses [44].

It is likely that mutation in *TP53* gene is an enabling event. Lineage tracing using millions of sub-clonal passenger mutations present in SOC tumors suggest that *TP53* mutation arises very early in the proliferation of pre-tumor cells [14]. While few studies focus on normal tissue, a publication on aged skin samples found that islands of cells had developed p53 mutations and achieved local proliferation. Exceptionally few copy number alterations were revealed, with the exception of deletions in *NOTCH1*, and these lesions did not progress to malignancy [45]. In murine models, too, SCNAs follow initiating mutational stimuli [46]. The findings support the idea that p53 is likely to become mutated prior to SCNA accumulation, and acts permissively to enable SCNA accumulation.

5. BRCA1/2 mutations and homologous repair defects

Though few SNVs in 'classic' tumor genes are found in SOC relative to other cancer types, BRCA1/2 mutations are among the most frequent at ~10% [12]. BRCA genes work in coordination with dozens of other proteins to perform genome maintenance via homologous recombination [4]. The double-stranded break repair pathway begins with PARylation of the break site by PARP1, megabases of phosphorylation of H2AX and subsequent formation of Rad51 filaments. Brca1 & Brca2 bind Rad51 to stimulate strand invasion of sister chromatids during homology directed repair. While only ~10% of SOC are mutated in BRCA1 or BRCA2, it is noteworthy that 75% of patients have lost one of two alleles of BRCA1 and 57% have lost an allele of BRCA2. Very few tumors (~1.5%) have homozygous deletions in BRCA1 [12], suggesting a system of compromised (but not lost) function. In fact, mRNA expression level does not track linearly with such deletions. It remains somewhat unclear if these monoallelic deletions do have a phenotype under genotoxic stress in human cells.

Mutations in homologous repair coordinating factors are often found in serous, clear cell, endometrioid, and carcinosarcoma ovarian cancers [47, 48]. Specific mutation patterns are found within BRCA1/2 or otherwise homologous repair deficient cells. Without functional homologous repair, cells default to non-homologous end joining (NHEJ) to repair double-stranded DNA (dsDNA) lesions. NHEJ does not perfectly repair DNA, but rather often introduces small insertions or deletions along with single-nucleotide variants at the break site. These mutational marks are frequently found in non-serous ovarian cancers, yet are unlikely the main drivers of SCNA instability in serous ovarian cancer. However, NHEJ factors involved in repairing unresolved dsDNA breaks across different chromosomes, or creating translocations and other complex rearrangements, are compromised in 40% *ex vivo* ovarian cancer isolates [13, 49]. This can lead to resistance to PARP inhibitors and promote inappropriate translocation or "repair" events [50]. Such defects in NHEJ may explain why the majority of SOC initially respond to cisplatin-based chemotherapy. Complex dsDNA lesions incurred by cisplatin target NHEJ and promote mitotic catastrophe [51].

Genetic and epigenetic changes alter *BRCA1* and the homologous repair pathways in SOC. Gene breakage is commonly observed within *RB1*, *NF1*, *RAD51B*, and *PTEN* [13]. While suppression of homologous recombination may lead to initial disease formation, there is evidence of *BRCA1/2* reversion mutations in tumors which become chemoresistant. This phenomenon follows the strong selective effects of carboplatin and taxanes which require cellular DNA repair pathways to enable cell division. Clinically, these findings should be considered in the context of the search for patient populations for PARP inhibitors. A primary hypothesis for how PARP inhibitors like Olaparib and Niraparib work is by targeting a DNA repair pathway which compensates for homologous repair, thereby presenting synthetic lethality specifically in cancer cells [52]. In a Phase III trial of Niraparib, clinicians treated both BRCA1 or BRCA2 mutant tumors as well as patients who were not found to have mutations in homologous repair genes in their tumors. Unexpectedly, all groups responded to Niraparib therapy [53], although patients with mutated BRCA1/2 or otherwise were defective in homologous repair were further delayed in cancer progression. While this is certainly an exciting development in the treatment possibilities for SOC patients, some caution is warranted. Reversion mutations enabling resistance to Niraparib may actually confer resistance to subsequent chemotherapeutics normally used upon disease recurrence [54].

Loss in BRCA1 enables microsatellite instability in mouse models and in colorectal cancer [55], though not in ovarian cancer [56, 57]. Microsatellite instability directly leads to centrosome amplification, but SCNA instability, which may explain why it is observed in only a small minority of ovarian cancer patients, and is not linked to BRCA mutation status. Nonetheless, BRCA genes are inactivated through allelic deletions and expression modulation in ovarian cancer. Inactivation of *TP53* also suppresses BRCA1 expression [58]. BRCA1 interacts with ATM, directing it to phosphorylate p53 to enable p21 induction and G1/S phase cell cycle arrest [59, 60]. Without these complementary functions, tumors spontaneously form in BRCA1−/− p53+/− mice [61]. Centrosome duplication correlates with BRCA1 deletion [60]. This complex is thus a critical factor determining proper chromosome segregation during mitosis, and upon centrosome duplication aneuploidy is assured to form upon cell division [62, 63]. This is facilitated by prior mutations of p53 that abolish its checkpoint control function, again stressing the role for early mutation of TP53 in SOC.

Coincident SCNA events enable subsequent SCNA catastrophe. BRCA1 is located within kilobases of the neighboring autophagy gene BECN1. Autophagy is a critical catabolic infrastructure that enables cellular survival, requiring only 10% or less of normal autophagy gene dose [64]. Monoallelic loss of *BECN1* promotes centrosome amplification and aneuploidy among apoptosis-resistant cells [65]. An activator of the BECN1–PIK3C3 autophagy initiating complex, UVRAG, displays a similar phenotype [66]. Remarkably, this centrosome amplification promotes cell migration independent of its function in aneuploidy via indirect, hyperactivation of Rac1 [67]. LC3B, a ubiquitin-related protein which marks autophagosomal membranes, also acts in microtubule quality control [68]. One allele of the LC3B gene, *MAP1LC3B*, is genetically deleted in over 75% of SOC, independent of changes to *BRCA1* and *BECN1*. These three aneuploidy-accelerating lesions are likely to play key roles in serous ovarian cancer tumor initiation: mutant p53 expression, along with *BRCA1* and *BECN1* loss. Additional tumor suppressors may synergize to foster genomic instability: *NF1* is on the same chromosome arm as *BRCA1* and *RB1* lies nearby to *BRCA2*. Cumulative haploinsufficiency associated with prime targets and nearby neighbors certainly contribute to SOC aneuploidy [9] (**Figure 3**).

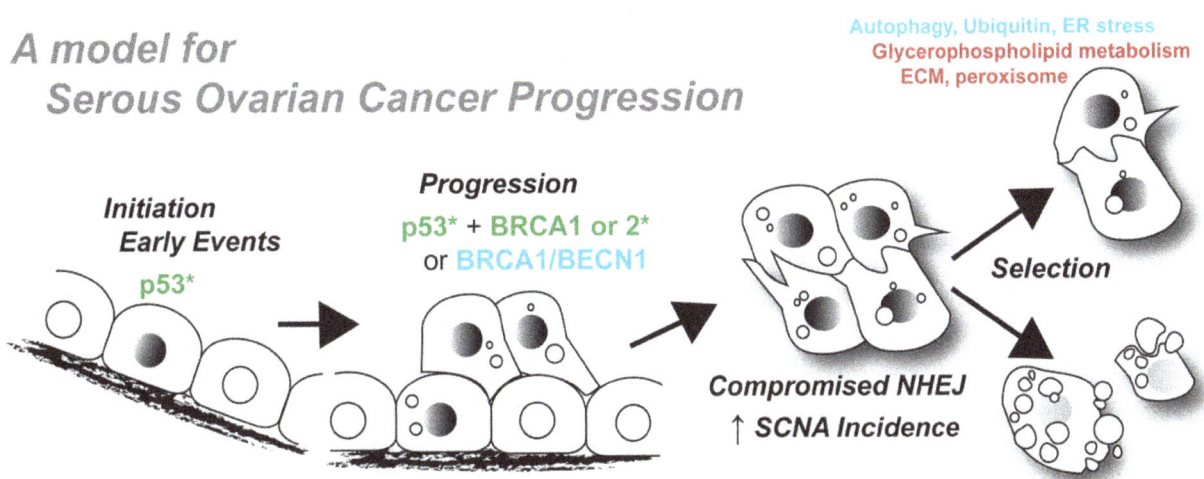

Figure 3. A model consistent with the ubiquitous mutation of p53 (SNV, indicated by green text) together with early SNV or haploid loss (indicated by light blue text) of repair enzymes, permitting a self-sustaining cascade of SCNAs and subsequent *in situ* selection for the observed SOC phenotypes.

In summary, *BRCA1/2* and homologous repair components are often suppressed by genetic deletions in SOC. This leads to further increases in SCNA formation and potentially independent metastatic phenotypes. However, SOC patients may benefit from the cancer's reliance on DNA repair pathways, as inhibition of PARPs prolongs progression free survival.

6. Pathways affected by SCNAs in serous ovarian cancer

Each cancer probably evolves at least 6–10 independent oncogene or tumor suppressor alterations [69] to circumvent natural homeostatic controls known as the "Hallmarks of Cancer" [70, 71]. These hallmarks include the evasion of regulated cell death, immortalization through telomere maintenance, defects in cell cycle control, immune system suppression, and enabling of metastatic capacity through physical and metabolic means. Traditionally, it has been assumed that single gene mutations are responsible for many of these oncogenic changes. Altered p53 function promotes escape to half of these hallmarks on its own, and mutations in strong oncogenes such as Ras family members, or growth factor receptor genes such as FGFRs, Her2 and even Met supplement many of the remaining hallmarks.

Individual gene amplifications can impact serous ovarian cancer. Aside from *TP53* and *BRCA1/2* mutations already discussed, tumors appear to be selected for specific chromosomal aberrations. Amplification of chromosomal region 8q, which contains the oncogenes *MYC* and *PTK2*, is a commonly found SCNV is SOC Myc overexpression promotes cell cycle progression, angiogenesis, and expression of target genes downstream of many other oncogenic factors such as NF-kB, β-catenin, and growth factor receptors [72]. Myc activation coordinately drives proliferation and promotes apoptosis, though since Myc-mediated apoptosis is p53-dependent, the pathway is averted. *PTK2*, the gene encoding focal adhesion kinase (FAK), enables metastatic phenotypes, cancer stem cell self-renewal, and neovascularization [73]. It is often co-amplified with *MYC*, as they both lie within cytoband 8q24. Myc overexpression is difficult to target therapeutically, although there are clinical trials underway for FAK inhibitors [74].

Recently, we analyzed single nucleotide and short 'in frame' deletion mutations across 120 validated oncogenes and tumor suppressors, finding that as many as 48% of serous ovarian primary tumors do not contain mutations in *any known* tumor suppressor or oncogene other than *TP53* [8]. Nonetheless, the average tumor has two-thirds of its genome altered by SCNAs. These findings support the notion that the actions of single oncogenes and tumor suppressors can only explain a portion of the genetics of ovarian cancer.

To analyze this, we developed new pathway network analytics tools to identify disrupted pathways in serous ovarian cancer in this unusually unstable genetic background. Despite the high levels of heterogeneity across patients, we found that coincident gene disruptions fell along surprisingly consistent patterns tumor-to-tumor, specifically suppressing or amplifying specific cellular pathways.

6.1. Autophagy

By far the most significantly suppressed pathway which stood out as unique in serous ovarian cancer and triple negative breast cancer was macroautophagy, which is most commonly known, simply, as autophagy. The term autophagy (*"self-eating"*) appropriately defines the process that cells use to recycle various macromolecular components, such as protein aggregates, lipids, and even entire organelles [75]. Autophagy is a primary method for the cellular catabolism, complementing turnover of proteins by the ubiquitin-proteosome system. Autophagy is described in terms of flux, which is the throughput of cellular *'detritus'* into autophagosomes, their transport to lysosomes, and subsequent enzymatic digestion. Ovarian cancer autophagy deletions impact the process primarily through deletions in *BECN1* (>75% of serous ovarian cancers) and in *MAP1LC3B* (>80% of serous ovarian cancers), though other genes are frequently affected. The average SOC tumor is 1 N across at least five different alleles; 95% of all serous ovarian cancers are deleted in BECN1 or *MAP1LC3B* and two others. The deficiency is as characteristic of SOC as p53 mutation. In addition to their roles in regulating chromosomal instability outlined above, *MAP1LC3B* and BECN1 (with the class three PI3 Kinase VPS34) play key roles in the formation of the early autophagosome, the phagophore, and recruitment autophagosome expansion proteins [76, 77].

Given this critical cellular function, we considered it counter-intuitive that cancer cells would delete a wide array of autophagy genes. In fact, KRAS mutant cancers have been described as "addicted" to autophagy, particularly in hypoxic or otherwise nutrient-stressed microenvironments [78]. This interpretation has been debated [79, 80], but the fact that autophagy has been established as a tumor suppressor system [81, 82], it is not exclusive of the possibility that specific tumor genotypes can promote addiction to autophagy [78]. Mono-allelic losses in the autophagy gene *BECN1* (homozygous deletions occur in only 0.9% of SOC cases) potentiate early development of tumors in mouse models [83, 84]. In this context, it is not at all counter-intuitive to consider that these gene losses likely synergize with defects in the BRCA1/2 pathway, the p53 pathway, and other initial SCNAs, thus producing the unique extreme level of aneuploidy associated with SOC. Moreover, the loss of gene copies does not completely "turn-off" autophagy. In fact, ovarian tumor cells, like other cells, require autophagy to provide clearing of protein aggregates, metabolic byproducts (especially in hypoxic environments), and possibly even to permit cell division, given their aneuploid state and relative chromosomal instability. This, in turn, may provide a second selection criteria for depressed autophagy. Autophagy is induced by missegregating chromosomes, chromosomal instability is a hallmark of SOC, and extreme induction of autophagy can promote cell death [85]. Therefore, it may be more appropriate to use the term "disrupted" rather than "suppressed" to define how ovarian cancer autophagy varies from that seen in normal somatic cells. The state renders SOC sensitive to agents that perturb autophagy by inhibiting the autophagic flux, or via the creation of proteotoxic stresses which must be resolved by autophagy (as discussed below).

6.2. Proteosome

Interestingly, a number of other proteostasis control pathways were suppressed in serous ovarian cancer, and foremost among these is complementary to autophagy, the ubiquitin-proteasome system. The core subunits, encoded by *PSMA1*, *PSMB1*, and *PSMC1*, are monoallelically deleted in 49, 62, and 41% of patients, respectively. Interestingly, the most interactive and deleted components of the proteasomal degradation pathway in ovarian cancer are enriched for cell cycle control related E3 ligases, including Park2, Fzr1, and Ube2d3. This suggests that not only is the core recycling process partly compromised by the core component deletions, but that the pathway is redirected to allow for cell cycle progression proteins to persist and push the cell through division. The latter finding is perhaps to be expected, given that this has been established as a mechanism for tumor formation in many reviews [86–88]. Yet the proteasome may have a similar function to autophagy in suppressing aneuploidy. In a screen for mutations which are enabling for cell cycle progression in aneuploidy cells, ubiquitin-proteasomal degradation components were a top hit [89].

6.3. p53 Interactome

In addition to *TP53* gene mutation, serous ovarian cancer exhibits a number of p53-interacting components that are also suppressed by deletions. Among the top hits by HAPTRIG [8] include *CHEK2*, *BAX*, and *GADD45A/B* gene deletions, along with *CCNE1* and *ATR* amplification. Chk2 is a kinase which coordinates DNA repair and cell cycle arrest, in part by stabilizing p53. Bax is a pro-apoptotic Bcl-2 family member which associates with p53 to induce apoptosis [90]. The Gadd45 proteins mediate DNA damage signaling to p53 and act as tumor suppressors by leading to damage-induced senescence [91]. Conversely, an upregulated ATR network allows for potential enhancement of DNA repair pathways which lead to aneuploidy and may also lead to centrosome duplications [92]. This is further supported by a common suppression of Rad51 networks in SOC.

6.4. Metabolism

Metabolism is fundamentally disrupted in serous ovarian cancer. This may be predicted by the observation that patients with metabolic disruptions are at risk for disease, or have a predisposition to tumors to undergo metastatic growth to adipose tissue [93, 94]. A shift to glycolysis, the Warburg effect, is a general hallmark of cancer. Glycolytic shift is considered essential to provide the many constituent molecules required for cell division: nucleotides, lipids, and amino acids, moreso than simply ATP which is produced in higher quantities by oxidative phosphorylation [95]. A metabolic pathway found to be suppressed with almost equal magnitude to autophagy was the arginine and proline metabolism pathway, particularly through deletions in *SAT1* and *SAT2* and guanidinoacetate N-methyltransferase. Such deletions are predicted to reduce spermidine metabolism and polyamine formation, which is normally upregulated in tumors [96]. The reason for their ubiquitous suppression may lie in the increase in glutamate which would come from an inhibition of arginine biosynthesis, which can then be used in the TCA cycle [97].

6.5. Adipocytokine

Adipocytokine signaling and *fatty acid* metabolism was also altered, led by suppressed networks with the *CPT1B* gene and *ADH4,6,7*, and *1A*. Again, this result is unique and unexpected: *CPT1* isoforms are often upregulated in prostate cancer [98] as are ADH enzymes [99]. Dysregulation of ADH isoforms may enable acetaldehyde formation, which is oncogenic, or favor class I alcohol dehydrogenases, which are upregulated in cancerous ovarian tissue [100]. Conversely, one of the most upregulated metabolic pathways in serous ovarian cancer is glycerolipid metabolism. Upregulation is led by amplification of the *DGAT1* gene, encoding diglyceride acyltransferase, the committing step for synthesis of triglycerides and an essential reaction for the formation of adipose tissue. The pathway is further reinforced by overexpression of *LPIN1* and *LPIN3* genes. While targeting metabolism has not historically been successful in cancer treatment, overexpression of these genes may act as early identifiers of ovarian cancer.

6.6. Peroxisome

An unusually altered pathway in serous ovarian cancer bridges metabolism, fatty acid oxidation and proteostasis disruption: *peroxisome* biogenesis. Peroxisomes are subcellular organelles whose primary function is to metabolize reactive-oxygen species and provide lipids to other organelles [101]. This pathway is amplified in serous ovarian cancer, and lung adenocarcinoma only [8]. *PEX5*, *PEX5L*, and *PEX19* are all commonly amplified. Pex5 and Pex19 bind to peroxisome enzymes in the cytosol and direct them to the peroxisome matrix [102, 103]. In fact, amplification of PEX5 is associated with poorer outcome in SOC. Peroxiredoxin-1 is also strongly amplified, and can be detected at increased levels in ovarian cancer patients' serum [104], and is also associated with lung cancer malignancy [105]. Upregulation of this pathway, and those associated with phospholipid metabolism may provide to a means to overcome oxidative stress, perform fatty acid beta-oxidation, and resist lipotoxicity associated with invasion of adipocyte-rich regions of the omentum.

While each of these pathways can help to define phenotypes associated with SOC, they also have the capacity to enable development of new classes of pathway-targeted therapeutics. It may be possible in future for SCNA-modified pathways to serve as targets the same way that SNVs do, now.

7. Potential for new treatments by targeting copy number alterations

SNVs have a proven track record of targetability using small molecules. Nonetheless, in the case of SOC, new cures are unlikely to be found unless somatic copy number alterations (SCNAs) are considered. Defining this interplay will be a difficult task. It remains unclear exactly which SCNAs are most critical to SOC proliferation and metastasis. The creation of cell line models will require new methods of whole-chromosome manipulation, even as attracting pharmaceutical company support will be harder due to limited experience which such targeting strategies, as well as conservative business approaches towards eventual clinical adaptation. Nonetheless, there are reasons to be optimistic that SCNA-targeted therapeutics can be effective and that some could enter the clinic in the near future.

Consider the abundance of SCNAs in advanced SOC relative to other cancer. The successful tumors have undergone selection. The phenotypes produced include well-known hallmarks of cancer: including cell cycle defects, heightened glucose uptake [106], spontaneous proliferative immortality [107], and dysregulated autophagy [108]. The same studies identify aneuploidy-associated characteristics which present vulnerabilities particular to these unstable cells. Perhaps the most promising vulnerability is an increased reliance on protein quality control processes such as ribosome biogenesis and maintenance factors and the cellular recycling process, autophagy. Aneuploid cells require these systems to function, and may result in a general reliance on catabolic function due to the proteotoxic effect of protein-complex subunit imbalance. Early studies recognized a general, if partial, sensitivity of these cells to rapamycin [106].

Chromosome instability can incur resistance to taxanes, a common front line therapeutic for SOC [109]. Chromosomal instability endowed by docetaxel may in fact lead to subsequent additional chemoresistance [110], though it is clear that the resistant phenotype is at least initially offset by an increased sensitivity to carboplatin, the second primary chemotherapeutic co-administered with a taxane as standard of care. Although aneuploidy enables oncogenic characteristics, it offers targetable vulnerabilities as well.

The mapped SCNA patterns in SOC revealed a general fault in proteostasis control, centered on autophagy [8]. Yet these cells require autophagy to maintain viability. The delicate balance within SOC relative to normal tissue, appears to provide a therapeutic window for proteostasis-targeting agents. Since SOC cells are already severely disrupted in their proteostasis-regulatory mechanisms, further disturbance can greatly compromise survival even as normal cells readily process the insult. Given this premise, we developed the Combination of Autophagy Selective Therapeutics (COAST) method to effectively manage SOC in the lab [8]. The general approach involves directly stressing the proteostasis system, while inhibiting autophagy resolution (**Figure 4**).

Mice given the cocktail of five proteostasis drugs did not lose weight nor negatively alter their blood chemistry panel [111], tolerating these drugs for months of daily treatment [8]. In mouse models using recurrent human SOC cells, the proteostasis drugs out-performed platinum-taxane dual treatment. The results are consistent with previous approaches pursuing a "cyclops" hypothesis: that monoallelic deletions in cancer sensitize cancer cells to further disruption of that gene's function [112]. As normal cells bear a full complement of

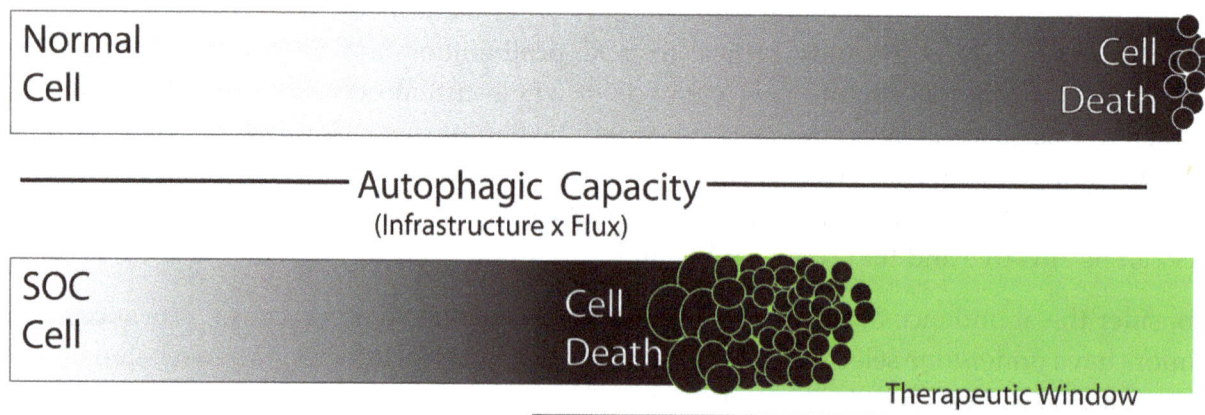

Figure 4. SCNA can compromise key cellular infrastructure. The figure shows how the disruption of autophagy capacity that is observed in SOC can render the cells more sensitive to agents that modulate autophagy. The lack of genetic infrastructure, combined with a constant requirement for autophagy, opens a therapeutic window for these agents. Nonetheless, the heterogeneity within tumors and between patients insures that no single agent, used alone, will provide a complete benefit.

all pathway genes, they are typically less sensitive to such stresses, which opens therapeutic windows for treatment.

Given that proteostasis pathways are only one type of disruption caused by SCNAs in SOC, what other SCNA-disrupted pathways might be targetable? Alluring targets may include the proteins downstream of the E3 ligases commonly deleted in SOC; inhibition of cell-cycle regulators may selectively target SOC cells even without any mutation or than copy number changes. Strong amplification of peroxisome transporters and the glycerophospholipid metabolism pathways suggest that metabolic targeting may be worthwhile. *GSK3B* controls signaling between varying development and stem cells pathways [113], and was marked as the most cumulatively impactful amplified gene in SOC by HAPTRIG [8]. Interestingly, inhibition of GSK3β in preclinical models of SOC showed strong tumor inhibition [114], and a number of drugs targeting GSK3β are in development for cancer, diabetes, and neurodegeneration [115]. Finally, the 8q24 region is the most commonly amplified genomic region in SOC, containing MYC and FAK. Inhibitors to FAK, such as defactinib, are already being tested in the clinic [116], and will hopefully provide some positive results in the near future.

A caveat of such designs is heterogeneity inherent in disease. Copy number instability is the result of SOC cells' extraordinary ability to create, tolerate, and expand genomic variation. Mathematical modeling of real tumor genetic data suggests that even small tumors with low mutation rates are statistically likely to contain multiple independent clones able to resist a particular drug treatment [117, 118]. Current SOC chemotherapeutics stimulate aneuploidy. Taxanes result in chromosome missegregation and platinum agents promote translocation events due to cross-strand DNA lesions. While it is absolutely true that common chemotherapeutics have limited combination potential due to dose limiting toxicities, that does not preclude the use of highly specific drugs to be used in combination or as maintenance therapy in SOC treatment regimens. Most likely, drugs independently targeting the many SCNA-disrupted pathways may be required to completely cure a patient.

While most patients are caught late in the evolution of their disease, it may not be "too late" to treat them. A genomic analysis in highly metastatic recurrent SOC patients found that the tumors likely form a metastasis-to-metastasis spread [14]. This may explain why round after round of different chemotherapy can extend the life of SOC patients [119]. This implies that current chemotherapy is quite effective at destroying a great majority of cells, and the challenge that remains is how to complement it. The COAST strategy studied in our lab functioned equally well or better for cisplatin resistant forms of SOC [8]. Autophagy has been widely implicated in the ability of quiescent cells to survive, including in SOC [120], and has been directly shown to enable growth of Doxil resistant disease [121]. However, given that one COAST agent, chloroquine is often prescribed for the same patient for decades in high-risk malaria areas, while another, nelfinavir, is a daily long-term HIV medication with no serious side-effects, the use of COAST is warranted based on the decades of use of COAST drugs, in humans, for diseases other than cancer. The side effects are well established to be below current chemotherapeutics carboplatin, paclitaxel, and Doxil [111]. The greatest health concern may lie in kidney cells, which are also exquisitely sensitive to autophagy drugs [122].

Since the drugs target different but complementary pathways, it is feasible to design clinical trials involving either simultaneous treatment or sequential treatment, enabling a greater chance of minimized side effects. Compromised DNA repair feeds into this pathway, suggesting that the recent successes of the PARP inhibitors are not simply due to BRCA1 complementation. An expanded range of options must be aggressively explored in the near future if we are to understand how to exploit the SCNA genetics of ovarian cancer in a timely fashion.

Abbreviations

AOC   Australian Ovarian Cancer (study)

N   the number of copies of a given gene present in a cell (e.g., 3N)

SCNA   somatic copy number alteration

SNV   single nucleotide variant (a point mutation)

SOC   serous ovarian carcinoma

TCGA   the Cancer Genome Atlas

TP53   tumor protein 53 kDa gene (protein is p53)

Author details

Joe R. Delaney and Dwayne G. Stupack*

*Address all correspondence to: dstupack@ucsd.edu

Division of Gynecologic Oncology, UCSD Department of Reproductive Medicine, UCSD Moores Cancer Center, USA

References

[1] Pon JR, Marra MA. Driver and passenger mutations in cancer. Annual Review of Pathology. 2015;**10**:25-50

[2] Olivier M, Hollstein M, Hainaut P. TP53 mutations in human cancers: Origins, consequences, and clinical use. Cold Spring Harbor Perspectives in Biology. 2010;**2**(1):a001008

[3] Tschaharganeh DF, Bosbach B, Lowe SW. Coordinated tumor suppression by chromosome 8p. Cancer Cell. 2016;**29**(5):617-619

[4] Ciccia A, Elledge SJ. The DNA damage response: Making it safe to play with knives. Molecular Cell. 2010;**40**(2):179-204

[5] Storlazzi CT et al. Gene amplification as double minutes or homogeneously staining regions in solid tumors: Origin and structure. Genome Research. 2010;**20**(9):1198-1206

[6]   Vogt N et al. Molecular structure of double-minute chromosomes bearing amplified copies of the epidermal growth factor receptor gene in gliomas. Proceedings of the National Academy of Sciences of the United States of America. 2004;**101**(31):11368-11373

[7]   Cai Y, Sablina AA. Cancer-associated chromosomal deletions: Size makes a difference. Cell Cycle. 2016;**15**(21):2850-2851

[8]   Delaney JR et al. Haploinsufficiency networks identify targetable patterns of allelic deficiency in low mutation ovarian cancer. Nature Communications. 2017;**8**:14423

[9]   Davoli T et al. Cumulative haploinsufficiency and triplosensitivity drive aneuploidy patterns and shape the cancer genome. Cell. 2013;**155**(4):948-962

[10]   Cai Y et al. Loss of chromosome 8p governs tumor progression and drug response by altering lipid metabolism. Cancer Cell. 2016;**29**(5):751-766

[11]   Zhang H et al. Integrated proteogenomic characterization of human high-grade serous ovarian cancer. Cell. 2016;**166**(3):755-765

[12]   Cancer Genome Atlas Research, N. Integrated genomic analyses of ovarian carcinoma. Nature. 2011;**474**(7353):609-15

[13]   Patch AM et al. Whole-genome characterization of chemoresistant ovarian cancer. Nature. 2015;**521**(7553):489-494

[14]   Schwarz RF et al. Spatial and temporal heterogeneity in high-grade serous ovarian cancer: A phylogenetic analysis. PLoS Medicine. 2015;**12**(2):e1001789

[15]   Kurose K et al. Frequent loss of PTEN expression is linked to elevated phosphorylated Akt levels, but not associated with p27 and cyclin D1 expression, in primary epithelial ovarian carcinomas. The American Journal of Pathology. 2001;**158**(6):2097-2106

[16]   Baker VV et al. C-myc amplification in ovarian cancer. Gynecologic Oncology. 1990; **38**(3):340-342

[17]   Li SB et al. Allele loss at the retinoblastoma locus in human ovarian cancer. Journal of the National Cancer Institute. 1991;**83**(9):637-640

[18]   Sasano H et al. An analysis of abnormalities of the retinoblastoma gene in human ovarian and endometrial carcinoma. Cancer. 1990;**66**(10):2150-2154

[19]   Fukumoto M et al. Association of Ki-ras with amplified DNA sequences, detected in human ovarian carcinomas by a modified in-gel renaturation assay. Cancer Research. 1989;**49**(7):1693-1697

[20]   Slamon DJ et al. Studies of the HER-2/neu proto-oncogene in human breast and ovarian cancer. Science. 1989;**244**(4905):707-712

[21]   Zhang X et al. Amplification and rearrangement of c-erb B proto-oncogenes in cancer of human female genital tract. Oncogene. 1989;**4**(8):985-989

[22]   Bourhis J et al. Expression of a human multidrug resistance gene in ovarian carcinomas. Cancer Research. 1989;**49**(18):5062-5065

[23] Mayr D et al. Analysis of gene amplification and prognostic markers in ovarian cancer using comparative genomic hybridization for microarrays and immunohistochemical analysis for tissue microarrays. American Journal of Clinical Pathology. 2006;**126**(1):101-109

[24] Nakayama K et al. Amplicon profiles in ovarian serous carcinomas. International Journal of Cancer. 2007;**120**(12):2613-2617

[25] Krogan NJ et al. The cancer cell map initiative: Defining the hallmark networks of cancer. Molecular Cell. 2015;**58**(4):690-698

[26] Zack TI et al. Pan-Cancer patterns of somatic copy number alteration. Nature Genetics. 2013;**45**(10):1134-1140

[27] Waclaw B et al. A spatial model predicts that dispersal and cell turnover limit intratumour heterogeneity. Nature. 2015;**525**(7568):261-264

[28] Burrell RA et al. The causes and consequences of genetic heterogeneity in cancer evolution. Nature. 2013;**501**(7467):338-345

[29] Mutation C, Pathway Analysis C. Working group of the international cancer genome, pathway and network analysis of cancer genomes. Nature Methods. 2015;**12**(7):615-621

[30] Huang RY et al. Histotype-specific copy-number alterations in ovarian cancer. BMC Medical Genomics. 2012;**5**:47

[31] Tapper J et al. Evidence for divergence of DNA copy number changes in serous, mucinous and endometrioid ovarian carcinomas. British Journal of Cancer. 1997;**75**(12):1782-1787

[32] Uehara Y et al. Integrated copy number and expression analysis identifies profiles of whole-arm chromosomal alterations and subgroups with favorable outcome in ovarian clear cell carcinomas. PLoS One. 2015;**10**(6):e0128066

[33] Project GENIE Goes Public. Cancer Discovery. 2017;**7**(2):118

[34] Marks JR et al. Overexpression and mutation of p53 in epithelial ovarian cancer. Cancer Research. 1991;**51**(11):2979-2984

[35] Lane DP. Cancer. p53, guardian of the genome. Nature. 1992;**358**(6381):15-16

[36] Levine AJ. p53, the cellular gatekeeper for growth and division. Cell. 1997;**88**(3):323-331

[37] Zilfou JT, Lowe SW. Tumor suppressive functions of p53. Cold Spring Harbor Perspectives in Biology. 2009;**1**(5):a001883

[38] Davis MA et al. Nelfinavir is effective against human cervical cancer cells in vivo: A potential treatment modality in resource-limited settings. Drug Design, Development and Therapy. 2016;**10**:1837-1846

[39] Manning AL, Benes C, Dyson NJ. Whole chromosome instability resulting from the synergistic effects of pRB and p53 inactivation. Oncogene. 2014;**33**(19):2487-2494

[40] Delaney JR, Stupack DG. Whole genome pathway analysis identifies an association of cadmium response gene loss with copy number variation in mutant p53 bearing uterine endometrial carcinomas. PLoS One. 2016;**11**(7):e0159114

[41] Janssen A et al. Chromosome segregation errors as a cause of DNA damage and structural chromosome aberrations. Science. 2011;**333**(6051):1895-1898

[42] Thompson SL, Compton DA. Proliferation of aneuploid human cells is limited by a p53-dependent mechanism. The Journal of Cell Biology. 2010;**188**(3):369-381

[43] Sheltzer JM et al. Single-chromosome gains commonly function as tumor suppressors. Cancer Cell. 2017;**31**(2):240-255

[44] Liu DP, Song H, Xu Y. A common gain of function of p53 cancer mutants in inducing genetic instability. Oncogene. 2010;**29**(7):949-956

[45] Martincorena I et al. Tumor evolution. High burden and pervasive positive selection of somatic mutations in normal human skin. Science. 2015;**348**(6237):880-886

[46] McCreery MQ et al. Evolution of metastasis revealed by mutational landscapes of chemically induced skin cancers. Nature Medicine. 2015;**21**(12):1514-1520

[47] Pennington KP et al. Germline and somatic mutations in homologous recombination genes predict platinum response and survival in ovarian, fallopian tube, and peritoneal carcinomas. Clinical Cancer Research. 2014;**20**(3):764-775

[48] Wang YK et al. Genomic consequences of aberrant DNA repair mechanisms stratify ovarian cancer histotypes. Nature Genetics. 2017;**49**(6):856-865

[49] Lieber MR et al. Nonhomologous DNA end joining (NHEJ) and chromosomal translocations in humans. Sub-Cellular Biochemistry. 2010;**50**:279-296

[50] McCormick A et al. Ovarian cancers harbor defects in nonhomologous end joining resulting in resistance to Rucaparib. Clinical Cancer Research. 2016

[51] Sears CR, Turchi JJ. Complex cisplatin-double strand break (DSB) lesions directly impair cellular non-homologous end-joining (NHEJ) independent of downstream damage response (DDR) pathways. The Journal of Biological Chemistry. 2012;**287**(29):24263-24272

[52] Aly A, Ganesan S. BRCA1, PARP, and 53BP1: Conditional synthetic lethality and synthetic viability. Journal of Molecular Cell Biology. 2011;**3**(1):66-74

[53] Mirza MR et al. Niraparib maintenance therapy in platinum-sensitive, recurrent ovarian cancer. The New England Journal of Medicine. 2016;**375**(22):2154-2164

[54] Niraparib in recurrent ovarian cancer. New England Journal of Medicine. 2017;**376**(8): 801-2

[55] Romanowicz-Makowska H et al. Analysis of microsatellite instability and BRCA1 mutations in patients from hereditary nonpolyposis colorectal cancer (HNPCC) family. Polish Journal of Pathology. 2005;**56**(1):21-26

[56] Segev Y et al. Risk factors for ovarian cancers with and without microsatellite instability. International Journal of Gynecological Cancer. 2013;**23**(6):1010-1015

[57] van der Looij M et al. Allelic imbalance and microsatellite instability in BRCA1 associated breast and ovarian tumors. International Journal of Oncology. 2001;**18**(4):775-780

[58] Arizti P et al. Tumor suppressor p53 is required to modulate BRCA1 expression. Molecular and Cellular Biology. 2000;**20**(20):7450-7459

[59] Wu LC et al. Identification of a RING protein that can interact in vivo with the BRCA1 gene product. Nature Genetics. 1996;**14**(4):430-440

[60] Deng CX. BRCA1: Cell cycle checkpoint, genetic instability, DNA damage response and cancer evolution. Nucleic Acids Research. 2006;**34**(5):1416-1426

[61] Xu X et al. Genetic interactions between tumor suppressors Brca1 and p53 in apoptosis, cell cycle and tumorigenesis. Nature Genetics. 2001;**28**(3):266-271

[62] Xu X et al. Centrosome amplification and a defective G2-M cell cycle checkpoint induce genetic instability in BRCA1 exon 11 isoform-deficient cells. Molecular Cell. 1999;**3**(3):389-395

[63] Deng CX. Tumorigenesis as a consequence of genetic instability in Brca1 mutant mice. Mutation Research. 2001;**477**(1-2):183-189

[64] Levine B, Yuan J. Autophagy in cell death: An innocent convict? The Journal of Clinical Investigation. 2005;**115**(10):2679-2688

[65] Mathew R et al. Autophagy suppresses tumor progression by limiting chromosomal instability. Genes & Development. 2007;**21**(11):1367-1381

[66] Zhao Z et al. UVRAG: At the crossroad of autophagy and genomic stability. Autophagy. 2012;**8**(9):1392-1393

[67] Godinho SA et al. Oncogene-like induction of cellular invasion from centrosome amplification. Nature. 2014;**510**(7503):167-171

[68] Mackeh R et al. Autophagy and microtubules—New story, old players. Journal of Cell Science. 2013;**126**(Pt 5):1071-1080

[69] Kandoth C et al. Mutational landscape and significance across 12 major cancer types. Nature. 2013;**502**(7471):333-339

[70] Hanahan D, Weinberg RA. The hallmarks of cancer. Cell. 2000;**100**(1):57-70

[71] Hanahan D, Weinberg RA. Hallmarks of cancer: The next generation. Cell. 2011;**144**(5): 646-674

[72] Nilsson JA, Cleveland JL. Myc pathways provoking cell suicide and cancer. Oncogene. 2003;**22**(56):9007-9021

[73] Sulzmaier FJ, Jean C, Schlaepfer DD. FAK in cancer: Mechanistic findings and clinical applications. Nature Reviews. Cancer. 2014;**14**(9):598-610

[74] Jones SF et al. A phase I study of VS-6063, a second-generation focal adhesion kinase inhibitor, in patients with advanced solid tumors. Investigational New Drugs. 2015;**33**(5): 1100-1107

[75] Yorimitsu T, Klionsky DJ. Autophagy: Molecular machinery for self-eating. Cell Death and Differentiation. 2005;**12**(Suppl 2):1542-1552

[76] Mizushima N. Autophagy: Process and function. Genes & Development. 2007;**21**(22): 2861-2873

[77] Noda T, Suzuki K, Ohsumi Y. Yeast autophagosomes: De novo formation of a membrane structure. Trends in Cell Biology. 2002;**12**(5):231-235

[78] Guo JY, White E. Autophagy is required for mitochondrial function, lipid metabolism, growth, and fate of KRAS(G12D)-driven lung tumors. Autophagy. 2013;**9**(10):1636-1638

[79] Nyfeler B, Eng CH. Revisiting autophagy addiction of tumor cells. Autophagy. 2016; **12**(7):1206-1207

[80] Kroemer G, Levine B. Autophagic cell death: The story of a misnomer. Nature Reviews. Molecular Cell Biology. 2008;**9**(12):1004-1010

[81] Avalos Y et al. Tumor suppression and promotion by autophagy. BioMed Research International. 2014;**2014**:603980

[82] Jin S. p53, autophagy and tumor suppression. Autophagy. 2005;**1**(3):171-173

[83] Yue Z et al. Beclin 1, an autophagy gene essential for early embryonic development, is a haploinsufficient tumor suppressor. Proceedings of the National Academy of Sciences of the United States of America. 2003;**100**(25):15077-15082

[84] Qu X et al. Promotion of tumorigenesis by heterozygous disruption of the beclin 1 autophagy gene. The Journal of Clinical Investigation. 2003;**112**(12):1809-1820

[85] Nezis IP et al. Autophagy as a trigger for cell death: Autophagic degradation of inhibitor of apoptosis dBruce controls DNA fragmentation during late oogenesis in Drosophila. Autophagy. 2010;**6**(8):1214-1215

[86] Devoy A et al. The ubiquitin-proteasome system and cancer. Essays in Biochemistry. 2005;**41**:187-203

[87] Devine T, Dai MS. Targeting the ubiquitin-mediated proteasome degradation of p53 for cancer therapy. Current Pharmaceutical Design. 2013;**19**(18):3248-3262

[88] Chen D, Dou QP. The ubiquitin-proteasome system as a prospective molecular target for cancer treatment and prevention. Current Protein & Peptide Science. 2010;**11**(6):459-470

[89] Torres EM et al. Identification of aneuploidy-tolerating mutations. Cell. 2010;**143**(1):71-83

[90] Chipuk JE et al. Direct activation of Bax by p53 mediates mitochondrial membrane permeabilization and apoptosis. Science. 2004;**303**(5660):1010-1014

[91] Tamura RE et al. GADD45 proteins: Central players in tumorigenesis. Current Molecular Medicine. 2012;**12**(5):634-651

[92] Katsura M et al. The ATR-Chk1 pathway plays a role in the generation of centrosome aberrations induced by Rad51C dysfunction. Nucleic Acids Research. 2009;**37**(12):3959-3968

[93] Lengyel E. Ovarian cancer development and metastasis. The American Journal of Pathology. 2010;**177**(3):1053-1064

[94] Clark R et al. Milky spots promote ovarian cancer metastatic colonization of peritoneal adipose in experimental models. The American Journal of Pathology. 2013;**183**(2):576-591

[95] Vander Heiden MG, Cantley LC, Thompson CB. Understanding the Warburg effect: The metabolic requirements of cell proliferation. Science. 2009;**324**(5930):1029-1033

[96] Gerner EW, Meyskens FL Jr. Polyamines and cancer: Old molecules, new understanding. Nature Reviews. Cancer. 2004;**4**(10):781-792

[97] Altman BJ, Stine ZE, Dang CV. From Krebs to clinic: Glutamine metabolism to cancer therapy. Nature Reviews. Cancer. 2016;**16**(10):619-634

[98] Wu X et al. Lipid metabolism in prostate cancer. American Journal of Clinical and Experimental Urology. 2014;**2**(2):111-120

[99] Jelski W, Szmitkowski M. Alcohol dehydrogenase (ADH) and aldehyde dehydrogenase (ALDH) in the cancer diseases. Clinica Chimica Acta. 2008;**395**(1-2):1-5

[100] Orywal K et al. The activity of class I, II, III and IV alcohol dehydrogenase isoenzymes and aldehyde dehydrogenase in ovarian cancer and ovarian cysts. Advances in Medical Sciences. 2013;**58**(2):216-220

[101] Lodhi IJ, Semenkovich CF. Peroxisomes: A nexus for lipid metabolism and cellular signaling. Cell Metabolism. 2014;**19**(3):380-392

[102] Erdmann R, Schliebs W. Peroxisomal matrix protein import: The transient pore model. Nature Reviews. Molecular Cell Biology. 2005;**6**(9):738-742

[103] Fang Y et al. PEX3 functions as a PEX19 docking factor in the import of class I peroxisomal membrane proteins. The Journal of Cell Biology. 2004;**164**(6):863-875

[104] Hoskins ER et al. Proteomic analysis of ovarian cancer proximal fluids: Validation of elevated peroxiredoxin 1 in patient peripheral circulation. PLoS One. 2011;**6**(9):e25056

[105] Jiang H et al. Expression of peroxiredoxin 1 and 4 promotes human lung cancer malignancy. American Journal of Cancer Research. 2014;**4**(5):445-460

[106] Torres EM et al. Effects of aneuploidy on cellular physiology and cell division in haploid yeast. Science. 2007;**317**(5840):916-924

[107] Williams BR et al. Aneuploidy affects proliferation and spontaneous immortalization in mammalian cells. Science. 2008;**322**(5902):703-709

[108] Stingele S et al. Global analysis of genome, transcriptome and proteome reveals the response to aneuploidy in human cells. Molecular Systems Biology. 2012;**8**:608

[109] Swanton C et al. Chromosomal instability determines taxane response. Proceedings of the National Academy of Sciences of the United States of America. 2009;**106**(21):8671-8676

[110] Ogden A et al. Docetaxel-induced polyploidization may underlie chemoresistance and disease relapse. Cancer Letters. 2015;**367**(2):89-92

[111] Delaney JR et al. A strategy to combine pathway-targeted low toxicity drugs in ovarian cancer. Oncotarget. 2015;**6**(31):31104-31118

[112] Nijhawan D et al. Cancer vulnerabilities unveiled by genomic loss. Cell. 2012;**150**(4):842-854

[113] McCubrey JA et al. GSK-3 as potential target for therapeutic intervention in cancer. Oncotarget. 2014;**5**(10):2881-2911

[114] Hilliard TS et al. Glycogen synthase kinase 3beta inhibitors induce apoptosis in ovarian cancer cells and inhibit in-vivo tumor growth. Anti-Cancer Drugs. 2011;**22**(10):978-985

[115] Cohen P, Goedert M. GSK3 inhibitors: Development and therapeutic potential. Nature Reviews. Drug Discovery. 2004;**3**(6):479-487

[116] Shimizu T et al. A first-in-Asian phase 1 study to evaluate safety, pharmacokinetics and clinical activity of VS-6063, a focal adhesion kinase (FAK) inhibitor in Japanese patients with advanced solid tumors. Cancer Chemotherapy and Pharmacology. 2016; **77**(5):997-1003

[117] Bozic I et al. Evolutionary dynamics of cancer in response to targeted combination therapy. eLife. 2013;**2**:e00747

[118] Diaz LA Jr et al. The molecular evolution of acquired resistance to targeted EGFR blockade in colorectal cancers. Nature. 2012;**486**(7404):537-540

[119] Luvero D, Milani A, Ledermann JA. Treatment options in recurrent ovarian cancer: Latest evidence and clinical potential. Therapeutic Advances in Medical Oncology. 2014;**6**(5):229-239

[120] Zhang Y et al. NAC1 modulates sensitivity of ovarian cancer cells to cisplatin by altering the HMGB1-mediated autophagic response. Oncogene. 2012;**31**(8):1055-1064

[121] Lu Z et al. The tumor suppressor gene ARHI regulates autophagy and tumor dormancy in human ovarian cancer cells. The Journal of Clinical Investigation. 2008;**118**(12): 3917-3929

[122] Kimura T et al. Chloroquine in cancer therapy: A double-edged sword of autophagy. Cancer Research. 2013;**73**(1):3-7

4

Immune Regulatory Network in Cervical Cancer Development: The Expanding Role of Innate Immunity Mechanisms

Olga Kurmyshkina, Pavel Kovchur,
Ludmila Schegoleva and Tatyana Volkova

Abstract

There is increasing evidence of a pivotal regulatory role of innate immune mechanisms in tumor-immune interplay. Among these diverse mechanisms, tumor-derived nucleic acids' sensing has recently emerged as one of the fundamental pathways linking innate and adaptive immunity, with DNA-sensor STING being the crucial member of this pathway. Another clear trend is understanding the striking diversity of innate and innate-like immune cell populations implicated in suppression or promotion of tumor growth. Papillomavirus-associated cervical cancer appears to represent a complex network of antiviral and antitumor innate immune mechanisms, whose regulation can be significantly influenced by developing neoplasia. In this chapter, we address new data on the problem of regulation of innate and acquired immunity in cervical cancer patients published in the past 2 years. To support the idea of multilevelness and diversity of changes in the innate arm of immunity, we also report our findings about (a) the expression of endogenous immune sensor STING in neoplastic tissue and peripheral blood lymphocytes, (b) altered frequencies of circulating natural killer and natural killer-like cell populations, as well as regulatory T lymphocytes from patients with precancerous or early cancerous lesions. Revisiting this problem may provide new insights into therapeutic options for cervical cancer.

Keywords: cervical neoplasia, innate immune system, antitumor immune response, innate-like lymphocytes, regulatory lymphocytes, immune suppression, DNA-sensing mechanisms

1. Introduction

Human papillomavirus (HPV)-associated cervical cancer is a type of oncopathology, one can consider as an example of a unique natural phenomenon of virus-related carcinogenesis, which realization is defined by dynamic interactions within a complex system "pathogen ('alien')-tumor ('altered-self')-host immunity." And while for the systems of "viral infection-immunity" and "tumor-immunity" interactions, the models well-describing molecular mechanisms supporting these interactions have been proposed, the situation when both pathological factors coexist seems to be much more complex. It is in these types of pathology that the dual (positive and negative) role of the immune system is most evident [1, 2], and it is for this reason that, obviously, despite a long history of studies, immunology of virus-related cancers still has a lot of blind-spots. The fact that clinical trials of immunotherapy methods to treat cervical cancer and other HPV-related cancers, which typically use unimodal approach, do not show the desired effect, particularly in advanced disease, underlines diverse multidirectional role of cellular, and molecular components of the immune system at different stages of disease development and points the need to study the combined multimodal approaches [3].

A large number of fundamental discoveries made recently in the area of oncoimmunology and immunology of infectious diseases have led to a substantial revision of the priorities in the studies of the antitumor immune response regulation mechanisms, including: (1) redefining the role for cellular components of the innate immune system, as well as the role for cells that represent a link between the innate and adaptive systems, in implementing an effective antitumor response; (2) understanding high phenotypic and functional heterogeneity (plasticity) of these components; (3) realization of the leading role of intrinsic (genetically encoded) mechanisms for stress-/damage-associated molecular pattern-dependent (neoantigen-independent) recognition and induction of immune response against transformed or virus-infected cells; (4) gaining insight into the expanding role of the immune checkpoint mechanisms (which normally have a protective, homeostatic function) tumors can adopt to resist antitumor immune response. It is clear that any attempts to activate (in clinical or experimental settings) specific T cell-mediated immunity, which is based on the T cell receptor (TCR) recognition of tumor-associated antigens (TAAs) presented by the major histocompatibility complex (MHC), to naught under the influence of immunosuppressive tumor micro- and macroenvironment. In this regard, current research has an explicit priority to study innate (genetically encoded) mechanisms of activation and suppression (i.e., immune regulation) of antitumor (and antiviral) response and cell subsets responsible for these mechanisms, as illustrated by thematic searching PubMed database for papers published in the last 2 years.

Among the innate mechanisms of immune recognition and immune regulation, the recognition of cell stress associated with the key hallmarks of carcinogenesis (such as uncontrolled cell mass accumulation, metabolic abnormalities, oxidative stress, and cell death program impairment) deserves special attention. These innate sensing mechanisms can be exploited not only in cells of the innate immune system itself, but also directly in neoplastic cells [4] and presumably even in adaptive immune cells of the system (see below). In general, they serve to detect mislocalized, normally non-immunogenic, molecules that can be regarded as damage-associated molecular patterns (DAMP), with the involvement of specific cell sensors that trigger downstream signaling to produce cytokines and other factors necessary for activation of effector functions of innate immune cells [4]. Among these signaling pathways, the innate response to extranuclear/cytosolic or extracellular DNA activated by various molecular DNA sensors (expressed virtually in all cell types) is an example of the most actively studied mechanisms, with the cGAS-STING molecular pair playing the main part. It is important to note that the mechanism of immune response to mislocalized/cytosolic DNA within the tumor site largely overlaps with the mechanism of recognition of viral infection (especially, in the case of DNA viruses such as HPV). However, even for such a common pathway of antitumor response induction, a dual (tumor-suppressing or tumor-promoting) role defined by the etiology or the stage of a disease has been reported.

More specialized populations of innate immune cells are also equipped with a large variety of receptors to detect mislocalized/ectopically expressed biomolecules in cancerous or virus-infected cells. Lymphoid cells (natural killer (NK) cells, NK-like T cells, and $T\gamma\delta$ lymphocytes), tumor-associated macrophages (TAMs, M1, and M2-polarized), tumor-associated neutrophils/myelocytes (TANs, N1, and N2-polarized), myeloid-derived suppressor cells (MDSCs), and other immature dendritic cells—all these cell populations (both tumor-infiltrating and circulating) are the main object of studies published recently. For most of them (including some innate-like T cell subpopulations), it has been established that they can significantly contribute to tumor progression, and at the same time, a crucial role in the elimination of malignant cells has been proved for innate-like lymphocytes (see below). The most difficult aspect of the functioning of these types of cells is their ability to produce the widest spectrum of cytokines that depends on the surrounding "context," thus defining their regulatory properties. In this sense, their activity should be considered in conjunction with the activity of regulatory/suppressor T and B cells (Treg, Breg) and different T helper subtypes, including pro-inflammatory Th17/Th22 cells, especially in light of the fact that the inflammation is appreciated as one of the most important tumor-promoting factors. Despite significant progress in the study of innate mechanisms of response to a developing tumor, which is implemented by the cell populations named above, many researchers point out that most of the information on this problem is obtained using laboratory mouse strains, which are certainly indispensable as experimental models, but this information cannot be simply extrapolated to the human body and thus requires a separate verification. This is especially important in case of virus-associated carcinogenesis because, due to high species-specificity of oncoviruses and their strong cell-type tropism, the range of *in vivo* models adequately reproducing the terms of the long-lasting, chronic infection, and gradual development of neoplasia in humans (which can take months and years), is limited [5].

HPV-associated cervical cancer as an object for studying the dynamics of "pathogen-tumor-immunity" interactions draws increasingly more attention due to the newly emerging findings demonstrating that during HPV-associated carcinogenesis, the immune system (and its innate components, in particular) acts as a double-edged sword and its role dramatically changes during the course of disease development [2]. Most HPV infections and low-grade lesions regress spontaneously in a short time; these cases are proposed to be considered as an "acute" infection [3], which is accompanied with the activation of inflammatory response superior in strength to a variety of mechanisms exploited by HPV to suppress inflammation and escape from immune recognition. However, in a number of cases, the infection turns into a persistent form, thereby

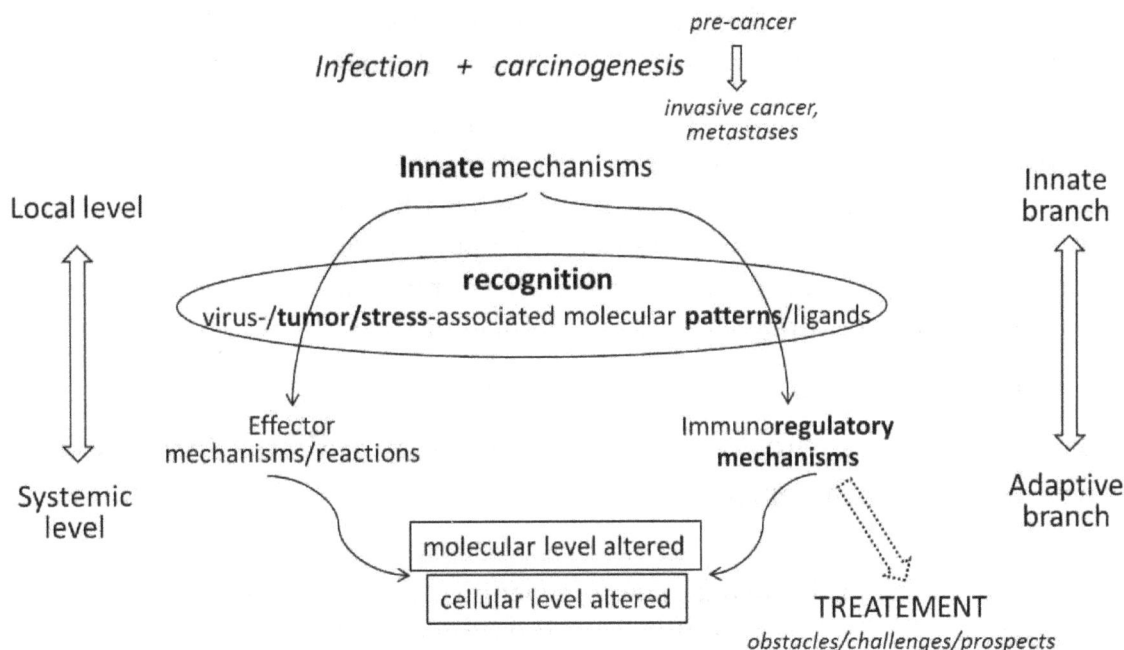

Figure 1. Scheme illustrating general relations between the key levels of immune response to cervical cancer that are addressed in the chapter.

increasing the risk of malignant transformation. In the later stages of carcinogenesis, in contrast to the stage of productive infection, HPV-transformed cells reprogram their environment in such a way that they gain the ability to recruit different populations of immune cells and to initiate chronic stromal inflammation, which contributes to further progression of precursor lesions into invasive cancer, facilitates tumor growth and metastatic spreading, and simultaneously promotes exhaustion of effector immune cells populations [2].

As a result of the fact that cervical cancer development is characterized by high genomic instability, the accumulated somatic mutations generate the enormous variety of neoantigens, which, together with the HPV-antigens, represent the potential targets for the T cell-mediated adaptive (TCR-restricted) response [6]. The range and immunogenicity (the ability to be presented to cytotoxic and helper T cells) of these antigens have been proved in high-throughput studies using integrated approaches to genome/transcriptome sequencing data analysis (see, for example, [7]). At the same time, the study by Qin et al. shows that increased mutation burden and neoantigen load correlates with HPV-dependent activation of master regulator genes that abrogate antitumor immune responses these neoantigens could cause by mobilizing immune regulatory, suppressive mechanisms. This again proves the rationale of studying the innate and innate-like lymphocytes, regulatory T/B lymphocytes, cells of myeloid lineage, as well as the mechanisms of antigen-independent innate immune response (including those involving DNA sensors) and the processes of immune regulation at different stages of cervical neoplasia development. In present chapter, the results of studies on these specific cell populations, mechanisms and processes published in last 2–3 years are described, with simultaneous discussion of our own experimental data on this problem, obtained from the patients with the diagnosis of pre- and microinvasive cervical cancer. Since a large number of constantly updated reviews are available on the issue of molecular strategies used by HPV to avoid immune response or other so-called cell restriction factors (see, for example, [8]), this question is not presented in the Chapter. In addition, we do not discuss the preventive and therapeutic vaccines developed for cervical cancer, as one can find many specialized detailed articles devoted to this applied question (for example, [9–11]).

The issues which are accentuated in this Chapter are showed schematically in **Figure 1**. Those are: the relationships between local and systemic changes, cells of innate and adaptive arms of immunity, their regulatory and effector properties, their phenotypic and quantitative changes—at different stages of cervical cancer development. We give special attention to pre- and microinvasive cervical carcinoma when reporting our findings is due to the idea that these stages can be considered as tipping points in re-formatting of the host immune system.

2. Intrinsic molecular mechanisms bridging antiviral and antitumor immune responses in cervical cancer

2.1. The role of nucleic acid-sensing pattern-recognition receptors (PRRs) and related signaling pathways in controlling cervical cancer development: current concepts

To respond to ectopically localized nucleic acids of exogenous (infectious) or endogenous (tumor cell- or stressed cell-derived) origin, cells are "armed" with a set of nucleic acid-sensing pattern recognition receptors (PRRs). Members of this essential group of PRRs are expressed in cells of both immune (lymphoid/myeloid) and non-immune (for example, epithelial) origin and can recognize various forms of nucleic acids (single- and double-stranded DNA or RNA, DNA-RNA-heteroduplexes, CpG-islets, as well as specific chemical modifications or structures, typical for viral DNA/RNA, and messenger cyclic nucleotides) in different cellular compartments (cytosol, endosomes/phagosomes, and even in the nucleus). These include some representatives of Toll-like receptor family (TLRs: 3, 7, 8, 9), Absent in Melanoma 2 family, (AIM2, IFI16), RIG-I-like receptors (RLRs: RIG-I and MDA5), and other members of the DExD/H helicase family, as well as a "signaling pair" of cyclic GMP-AMP synthase (cGAS)—Stimulator of Interferon Genes (STING). In spite of the fact that these receptors/sensors activate different signaling pathways, they all eventually lead to the activation of transcription factors such as Interferon Regulatory Factors (IRFs) or Nuclear Factor kappa B (NF-kB), which are responsible for the production of type I interferons (IFN-I) or proinflammatory cytokines, respectively [12].

Among the listed molecular sensors, the STING protein is recognized as a signaling hub (**Figure 2A**): it can receive and redistribute signals coming from different upstream molecular partners, although the most well studied and, perhaps, most important for mammalian cells, is the cGAS-STING signaling axis [13]. Binding of cGAS with cytosolic DNA results in the synthesis of secondary messenger—cyclic dinucleotide cGAMP—a natural STING ligand; following interaction with cGAMP, STING (an endoplasmic reticulum membrane-resident protein) initiates assembly of a multiprotein complex (i.e., signaling platform) and, through activation of IRF3 transcription factor, triggers expression of a large number of genes, including IFN-I genes and IFN-stimulated genes (ISG). Moreover, the new data from high-throughput transcriptome analysis showed that depending on the cell type, STING can alter the expression of not only the immune response-associated genes, but also many other genes that govern crucial cellular processes (proliferation, apoptosis, and stress response) [14–16]. The existence of alternative pathways that lead to STING activation (possibly ligand/agonist-independent) is also assumed, although the mechanisms have not yet been sufficiently described [17]. The key role of STING in antiviral innate immune defense has been confirmed by numerous studies, and it is not surprising, therefore, that different groups of viruses have evolved a variety of strategies to avoid/inhibit STING-dependent response, and oncoviruses are no exception: for most of tumor-associated mammalian viruses, STING, and other components of the STING-dependent signaling pathway were found to be specifically targeted by viral oncoproteins (in our previous paper, we summarized known mechanisms that are used by the oncoviruses, in particular, HPV, to evade STING-mediated recognition [18]).

The involvement of STING in regulation of the relationship between the tumor and the immune system (both innate and adaptive branches) mediated through the recognition of tumor DNA has been experimentally corroborated, although there are still many unresolved contradictions regarding its precise role in carcinogenesis: in different mouse tumor models, stimulation of expression, and/or activity of STING resulted in either restriction of tumor growth or tumor progression. What reasons could underlie these contradictions? On one hand, the STING-induced production of type I IFNs and activation of inflammatory reactions are obviously indispensable for the proper functioning of antigen-presenting cells (APC) and for further induction of adaptive antitumor response (discussed in [13, 19, 20]). On the other hand, the increased activity of STING leads to chronic inflammation within the locus of neoplasia which is a driving force of immunosuppression and tumorigenesis. In addition, there is still no clear understanding of exactly which cells within a tumor are responsible for STING-dependent recognition of tumor DNA. A previously proposed model, according to which it is phagocytizing cells (primarily dendritic cells and macrophages) that can engulf tumor DNA from dead/apoptotic tumor cells and activate the STING-signaling pathway, causes many doubts as it is not clear how endosomal/phagosomal DNA can reach cytosolic cGAS. Another model has been recently proposed, whereby the primary recognition of tumor DNA and synthesis of cGAMP occurs in tumor cells themselves because of the "leakage" of nuclear DNA into the cytosol (as a result of genomic instability, DNA damage, increased proliferation rates); cGAMP can diffuse to neighboring cells, including immune ones—presumably during the formation of immunological synapse—which are more efficient IFN-I producers and thus are able to promote recruitment of dendritic cells (DCs) and effector T cells [21]. APCs are widely recognized as such efficient producers, but other types of cells, for instance, lymphoid cells, can also be the candidates, considering that the level of STING mRNA/protein expression in lymphocytes was shown to be significantly higher than in macrophages [14, 16]. This model assumes that the initial stages of carcinogenesis are accompanied by an increased expression/activity of cGAS-STING, but as the tumor progresses, a disruption of cGAS-STING signaling—as a way to counterattack anti-tumor immunity—can occur. However, in virus-associated cancers, including cervical cancer, where STING activity can potentially be modulated by virus-derived and tumor-derived DNA, there may be the opposite sequence of events: in the initial phase of the establishment of a chronic infection, viral oncoproteins inhibit cGAS-STING pathway in infected cells (**Figure 2B**) and then, after undergoing malignant transformation, tumor cells gain the ability to support up-regulated state of cGAS-STING signaling in order to generate inflammatory immunosupressive microenvironment. Immunohistochemical study of HPV-infected cervical epithelium and low-grade cervical lesions indeed showed reduced expression of STING in relation to normal epithelium [22], but what changes are characteristic of high grade lesions and cervical cancer are as yet unknown.

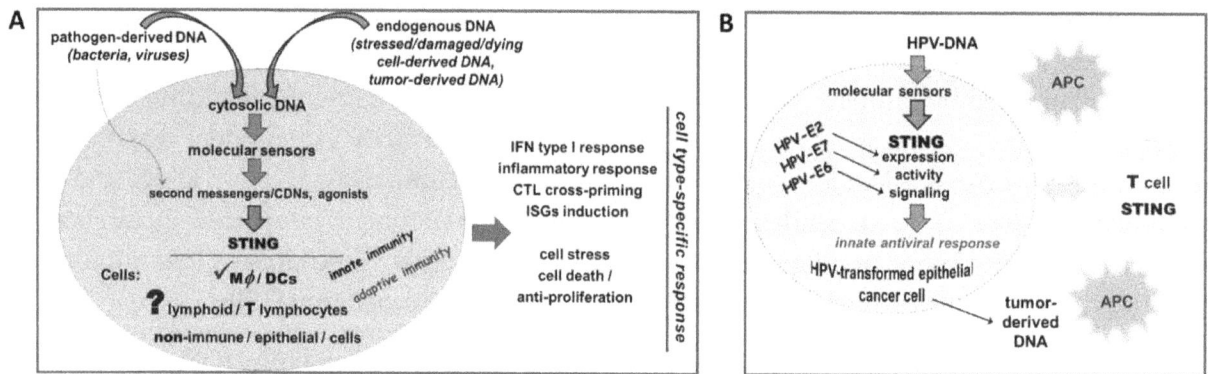

Figure 2. (A) Activating signals from various sources converge on STING to initiate cell type-specific innate response to cytosolic DNA. (B) In HPV-induced neoplastic lesions, STING can receive activating signals both from invading HPV-DNA and mislocalized self-DNA.

As mentioned before, STING-mediated signaling has been most thoroughly investigated in macrophages and dendritic cells while its role in other cell populations, specifically non-myeloid cells, is not fully understood. In this respect, recently published findings from *in vitro* and *in vivo* experiments (carried out using genetically engineered mice and STING ligands/agonists) demonstrating the functionality of canonical STING-dependent signaling in T cells [14–16] are of high importance. Surprisingly, besides activation of IFN-I response these experiments revealed T cell-specific ability of STING to modulate (inhibit) TCR-stimulated expansion and to induce cell death (through IRF3- and p53-dependent pathway), which is the fundamental difference from macrophages, in which stimulation of STING never leads to activation of death-associated genes [14–16]. The T cell-specific effect is extremely important for the prediction of therapeutic effect of STING agonists, which are currently undergoing extensive clinical trials as adjuvants in chemo-and immunotherapy of different types of cancer; however, in the case of cervical cancer the specificity of STING expression changes has not been investigated so far. At the same time, HPV-associated cervical cancer, in our opinion, can be used as a model object to study either cell type-specific or stage-specific involvement of STING in the innate/adaptive immune functioning at local and, most importantly, systemic level.

2.2. Altered patterns of STING expression indicate its putative role in cervical cancer

Based on the above facts, a study of the expression profile of STING (at mRNA/protein level) in tissue samples as well as in the major populations of peripheral blood T lymphocytes obtained from patients with preinvasive and microinvasive cervical cancer compared to healthy women (control group) has been started by our research team. We also took into account that: (1) increased expression of markers of apoptosis can be observed in circulating T lymphocytes in patients with early (pre-clinical) stages of cervical cancer [23]; (2) patients with early-stage cancer or precursor lesions display a variety of systemic alterations in the immune system including altered phenotype/activity and frequencies of different T cell populations, as evidenced by the large number of data (including those described below); (3) HPV-DNA (and possibly tumor DNA) circulates in the body and thus can be detected in various tissues and lymphoid organs long before the first detectable signs of metastases [24], whereby it potentially exerts a systemic effect on the activity of the STING.

2.2.1. STING protein levels in different subsets of circulating lymphocytes from early-stage cervical cancer patients

Intracellular STING level was measured in circulating CD4 and CD8 T cells, as well as in CD4CD25 subset (**Figure 3**) by flow cytometry using anti-human STING monoclonal antibody (MAb; clone 723505). Since the majority of lymphocyte population were stained positively for STING (which is in compliance with previously reported data showing that STING is robustly expressed in lymphoid tissue, specifically in T cells [14]), making the percentage values less informative, the level of STING protein was expressed as relative Mean Fluorescence Intensity value (ΔMFI) normalized to MFI of isotype control (IgG) with correction for autofluorescence of corresponding T cell subsets (Fluorescence Minus One, or FMO, control) (**Figure 3**).

As we did not find published works reporting on the level of STING in peripheral blood lymphocytes analyzed by means of immunofluorescence techniques, we first compared different commercially available kits for intracellular protein staining. The results of intracellular STING evaluation in peripheral blood T cells appeared to be sensitive to the permeabilizing ability of a fixation/permeabilization buffer set used, specifically: when kits designed for staining of intracellular proteins (such as cytokines) were applied, the level of anti-STING MAb binding did not differ from isotype control (**Figure 4A**); whereas the use of a reagent kit intended for intracellular detection of antigens such as nuclear transcription factors resulted in significant anti-STING MAb binding compared to isotype control (**Figure 4B**). This might be due to specific localization of STING and availability of its epitopes: homodimeric STING resides in the ER membrane and upon activation may form aggregates and translocate to Golgi and perinuclear space [25] (according to the manufacturer, the immunogen aa215-379 for the clone 723505 of anti-STING MAb corresponds to the C-terminal cytoplasmic domain of human STING).

In early-stage cervical cancer patients (with carcinoma *in situ* or microinvasive carcinoma), the level of STING protein showed a decreasing trend in both CD4 and CD8 T subsets compared to

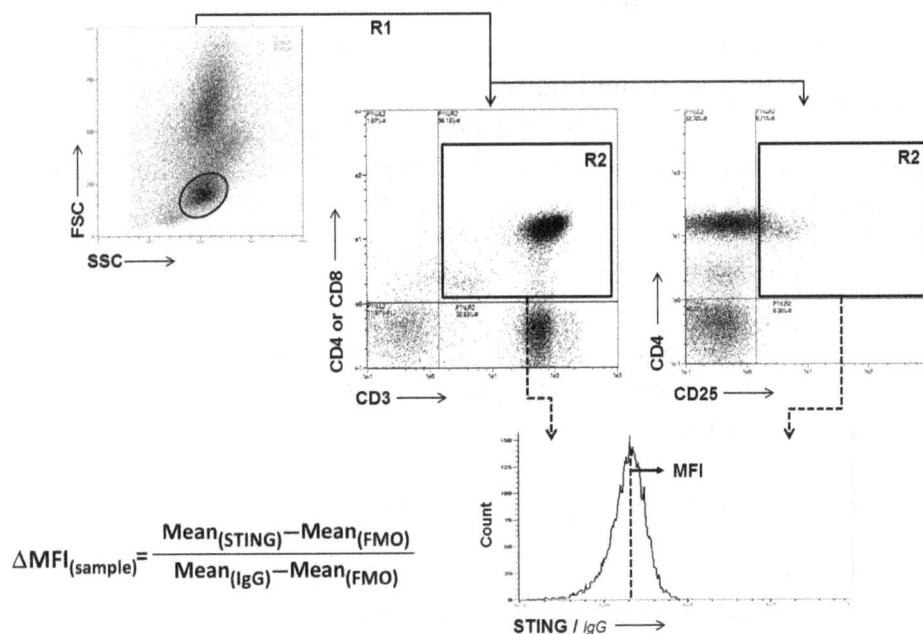

$$\Delta MFI_{(sample)} = \frac{Mean_{(STING)} - Mean_{(FMO)}}{Mean_{(IgG)} - Mean_{(FMO)}}$$

Figure 3. T cell gating and evaluation of STING protein level.

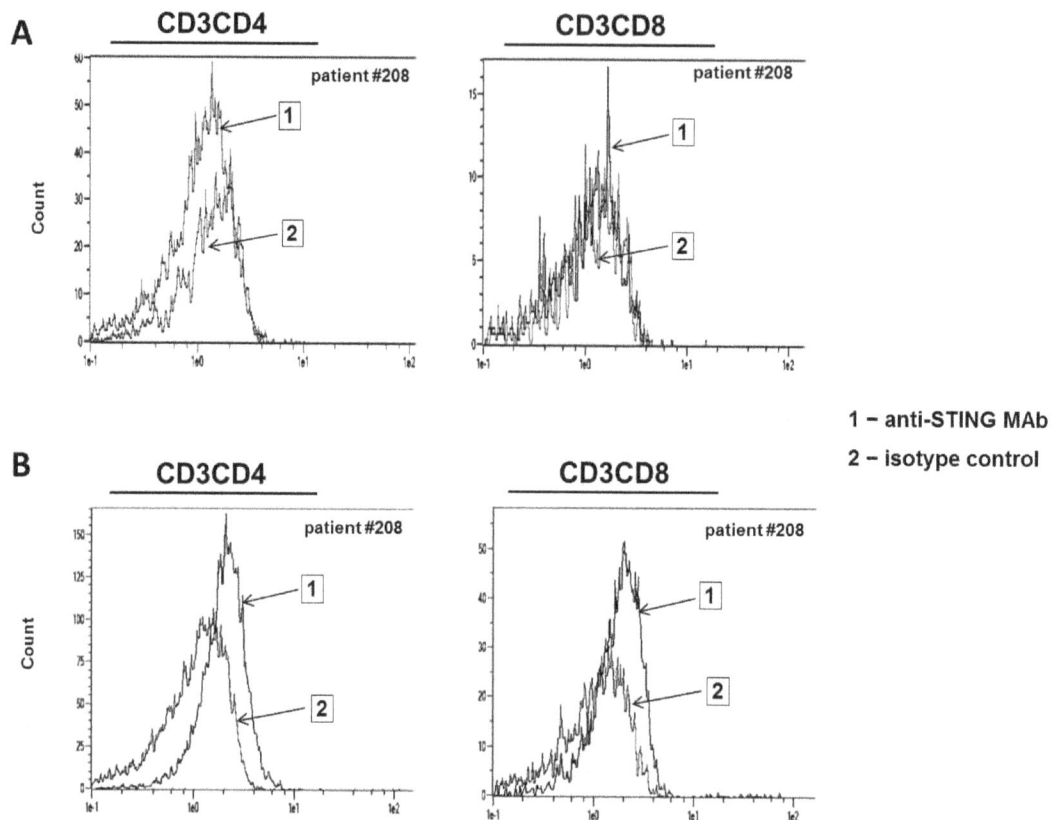

Figure 4. Representative examples of STING staining carried out using (A) a reagent buffer set for staining cytosolic proteins (e.g., cytokines), or (B) a reagent kit with stronger permeabilizing capacity for intracellular/nuclear protein staining.

healthy controls with this decrease being more pronounced in CD8 T lymphocytes (**Figure 5A**). No significant change was observed for CD4CD25 subpopulation. A notable increase in ΔMFI (CD4CD25)/ΔMFI (CD3CD8) ratio was revealed for circulating T cells from cancer patients (**Figure 5B**), implying that STING expression became more pronounced in CD4CD25 lymphocytes in relation to CD3CD8 subset. At the same time, the difference between STING levels in CD3CD4 and CD3CD8 cells from both controls and cancer patients was less significant; ΔMFI(CD3CD4)/ΔMFI (CD3CD8) ratios were close to 1 in all groups studied suggesting that the expression of STING is associated with both CD4 and CD8 T cell subsets. These results are, in a certain sense, in consistence with data reported previously by others for mouse models [14].

The percentage of STING-positive cells in total population of circulating lymphocytes from cervical cancer patients was on average lower than that in the control group, although this difference was not statistically significant (p > 0.05, U-test; **Figure 6**). When analyzing CD3 T cells, the same trend could be observed (while the total frequencies of T cells did not differ between patients and controls).

2.2.2. STING mRNA expression in peripheral blood mononuclear cells (PBMC) and neoplastic tissue samples

At the mRNA level, STING expression was analyzed in ficoll-isolated PBMC using semi-qPCR (RPLP0 and PGK1 genes were used as endogenous controls [26]): similar to flow cytometry results, in PBMC from patients with preinvasive/microinvasive cancer (stage 0-IA), STING-mRNA

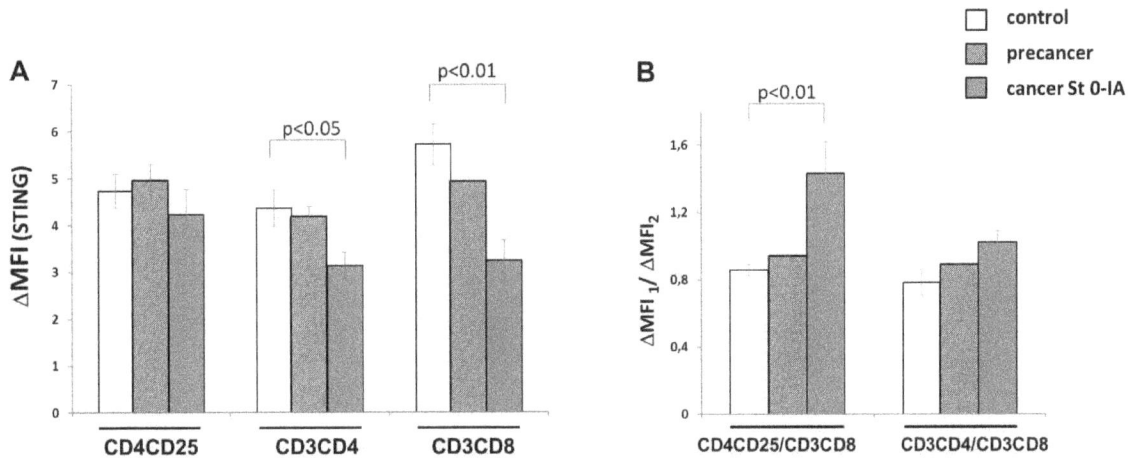

Figure 5. (A) The change of STING protein levels in major subsets of peripheral blood T cells from patients with precancerous cervical lesions or cancer (stage 0-IA, n = 20) relative to the control group of healthy donors (n = 15). (B) The ratio of the relative STING expression level in different T cell populations. Mean ± SEM values are displayed; p-value was assessed by U-test.

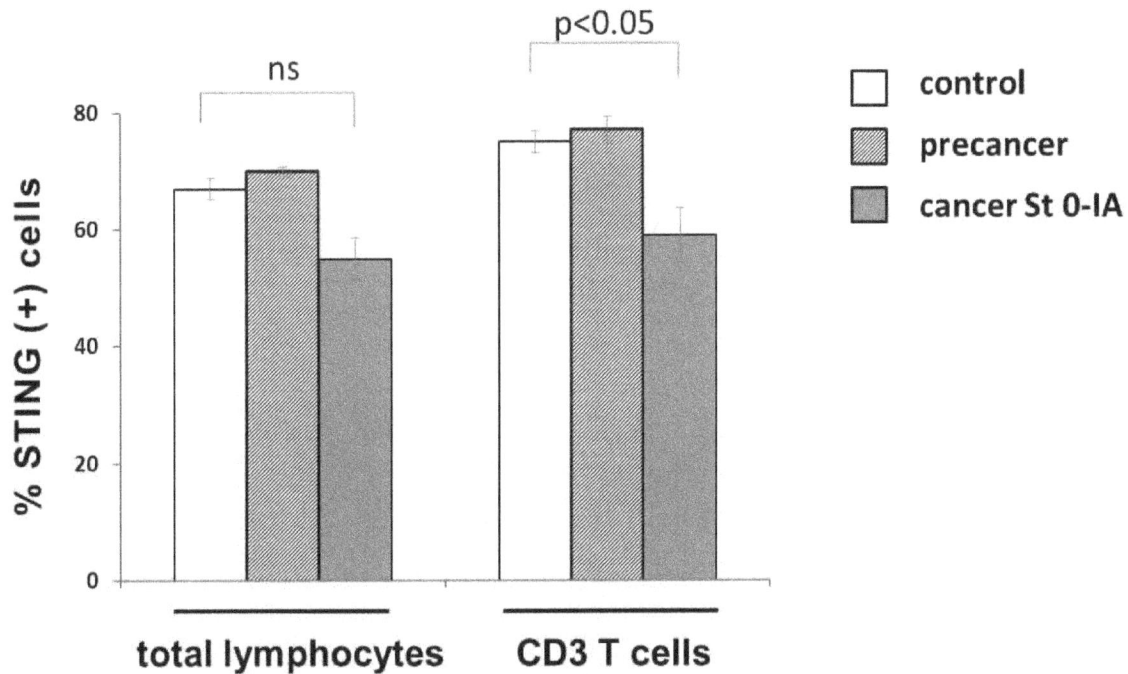

Figure 6. Percentage of peripheral blood lymphocytes stained positively for STING in patients with precancerous cervical lesions or cancer (stage 0-IA, n = 20) vs. healthy donors (control, n = 15). Mean ± SEM values are shown, ns—not significant.

level showed a slight decrease compared to the control group (p > 0.05, U-test; **Figure 7A**) suggesting the need for T cell (CD4/CD8) separation in further analysis. STING-mRNA expression was also assessed in samples of HPV-negative morphologically normal epithelium (control), HPV-positive precancerous lesions of the cervix, carcinoma in situ and microinvasive carcinoma (relative to four genes—EEF1A1, ACTB, GAPDH, and RPLP0—taken as endogenous controls due to their proved constitutive expression in cervical tissues [27]) (**Figure 7B**). In contrast to lymphocytes, a considerable (up to 50%) proportion of pathological samples

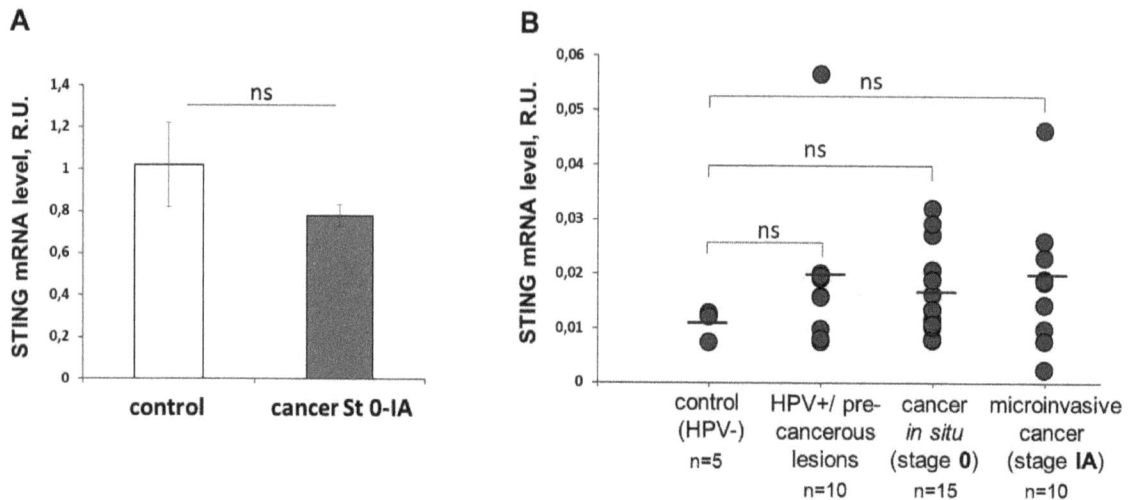

Figure 7. (A) The change of STING mRNA expression in PBMC isolated from cervical cancer patients compared to healthy women (controls); mean ± SEM values are shown. (B) The change of STING mRNA expression in cervical neoplastic lesions; group mean values are depicted as horizontal bars; ns—not significant.

in each patient group showed elevated STING expression as compared with normal non-infected epithelium (though the group mean values did not differ statistically). Up-regulation of STING at early stages of cervical carcinogenesis is consistent with some previous reports by other researchers and is, overall, in line with the conception of dichotomous role of STING-pathway in tumor development [28]. The data may also indicate STING's participation in as yet unexplored mechanisms promoting tumor development: for example, c-MYC proto-oncogene which overexpression is a hallmark of cervical cancer has been recently described as an essential transcription factor for the STING gene [29]).

Taking into account that cervical carcinogenesis can be associated with decreased proportion of STING-expressing T lymphocytes, as well as decreased level of STING protein in both T cell subsets (CD4 and CD8), one may assume the involvement of T cell STING in controlling papillomavirus infection and HPV-induced oncopathology. On the other hand, despite the lower level of STING observed in total CD3CD4 population of patients' peripheral blood lymphocytes, in CD25-positive subpopulation its expression was sustained at levels similar to the control: as CD25 is known to be a Treg marker, as well as a T-activation marker, this may be related to the processes of T cell activation/proliferation, interleukin (IL) 2-signaling, and T cell death. This assumption can be confirmed by recent findings [14, 15] demonstrating anti-proliferative or cell-death promoting activity of STING in TCR-stimulated T cells. Previously, we also showed up-regulation of apoptotic processes in circulating lymphocytes from early-stage cervical cancer patients [23], which was correlated with the expansion of CD25-positive cells (including FoxP3-expressing Treg) prompting further investigation of STING in T cells during virus-related carcinogenesis. Thus, the study of naturally occurred cervical neoplastic pathology that develops as a result of chronic viral infection suggests that STING being a key player in modulation of innate immune reactions may have an essential role in T cell functions. During the development of infection-related cancer, the importance of this specific role can be realized through redistribution of STING levels in different T cell subsets. Oppositely directed changes in STING expression observed in different compartments—blood T lymphocytes and neoplastic tissue—may illustrate the putative dual role of STING in virus-related carcinogenesis, which, in turn, may represent an important point in prognosing therapeutic outcome of STING stimulation. While administration of STING agonists may occur beneficial, for example, for patients with T cell-derived cancer (or other lymphoproliferative disorders) due to promotion of apoptosis in malignant T cells [16], mobilization of STING activity in solid tumors may have an opposite effect due to increased apoptosis of T effectors.

Summarizing, it is worth noting that the abundance of STING in T cells may imply; on one hand, their engagement in the innate immune mechanisms (as was revealed by a study of Larkin and co-authors who observed induction of intact antiviral IFN-I response in mouse T cells upon stimulation with STING agonists [14]) or, on the other hand, the plausibility of noncanonical functions exerted by human STING in cells of the adaptive immune system, these issues to be further investigated in the norm and in various pathological states, including virus-induced cervical cancer. In conclusion, it is worth mentioning that such noncanonical activity of STING, specifically, ability to switch on the apoptotic pathway has been unraveled not only in T cells, but in murine B lymphocytes (normal and malignant) as well [30]. However, in another study, the expression of STING in human B cells could be detected only upon Epstein-Barr virus-mediated transformation, while normal B lymphocytes were unable to elicit IFN-I response upon treatment with STING agonists due to the absence of STING expression [31]. Regarding other types of lymphocytes, for instance, NK cells, there is limited or no information. According to our flow cytometry data, the level of STING protein in circulating natural killer cells from patients with cervical carcinoma in situ is notably lower than in CD3CD4 and CD3CD8 (ΔMFI for CD3negCD16pos population was 2.16±0.16), but nonetheless 35 ± 4% of NK cells appear to be STING-positive suggesting potential involvement of STING in NK cell functions.

3. Cellular component of innate immunity (natural killer lymphocytes, myeloid cell populations): its role in regulation of T cell-mediated antitumor/antiviral immunity

3.1. Regulatory functions of innate immune cells in relation to cervical cancer development: current knowledge

The regulatory role of myeloid cells (monocytes—dendritic cells and macrophages, and especially granulocytes) has been undervalued for a long time; however, recently emerged data have prompted reconsideration of significance of these cells, classically regarded as professional phagocytes or professional APC, in mediating regulatory/suppressor effects of tumor cells on T-effectors [32]. In addition, the systemic effect of local neoplastic lesions on deviations within these innate immune cell populations, which can become detectable even earlier than the distribution of tumor-infiltrating cell populations is changed, is becoming increasingly apparent [32]. In respect of these abnormalities, a number of fundamentally important data have been obtained for cervical cancer.

According to the model described by Smola et al., IL-6 secreted by HPV-transformed cells acts as a triggering factor that leads to multiple impairments in the key functions of myelomonocytic cells during the intraepithelial stage of cervical cancer development. Under the influence of IL-6 and chemokines, myelocytes are actively recruited into the site of neoplasia, where they can differentiate into functionally impaired dendritic cells or M2-polarized macrophages to maintain pro-inflammatory environment. Despite they have mature phenotype, dendritic cells are not able to migrate to the lymph nodes to initiate adaptive response due to the lack of appropriate homing receptors; instead they accumulate within cervical cancer stroma and secrete pro-tumorigenic and Th2-polarizing factors. Cervical cancer-infiltrating M2-macrophages not only fail to produce IFNs at levels required for T cell activation and proliferation, but also express ligands for the immune checkpoint molecules, for example PD-1L, thereby promoting cytotoxic T cell exhaustion [6, 32–34]. Interestingly, according to Swangphon et al., cervical cancer patients exhibit altered ratio of M1/M2-polarized (CD64+/CD163+) monocytes not only at the local level, but in systemic circulation as well; notably, circulating M1/M2 ratio was shown to be correlated with the number of stroma- or peritumoral area-infiltrating M2-macrophages (CD163+), and with severity of the disease [35]. Similarly, cervical cancer patients displayed increased numbers of circulating dendritic cells (CD11b+) expressing PD-1L [36]. Moreover, an increase in the number of tumor-promoting M2-macrophages/ monocytes has been found to occur not only locally, i.e., in the tumor site, or systemically, i.e., in circulation, but also in tumor-draining lymph nodes (TDLN) of cervical cancer patients implying that the number of PD-1L+ M2-macrophages and metastasis are interrelated; this association allows to suppose that metastasizing cancer cells have the ability to recruit CD14+ monocytes and drive their conversion into M2-macrophages further contributing to the expansion of highly suppressive Treg cells [34].

Progression of precursor lesions into cervical cancer is also accompanied by an increase in the number of infiltrating neutrophils (TANs) displaying suppressive phenotype. A negative correlation found between the amount of TANs and CD8 T cells in high-grade lesions (cervical intraepithelial neoplasia grade 3, CIN3) or cervical cancer samples suggests that TANs can potentially contribute to inhibition of T cell activity and thereby facilitate tumor growth [32]. This assumption was confirmed experimentally in in vitro cell system using co-cultures of SiHa-spheroids, ex vivo-stimulated T lymphocytes, and neutrophils, with the ratio of T cell/neutrophil numbers appeared to be the determining factor for the degree of suppression of T cell proliferation, their expression of activation markers, secretion of IFNγ, and cytotoxic activity against SiHa cells [32]. At the systemic level—in the peripheral blood of cervical cancer patients—higher frequency of immature low density neutrophils has been also revealed, with elevated serum levels of granulocyte colony stimulating factor (G-CSF) discovered not only in cervical cancer patients, but also in women with precursor lesions (CIN2-3). Furthermore, patients diagnosed with cervical cancer are characterized by a systemic increase in the frequency of the tolerogenic monocyte-derived dendritic cells (MoDCs), the differentiation of which is modulated by G-CSF: MoDCs that were differentiated from monocytes taken from patients with CIN3 or cervical cancer and showing higher serum level of G-CSF were able to significantly more intensively inhibit proliferation of T cells from healthy donors and to promote Treg differentiation in the ex vivo system [32]. The effect of cervical neoplastic lesions on the process of MoDCs differentiation (expression of maturation markers, the profile of secreted cytokines) has been also demonstrated in a study by Lopes et al. [37]. Altogether, these data once again prove that early neoplastic lesions can be accompanied by systemic deviations in innate immunity, which in turn can influence redistribution of innate and adaptive cell populations and their interactions with each other within the tumor locus. The entirety of systemic and local immune changes is also an important point to consider when developing antitumor therapies based on adoptive DC transfer, because it is obviously these changes that determine the absence of the desired therapeutic effect (such developments aimed at overcoming the suppressive impact on DC are conducted using preclinical murine models of cervical cancer, see, for example, [38, 39]). In addition, a study performed by van Meir et al. showed that myeloid cells from cervical cancer patients can systematically respond to radio-therapy (RT): during the course of RT and 3–9 weeks after its completion (regardless the administration of cisplatin), increased frequencies of circulating CD3(-)CD19(-)HLA-DR(+) monocytes as well as CD3(-)CD19(-)HLA-DR(-) MDSCs were detected in parallel with the loss of T cell reactivity and stimulatory capacity of APC in *ex vivo* testing [40].

Unlike neutrophils and suppressor populations of myeloid cells, whose contribution to the progression of solid tumors has only recently come under intense investigation, the functions of natural killer cells have always been considered in the context of cancer immunosurveillance. However, in spite of the fact that for this group of innate lymphoid cells, a detailed spectrum of receptors allowing for recognition of transformed cells has been described and a vast diversity of mechanisms for their cytotoxic action has been established, attempts to use them in anticancer therapy occurred to be unsuccessful—the reasons for this situation are reviewed in [41], and among these reasons are the underappreciated regulatory properties of NK cells implementing via production of a wide range of cytokines, the specificity of which is largely determined by the surrounding molecular context. Nevertheless, recently there has been considerable revival of interest in NK cells brought about by the invention of chimeric antigen receptors (CAR) technology that made possible creation of engineered CAR-NKs with "improved" properties (e.g., increased migrating and proliferating ability, up-regulated expression of activating receptors) for their subsequent adoptive transfer into a cancer patient. Another promising concept seems to be the use of Cord-Blood NK cells that can retain a highly activated phenotype and whose expansion capacity substantially exceeds that of peripheral blood NK cells (successful implementation of this approach in the preclinical model system using cervical cancer cell lines has been recently reported in [42]).

Cervical cancer cells' ability to withstand NK cell-mediated response is clearly confirmed by the observation that the prevalence of NK cells in CD45(+)-infiltrating leukocytes is greatly reduced with the progression of intraepithelial neoplasia to invasive cancer [32]. In addition to the known mechanisms recruited by cervical cancer cells to escape from NK-mediated recognition (including down-regulation of activating NK-cell receptor ligands MICA/B, ULBPs, or aberrant expression of non-classical HLA-G [43]), inhibition of NK cell activity can be driven by intra-tumoral Tregs, as was confirmed in ex vivo experiments with Tregs and NK cells isolated from primary tumors of cervical cancer patients [44]. Whether these negative processes have any influence on circulating NK cells during the development of cervical cancer remains a poorly studied question.

Despite the high phenotypic heterogeneity of NK cells, they can be divided into two subsets depending on the level of expression of CD56 marker: CD56bright and CD56dim. These two populations differ not only phenotypically and functionally—they are differently represented in the systemic circulation and tissues [45]. CD56dim population comprises the vast majority (80–95%) of peripheral blood NK cells and is characterized by high expression of markers of mature phenotype (including CD16/FcγRIIIa required for activation of antibody-dependent cytotoxicity, perforin and granzyme B cytotoxic proteins); traditionally, this population is associated with anti-tumor response. Unlike CD56dim, CD56bright NK cells represent the minor population in peripheral blood, while in the secondary lymphoid organs and other tissues CD56bright cells account for the majority of peripheral NKs. In addition, they are characterized by the absence or low expression of CD16 (CD16dim/neg) and low cytotoxic activity, so their role in direct killing of tumor cells is less clear; on the other hand, CD56bright NK cells are known for their high cytokine and chemokine production capacity (including IFNγ, TNFα, GM-CSF, IL-10, IL-13, CCL3, and CCL4), and immunomodulation of activity of other innate or adaptive immune cells is therefore believed to be a key feature of CD56bright NK cell subset.

Presently, increasing attention is being paid to CD56bright NK cells as new facts are emerging suggesting that there is no strict functional dichotomy between the so called regulatory CD56bright and cytolytic CD56dim subsets, and that CD56bright cells are capable of acquiring cytotoxicity upon appropriate stimulation with specific combinations of cytokines [45]. Indeed, it has been recently shown that priming of CD56bright NK cells with IL-15 is accompanied by a burst of cytotoxic activity against tumor cells; however, this has only been confirmed so far for hematological malignancies [46]. Upon treatment with different stimuli, CD56bright NK cells exhibit ability of suppressing proliferation of autologous CD4 T cells via both cytotoxic and immunoregulatory mechanisms, e.g., by secreting the immunosuppressive molecule adenosine (these mechanisms are reviewed in detail in [47]). For some types of solid cancers, in particular lung cancer and breast cancer, the proportion of CD56bright cells in a total amount of tumor-infiltrating NK cells was found to be significantly higher than in the corresponding normal tissues, however, they express low perforin and rather play an immunoregulatory role, but not cytotoxic [48].

3.2. Analysis of NK cell subpopulations in peripheral blood lymphocytes of early-stage cervical cancer patients

Taking into consideration, the proposed model that describes the ability of CD56bright NK cells to circulate among tissues, lymphoid organs, and peripheral blood [45, 48], it can be assumed that altered frequencies of these cells in the blood of cancer patients are highly relevant to immune regulation at the tumor locus. Quantitative assessment of circulating CD56bright NK cell population has been performed for head and neck cancer [49], prostate [50], and breast cancer [51, 52]); we also recently reported our findings concerning circulating NK subsets in women with CIN3 (including carcinoma in situ) and microinvasive carcinoma (stage IA1) of the cervix [23].

Based on the intensity of CD16/CD56 staining, we could distinguish four main subsets of circulating NK cells within CD3-negative lymphocytes (gates P1–P4, **Figure 8**). As expected, we found no significant difference in the frequency of cells within CD16brightCD56dim gate (which encompasses the major pool of circulating cytotoxic NKs), as well as within CD16dim/negCD56dim and CD16brightCD56neg gates (comprising less abundant populations with poorly established functions) between patients and controls. As opposed to these subsets, a decrease in the frequency of CD16dim/negCD56bright NK cells and, accordingly, higher CD56dim/CD56bright ratio were observed in cervical cancer patients relative to the control group. We hypothesized this specific alteration reflects a systemic shift in the balance between effector and regulatory NK subsets that occur early in invasive cervical cancer development. One can also speculate this change, along with those described above for M2/M1, neutrophils and MoDC subsets, is part of a complex cervical cancer-related immunoregulatory network. As it is well known that activation of NK cells occurs locally, in our attempt to interpret the obtained data we therefore use the idea that circulating CD56bright NKregs are recruited to the lymphoid tissue (regional lymph nodes) and the primary tumor site, where they are thought to serve as precursors for cytotoxic/effector CD56dim NK cells [45]. This assumption encourages further investigation into the regulatory role of NK cells in cervical cancer progression.

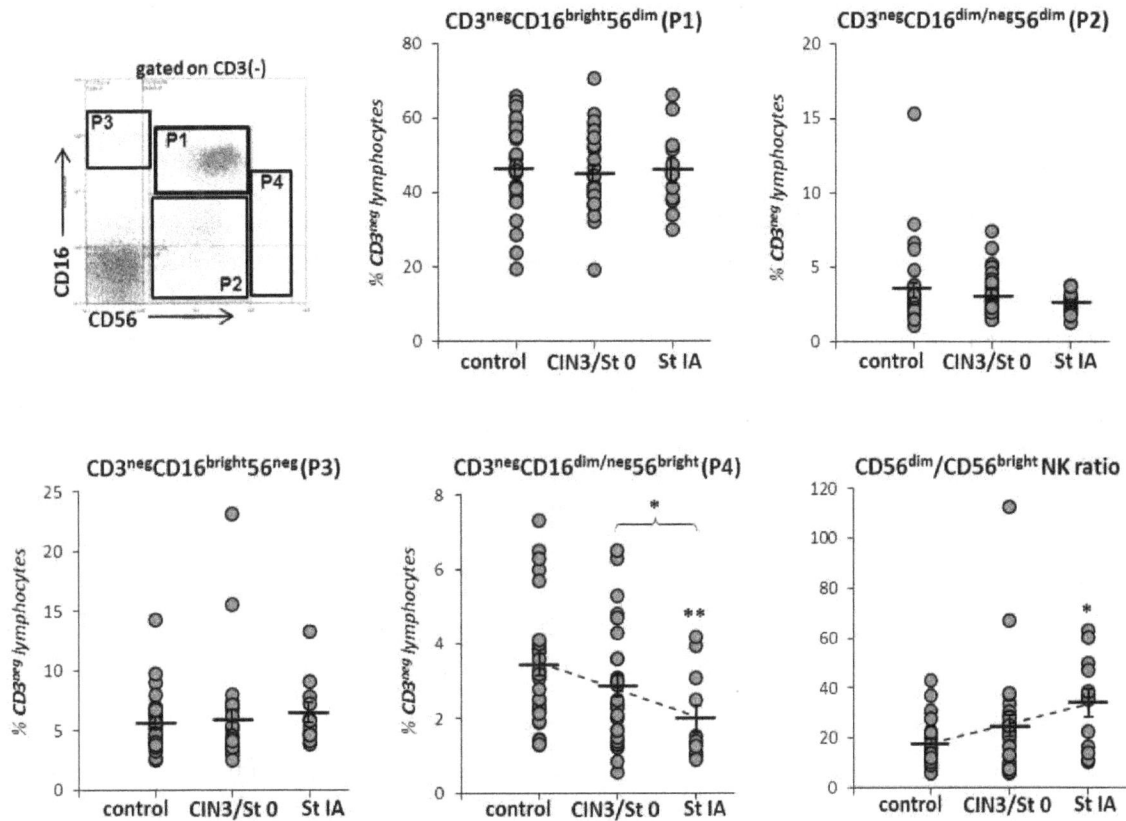

Figure 8. Percentage of peripheral blood CD56bright NK cells and CD56dim/CD56bright ratio within circulating NK cell population in patients (n = 30 for CIN3/stage 0, n = 15 for stage IA) vs. healthy controls (n = 30) as measured by flow cytometry. Lymphocytes were gated for CD3-negativity (a diagram on the left) and a population of interest was defined according to CD16/CD56 membrane expression levels (gates P1–P4). Here and below, individual values are shown as dots; bars correspond to the mean ± SEM values; statistically significant difference between the patient group and the control group are marked with asterisk: *p < 0.05, **p < 0.01 (U-test).

4. Innate-like T lymphocytes: pivotal players in the tumor: immunity interplay

4.1. The emerging role of NK-like T cells (NKT) and γδT lymphocytes in cervical cancer progression

Since recently, a heterogeneous group of innate-like T lymphocytes linking the two branches of immunity, innate and adaptive, is being increasingly acknowledged as a valuable source of novel opportunities for antitumor therapies development. This was facilitated by increasing realization of the pivotal role of innate-like T cells in tumor immune surveillance and their unique ability to recognize cancerous and virus-infected cells in a highly specific, though MHC-unrestricted, manner. Similar to innate immune cells, they are equipped with a rich set of germline-encoded receptors conferring them ability to undergo rapid activation upon interaction with ectopically expressed or stress-associated molecules on the surface of target cells. In addition, like conventional αβT cells, innate-like T lymphocytes (NKT and γδT) express T cell receptors (TCR), although their repertoire differs from αβT cells. The range of antigens the innate-like lymphocytes' TCRs are able to recognize is defined by their structural properties (for example, lipid antigens in the case of NKT cells or phosphoantigens in the case of γδT cells) and therefore is thought to be restricted and universal; at the same time, these antigens are present within a plenty of natural ligands, which is doubtless advantageous from a therapeutic standpoint. Quick activation in response to antigenic exposure followed by intense production of a broad range of cytokines is another valuable characteristic of innate-like lymphocytes they have in common with typical innate lymphocytes; it is known, for instance, that even in the absence of stimulation NKT cells permanently stay in pre-activated state. That is why innate-like lymphocytes supposedly perform "guarding" functions by being the first to respond efficiently to pathological changes (infection, transformation) and stimulate further activation of dendritic cells and adaptive response. However, in spite of their apparent beneficial properties, there are several features that greatly impede potential manipulations of innate-like lymphocytes, among them are: high structural and functional population heterogeneity, low abundance, heterogeneous distribution of different subpopulations in tissue and blood compartments, ability to provoke chronic inflammation and to secrete not only Th1-cytokines, but Th2 as well. If structural heterogeneity of innate-like lymphocytes is defined by their receptor repertoire, their functional heterogeneity is believed to be driven by polarizing factors coming from the environment. Importantly, conclusions about existing functional subtypes of innate-like lymphocytes were made based mostly on the results of in vitro stimulation [53–55].

Like conventional T lymphocytes, NKT cells express αβTCR, but can undergo activation only on interaction with lipid antigens presented by CD1b (a nonpolymorphic MHC-I-like molecule). In spite of such a relatively narrow specificity, NKT cells however exhibit an important feature—ability for TCR-independent activation upon stimulation with proinflammatory cytokines IL-12, IL-18, IL-25, and IL-23. According to the structure and binding specificity of TCRs, two NKT subsets can be distinguished: NKT-I, or iNKT—invariant NKT cells (with α-galactosylceramide being a prototypic ligand), and NKT-II cells—variant NKT having less restricted specificity. NKT-II cells are thought to be the most prevalent NKT subset in humans (in contrast to, for example, mice, where NKT-I cells are known to be more abundant), although their identification and characterization is still a challenging task due to the lack of distinctive NKT-II markers or agonists specifically targeting their receptors. In general, following the results of *in vivo* modeling of various cancers, NKT-I cells have been associated with the protective antitumor response, while NKT-II have been implicated in immunosuppression/immunoregulation and tumor promotion. The mechanisms of antitumor activity of NKT-I cells consist in their ability for both direct tumor lysis and generation of copious amounts of IFNγ (along with other Th1 cytokines) required for recruitment and activation/full maturation of APC, CD8 cytotoxic T lymphocytes, and NK cells. Immunosuppressive effect of NKT-II cells is thought to be due to their ability to produce high levels of IL-4 and IL-13 that shift immune response towards Th2 type. Nevertheless, this functional dichotomy is at present actively debated, and there is growing conviction that it is not so firmly associated with NKT-I or -II subset; rather, it is determined by the context (for example, tissue location) or microenvironment where activation of NKT cells occurs [53]. (Due to limited space, in our characteristic of NKT cells and γδT cells, here and below we refer to several recently published comprehensive reviews that contain links to original papers).

In spite of the relatively low abundance of NKT cells, there is constantly growing body of evidence showing this cell population undergoes quantitative and phenotypic changes (both in peripheral blood and within the tumor locus) in patients with different types of cancer, however there is only scares information available for cervical cancer. It has been found that

HPV can escape from NKT cell-mediated CD1d-restricted recognition of infected keratinocytes and low-grade cervical neoplastic lesions via HPV-E5 dependent inhibition of CD1d expression (while normal keratinocytes express high levels of CD1d molecule) [56]. Despite this evasion mechanism, CIN2-3 lesions were shown to be associated with increased numbers of infiltrating iNKT, with these numbers being higher for HPV-positive lesions than for HPV-negative [57]. Elevated frequency of circulating NKT have been revealed in peripheral blood of women with CIN1 and HPV infection, compared to the control group or HPV-positive women without signs of neoplastic abnormalities [58]. It can be inferred from these findings that the population of NKT cells may undergo early changes upon persistent HPV infection and progressing neoplasia, although there is no data available for more advanced stages of the disease.

γδT lymphocytes differ from both conventional T cells and NKT cells in their TCR chains composition and ability to recognize phosphoantigens, while many other features characteristic of NKT cells are shared by γδT as well, specifically: rapid activation, direct cytotoxicity against infected or transformed cells, reliance on natural killer receptors that enable fast (MHC-independent) response to stress-related ligands expressed on the surface of cancer cells, strong regulatory properties and ability to modulate activity of other immune cells via production of a wide range of cytokines. Further, similar to NKT cells, γδT also demonstrate functional heterogeneity (polarization) with regard to antitumor response, with this heterogeneity partially overlapping with the structural features of γδTCR, but nevertheless being mostly driven by differential environmental stimulation, as was mentioned for NKT cells. In humans, Vδ2 T cells were found to be the most frequent subpopulation of peripheral blood γδT cells (70%); Vδ1 T cells constitute the remaining 30% of γδT in circulation, although they represent the dominant γδT subset in epithelial and some other tissues. Antitumor activity of Vδ2 T cells is attributed to not only their ability to directly recognize (via congenital receptors) and kill tumor cells, but also their ability to effectively cross-present antigens to CD8 αβT effectors and NKT cells, as well as facilitate DC maturation and co-stimulate cytolytic activity of NK cells. Pro-tumor role of Vδ1 T cells can be explained by their IL-17-producing ability; at the same time, however, these cells show unique specificity for B7-H6 molecule expressed exclusively on tumor cells, being able thereby to exert antitumor effect. Immunoregulatory (suppressive) function of γδT cells in antitumor immunity is thought to be mediated by IL-10 and TGF-β, or adenosine secreted by tumor-infiltrating γδT cells [54, 55].

The impact of γδT cells on pathogenesis of cervical cancer is largely unexplored. Gosmann and co-authors analyzed total population of CD45+IL-17+ cells infiltrating CIN2-3 lesions and found them to be represented by not only CD3CD4 T helpers (Th17), but also by γδT cells, although the percentage of γδT cells was significantly lower than that of Th17 [59]; this observation may indicate their putative involvement in the promotion of proinflammatory suppressive microenvironment as CIN progresses to invasive cancer. The cytotoxic activity of γδT cells isolated from PBMC against cervical cancer cell lines (HeLa, SiHa, and CaSki) pre-treated with bisphosphonate pamidronate was also confirmed in [60]. A vast amount of clinical data on the role of γδT cells in viral infections, as well as their correlation with cancer prognosis allows speculation on γδT cell involvement in pathogenesis of virus-associated cervical cancer. Whether this cell population experiences any changes at different stages of cervical cancer, and if so, in which tissue compartments or depending on which clinical-pathological parameters—remains an open question.

Taken together, innate and innate-like (NK, NKT, and γδT) lymphocytes proved to have non-redundant functions in antitumor immune response, which makes them attractive objects for the development of adoptive cell transfer therapy combined with immune checkpoints blockade or neutralization of other immune-suppressive factors [55, 61]. At the same time, the results of preclinical studies and attempts to translate them to clinical settings explicitly point to our insufficient knowledge of the role of innate-like lymphocytes and the mechanisms, whereby they contribute to cancer progression [53, 55].

4.2. Analysis of CD3+CD56+ population and its CD3bright subset in PBMC from early-stage cervical cancer patients

CD56 is a natural killer prototypic marker, but, apart from NK cells, its expression is shared by T lymphocytes (NKT and γδT) and is commonly considered as a marker of an activated state, NK-like cytotoxicity and IFNγproduction [62]. Accordingly, CD3+CD56+ population comprises of both NKT and γδT lymphocytes, but within this population, a CD3bright subset can be observed [63]. Studies on phenotyping of CD3bright subpopulation have identified it as γδT lymphocytes [63, 64]. Furthermore, Paget and co-authors [64] established mouse CD3bright γδT cells were identical to Vδ1 sub-lineage (Vγ6/Vδ1+ TCR) and possessed high IL-17-producing capacity; the high CD3 expression (CD3bright phenotype) could hence be considered as a surrogate marker of γδT identity. In humans, the population of circulating CD3brightCD56+ cells has been analyzed in patients with chronic hepatitis B infection: it has been shown that, despite increased numbers, their activity and phenotype are substantially impaired, this impairment includes down-modulation of IFNγ and LAMP1 expression (i.e., markers of antiviral and killing activity) and, conversely, up-regulation of NKG2A [65].

Given, the described data on the ability of CD3bright T cells to respond to inflammation and chronic infection observed either in model animals or in humans, in the norm or under pathological conditions, we decided to examine whether changes of the frequency of this cell population could be detected in the circulation of patients at early stages of cervical cancer progression (**Figure 9**). Using clone UCHT1 of anti-human CD3 MAb, we were able to clearly identify subpopulation of CD3bright lymphocytes in peripheral blood of CUN3/cervical cancer patients and the controls. In spite of the relatively wide range of individual values in all studied groups, a trend towards a decreased number of circulating CD3brightCD56+ cells (p > 0.05) was observed for women with microinvasive carcinoma (gate P1, **Figure 9**); at the same time, no difference in the frequency of cells falling within gate P2 and the total frequency of CD3+CD56+ (including CD3+CD16+/-CD56+) cells was revealed (data not shown). Then, within the CD3bright population, we also analyzed the expression of CD16, a marker of antibody-mediated cytotoxicity, but did not find any significant difference between the controls and the patients groups (data not shown). According to Lambert et al., CD3bright T cells (i.e., γδT) do not express CD4, but express low levels of CD8 [63]. We compared the frequencies of CD3brightCD8low cells (gate P3) between the study groups, but again did not observe any difference. Therefore, in contrast to regulatory NK cells, the combination of CD3/CD16/CD56 markers is not sufficient to show if there are any significant changes occurring within the population of circulating innate-like T cells in early-stage cervical cancer. Although these results cannot be compared with the results reported by Pita-Lopez et al., who used the same combination of CD markers to analyze blood samples from women with low-grade lesions (CIN1), nevertheless, observations made for CD3brightCD56 cells, along with published data mentioned above underline the need for continuing investigation into innate-like lymphocytes at various stages of cervical cancer development and progression with the use of lineage-specific (e.g., anti-TCR) antibodies.

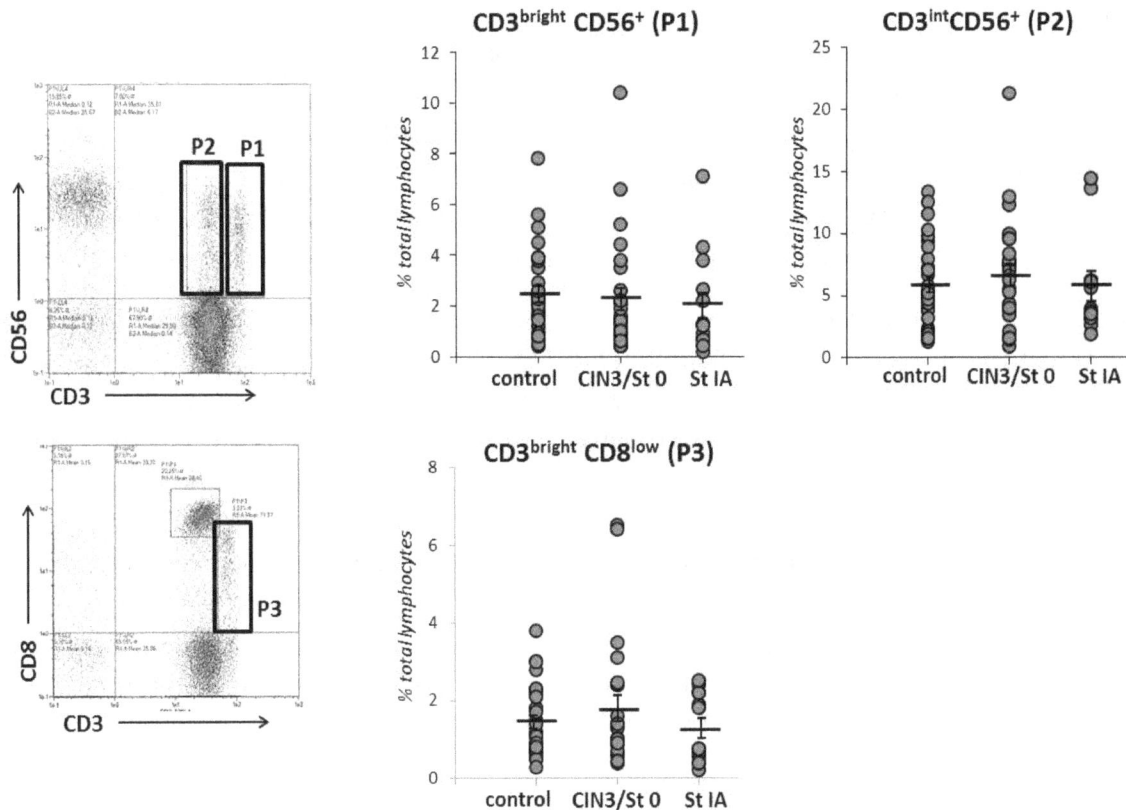

Figure 9. Percentage of peripheral blood T cells with NK-like phenotype in patients with CIN3 or microinvasive carcinoma (St IA) and healthy controls. Lymphocyte populations of interest were defined according to CD3/CD56 expression levels (gates P1-P3).

5. Regulatory T and B cells and immune checkpoint molecules in cervical cancer: at the crossroads of immune suppression mechanisms

Mobilization of intrinsic immune checkpoint mechanisms by a tumor to restrict antitumor immune response is one of the topical issues currently discussed; the phenomenon of effector cell exhaustion and the expression of checkpoint markers have been described for various innate/acquired immune cell populations, including innate-like cells. Regarding cervical cancer, one can observe an avalanche of new data emerged in recent 2 years on the expression of immune checkpoint markers, first of all PD-1/PD-1L, a hallmark of T cell exhaustion caused by chronic antigenic stimulation [66], as well as other members of B7 and CD28 protein families (e.g., B7-H3 [67] and B7-H4 [68]). For example, patients with CIN or cervical cancer show increased expression of PD-1 both in infiltrating lymphocytes and macrophages (TAMs) [69, 70], as well as in circulating CD4 and CD8 T cells [36], and, furthermore, in the sentinel lymph nodes [71]. Cervical neoplastic cells are considered as the primary source of PD-1 Ligand (PD-1L) [69, 70], with HPV16-E7 oncoprotein proved to be the driving force for elevated PD-L1 expression [72] and copy number gains of PD-L1 gene being one of the putative underlying reasons [73, 74]. Tumor-infiltrating and stromal M2 macrophages are another such source [34]. Finally, there is one more important source of PD-L1 among adaptive immune cells represented by regulatory T cells (Treg); a correlation between PD-L1 expression and FoxP3+Treg was reported by Ma et al. [75]. Moreover, CD4CD25 Tregs are able to upregulate PD-1 expression in patients with CIN/ cervical carcinoma [36], which, however, does not result in Treg exhaustion, but, conversely, favors upregulation of their immunosuppressive activity. Lastly, it has been reported that regional lymph nodes from stage IB1 cervical cancer patients, along with elevated PD-1, have increased expression of FoxP3 Treg-marker, which may shed light on the establishment of pre-metastatic niches [71], as well as on systemic expansion of suppressive mechanisms Tregs are engaged in.

Several studies have previously reported on increased frequency of circulating CD4 Tregs at initial stages of cervical cancer development [76–78]. Furthermore, we have recently confirmed systemic expansion of Tregs within not only CD4 cell subset, but within CD8 subset as well, at as early as preinvasive and microinvasive cancer (**Figure 10**); we have also revealed correlations between the number of circulating Tregs and the T cell expression of markers of apoptosis, whose induction is supposed to be one of the mechanisms mediating exhaustion of T effector pool during cervical cancer progression [23]. In parallel, the search of new mechanisms providing conditions for Treg expansion during the course of cervical cancer progression is continued: for example, it has been recently found that cervical cancer cells, as well as mesenchymal stromal cells isolated from cervical tumor tissue can upregulate CD73 ectonucleotidase to generate high amounts of adenosine, a potent inducer of Treg differentiation and recruitment [79, 80].

Apart from regulatory T cells, the potential involvement of regulatory B lymphocytes (Breg) in cervical cancer promotion should not be ignored. This can be supported by the results obtained

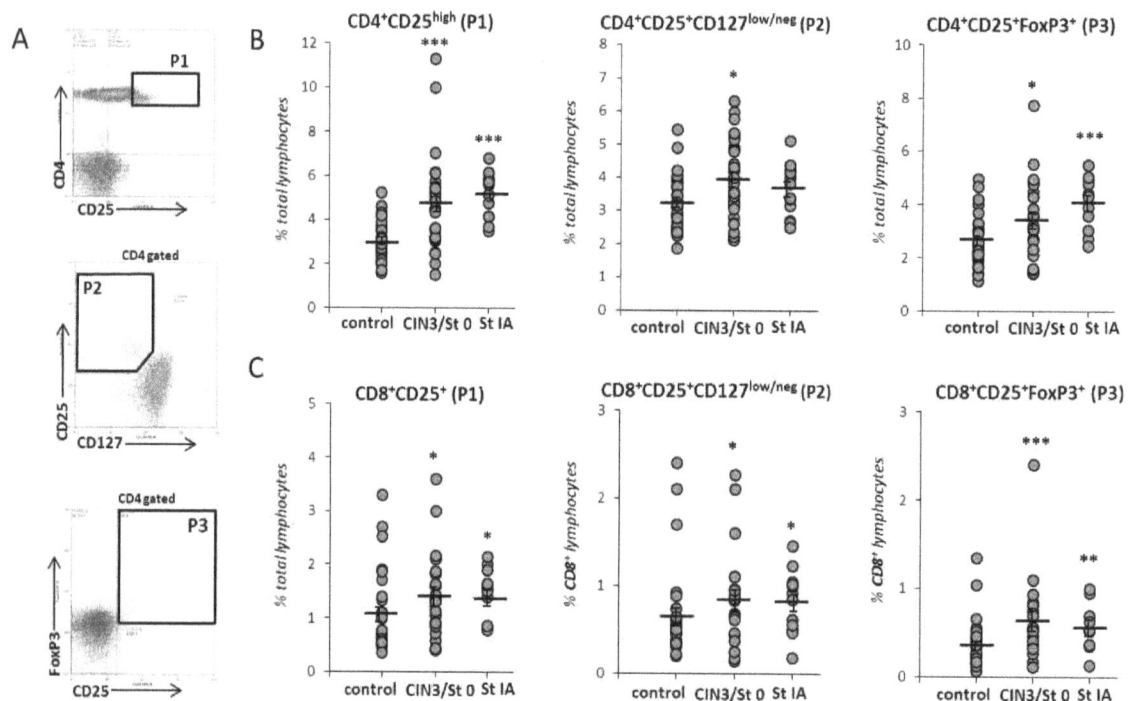

Figure 10. The frequencies of peripheral blood Treg lymphocytes in patients with CIN3 or microinvasive carcinoma (St IA) and healthy controls. (A) CD4 Tregs were gated according to the level of CD25, CD127, and FoxP3 expression; gating of CD8 Tregs was performed in a similar way. (B) The change in the frequency of circulating CD4 regulatory cells in patients compared to healthy donors. (C) The change in the frequency of circulating CD8 regulatory cells in patients compared to healthy donors: *p < 0.05, **p < 0.01, ***p < 0.001 (U-test).

by Tang et al. who used mouse model of HPV-related cancer to demonstrate that Bregs accumulate in tumor-draining lymph nodes, have altered phenotype (specifically, altered expression of cell surface markers, such as MHC II, PD-L1, and CD39), exhibit high regulatory potency, thus fostering tumor growth [81]. In humans, many types of solid tumors were found to be accompanied with increased numbers of both tumor-infiltrating and circulating Bregs capable of producing suppressor cytokines (e.g., IL-10) and immune checkpoint ligands, thus impairing T cell function (see reviews [82, 83]), suggesting this issue to be investigated for cervical cancer patients.

6. Conclusion

Further ways to develop approaches for the treatment of HPV-associated malignancies, including cervical cancer, belong to the area of combined therapies, where particular attention is to be paid to restoration the effectiveness of innate mechanisms of immune response, including those trigged by PRRs (e.g., STING). PRR agonists are expected to serve potent adjuvant function; another promising area is the use of agonists to stimulate NK, NKT, and γδT receptors. Despite substantial progress, there is clear understanding that stimulation of innate immune cells "per se" is senseless without concomitant inhibition of immunosuppressive factors (such as inhibitory molecules of immune checkpoint or other Treg-associated factors). Therefore, as illustrated by recent findings summarized in the chapter, there is obvious need for continuing comprehensive characterization of functional diversity of innate immune cells that organize cervical cancer immune regulatory network, exploration of noncanonical functions of innate immunity mediators, identification of precise resources of immune suppression and assessments of local and systemic changes in immune parameters.

Acknowledgements

The work was supported by the Russian Science Foundation, project No. 17-15-01024 (sections 1, 2, 4, 5); and the Russian Foundation for Basic Research, project No. 16-34-60019 (section 3).

Conflict of interest

Authors have no conflict of interest to declare.

Abbreviations

APC   Antigen-presenting cell

Breg   Regulatory B cells

CAR   Chimeric antigen receptor

CD	Cluster of differentiation
cGAMP	Cyclic GMP-AMP
cGAS	cGAMP synthase
CIN	Cervical intraepithelial neoplasia
DAMP	Damage-associated molecular patterns
DC	Dendritic cells
G-CSF	Granulocyte-colony stimulating factor
HPV	Human papillomavirus
IFN-I	Type I interferon
IL	Interleukin
IRF	Interferon regulatory factor
MAb	Monoclonal antibody
MDSC	Myeloid-derived suppressor cells
MFI	Mean fluorescence intensity
MHC	Major histocompatibility complex
MoDC	Monocyte-derived dendritic cells
NK	Natural killer cells
NKT	Natural killer-like cells
PBL	Peripheral blood lymphocytes
PBMC	Peripheral blood monocyte cells
PRR	Pattern recognition receptor
SEM	Standard error of the mean
STING	Stimulator of Interferon Genes
TAM	Tumor-associated macrophages
TAN	Tumor-associated neutrophils
TCR	T cell receptor
TDLN	Tumor-draining lymph nodes
TGFβ	Transforming growth factor beta

Th   Helper T cell

TLR   Toll-like receptor

Treg   Regulatory T cell

A. Appendices and nomenclature

A.1. Experimental procedures

Patients and specimens: Samples of peripheral blood and epithelial tissue were obtained from 55 patients who were diagnosed with CIN2-3 (including cancer *in situ*) or microinvasive carcinoma (FIGO stage IA1) and underwent surgery in Oncological Dispensary of the Republic of Karelia. CIN and cervical cancer diagnosis was based on comprehensive physical examination, extended colposcopy findings, cytology, and histopathology tests, in full compliance with the approved standards for the diagnosis and treatment of patients with gynecological malignancies. All women engaged in this this study were informed and gave voluntary written consent. The research was approved by the Committee on Medical Ethics of Petrozavodsk State University and the Ministry of Healthcare and Social Development of the Republic of Karelia, and was done in accordance with the Declaration of Helsinki and good clinical practice guidelines. All women from patient group were positive for oncogenic HPV types (with the prevalence of $HPV16 > 80\%$). Thirty healthy non-pregnant women without cervical abnormalities and HPV-infection at the time of blood sampling served as normal controls. Venous blood was collected immediately before the surgery or any other treatment and immediately processed for multicolor flow cytometry. Tissue samples were submerged in RNA stabilizing reagent right after excision and stored at −80.

Flow cytometry: The following fluorophore-conjugated monoclonal antibodies were used: CD3-APC (Clone: UCHT1), CD4-FITC (Clone: MT310), CD8-FITC (Clone: DK25), CD16-FITC (Clone: DJ130c), CD56-RPE (Clone: C5.9) (Dako, Austria), CD25-APC (Clone: 4E3), CD45-VioBlue (Clone: 5B1), CD127-RPE (Clone: MB15-18C9), FoxP3-RPE (Clone: 3G3) (Miltenyi Biotec, Germany), STING/TMEM173-RPE (Clone: 723505, R&D Systems, USA). For blocking of non-specific antibody binding, FcR Blocking Reagent (Miltenyi Biotec) was used. For intracellular detection, cells were fixed and permeabilized using "FoxP3 Staining Buffer Set" (Miltenyi Biotec). Cells were acquired on a MACSQuant Analyzer flow cytometer (Miltenyi Biotec) and analyzed using MACSQuantify software.

Real-time PCR: Total RNA was extracted from tissue samples or ficoll-isolated PBMC with Trizol Reagent (Invitrogen). cDNA was synthesized from DNAse I-treated RNA (1 mg RNA per 1 reaction volume) using ProtoScript II (New England BioLabs, UK) or RevertAid First Strand cDNA Synthesis Kit (Fermentas, ThermoScientific, USA). Amplification was performed in StepOnePlus thermal cycler (Applied Biosystems, USA) using qPCRmix-HS-SYBR+HighROX reaction mix (Evrogen, Russia).

Statistical analysis: Data analysis was performed using R software. Mann-Whitney U-test was used to evaluate the differences between the patient and the control groups; the difference was considered to be statistically significant at $p < 0.05$.

Author details

Olga Kurmyshkina[1], Pavel Kovchur[2], Ludmila Schegoleva[3] and Tatyana Volkova[4,5]*

*Address all correspondence to: volkovato@yandex.ru

1 Laboratory of Molecular Genetics of Innate Immunity, Institute of High-Tech Biomedicine, Petrozavodsk State University, Petrozavodsk, Russian Federation

2 Department of Hospital Surgery, ENT Diseases, Ophthalmology, Dentistry, Oncology, Urology, Institute of Medicine, Petrozavodsk State University, Petrozavodsk, Russian Federation

3 Department of Applied Mathematics and Cybernetics, Institute of Mathematics and Information Technologies, Petrozavodsk State University, Petrozavodsk, Russian Federation

4 Department of Biomedical Chemistry, Immunology and Laboratory Diagnostics, Institute of Medicine, Petrozavodsk State University, Petrozavodsk, Russian Federation

5 Institute of High-Tech Biomedicine, Petrozavodsk State University, Petrozavodsk, Russia

References

[1] Calì B, Molon B, Viola A. Tuning cancer fate: The unremitting role of host immunity. Open Biology. 2017;**7**(4):170006. DOI: 10.1098/rsob.170006

[2] Smola S. Immunopathogenesis of HPV-associated cancers and prospects for immunotherapy. Virus. 2017;**9**(9):E254. DOI: 10.3390/v9090254

[3] Alizon S, Murall CL, Bravo IG. Why human papillomavirus acute infections matter. Virus. 2017;**9**(10):E293. DOI: 10.3390/v9100293

[4] Seelige R, Searles S, Bui JD. Innate sensing of cancer's non-immunologic hallmarks. Current Opinion in Immunology. 2017;**50**:1-8. DOI: 10.1016/j.coi.2017.09.005

[5] Doorbar J. Model systems of human papillomavirus-associated disease. The Journal of Pathology. 2016;**238**(2):166-179. DOI: 10.1002/path.4656

[6] Smola S, Trimble C, Stern PL. Human papillomavirus-driven immune deviation: Challenge and novel opportunity for immunotherapy. Therapeutic Advances in Vaccines. 2017;**5**(3):69-82. DOI: 10.1177/2051013617717914

[7] Qin Y, Ekmekcioglu S, Forget MA, Szekvolgyi L, Hwu P, Grimm EA, Jazaeri AA, Roszik J. Cervical cancer neoantigen landscape and immune activity is associated with human papillomavirus master regulators. Frontiers in Immunology. 2017;**8**:689. DOI: 10.3389/fimmu.2017.00689

[8] Steinbach A, Riemer AB. Immune evasion mechanisms of human papillomavirus: An update. International Journal of Cancer. 2018;**142**(2):224-229. DOI: 10.1002/ijc.31027

[9] Miles B, Safran HP, Monk BJ. Therapeutic options for treatment of human papillomavirus-associated cancers – novel immunologic vaccines: ADXS11-001. Gynecologic Oncology Research and Practice. 2017;**4**:10. DOI: 10.1186/s40661-017-0047-8

[10] Vici P, Pizzuti L, Mariani L, Zampa G, Santini D, Di Lauro L, Gamucci T, Natoli C, Marchetti P, Barba M, Maugeri-Saccà M, Sergi D, Tomao F, Vizza E, Di Filippo S, Paolini F, Curzio G, Corrado G, Michelotti A, Sanguineti G, Giordano A, De Maria R, Venuti A. Targeting immune response with therapeutic vaccines in premalignant lesions and cervical cancer: Hope or reality from clinical studies. Expert Review of Vaccines. 2016;**15**(10):1327-1336. DOI: 10.1080/14760584.2016.1176533

[11] Lee SJ, Yang A, Wu TC, Hung CF. Immunotherapy for human papillomavirus-associated disease and cervical cancer: Review of clinical and translational research. Journal of Gynecologic Oncology. 2016;**27**(5):e51. DOI: 10.3802/jgo.2016.27.e51

[12] Radoshevich L, Dussurget O. Cytosolic innate immune sensing and signaling upon infection. Frontiers in Microbiology. 2016;**7**:313. DOI: 10.3389/fmicb.2016.00313.

[13] Corrales L, McWhirter SM, Dubensky Jr TW, Gajewski TF. The host STING pathway at the interface of cancer and immunity. The Journal of Clinical Investigation. 2016;**126**(7):2404-2411. DOI: 10.1172/JCI86892

[14] Larkin B, Ilyukha V, Sorokin M, Buzdin A, Vannier E, Poltorak A. Cutting edge: Activation of STING in T cells induces type I IFN responses and cell death. Journal of Immunology. 2017;**199**(2):397-402. DOI: 10.4049/jimmunol.1601999

[15] Cerboni S, Jeremiah N, Gentili M, Gehrmann U, Conrad C, Stolzenberg MC, Picard C, Neven B, Fischer A, Amigorena S, Rieux-Laucat F, Manel N. Intrinsic antiproliferative activity of the innate sensor STING in T lymphocytes. The Journal of Experimental Medicine. 2017;**214**(6):1769-1785. DOI: 10.1084/jem.20161674

[16] Gulen MF, Koch U, Haag SM, Schuler F, Apetoh L, Villunger A, Radtke F, Ablasser A. Signalling strength determines proapoptotic functions of STING. Nature Communications. 2017;**8**(1):427. DOI: 10.1038/s41467-017-00573-w

[17] Surpris G, Poltorak A. The expanding regulatory network of STING-mediated signaling. Current Opinion in Microbiology. 2016;**32**:144-150. DOI: 10.1016/j.mib.2016.05.014

[18] Poltorak A, Kurmyshkina O, Volkova T. Stimulator of interferon genes (STING): A "new chapter" in virus-associated cancer research. Lessons from wild-derived mouse models of innate immunity. Cytokine & Growth Factor Reviews. 2016;**29**:83-91. DOI: 10.1016/j.cytogfr.2016.02.009

[19] Musella M, Manic G, De Maria R, Vitale I, Sistigu A. Type-I-interferons in infection and cancer: Unanticipated dynamics with therapeutic implications. Oncoimmunology. 2017;**6**(5):e1314424. DOI: 10.1080/2162402X.2017.1314424

[20] Snell LM, McGaha TL, Brooks DG. Type I interferon in chronic virus infection and cancer. Trends in Immunology. 2017;**38**(8):542-557. DOI: 10.1016/j.it.2017.05.005

[21] Pépin G, Gantier MP. cGAS-STING activation in the tumor microenvironment and its role in cancer immunity. Advances in Experimental Medicine and Biology. 2017;**1024**:175-194. DOI: 10.1007/978-981-10-5987-2_8

[22] Sunthamala N, Thierry F, Teissier S, Pientong C, Kongyingyoes B, Tangsiriwatthana T, Sangkomkamhang U, Ekalaksananan T. E2 proteins of high risk human papillomaviruses down-modulate STING and IFN-κ transcription in keratinocytes. PLoS One. 2014;**9**(3):e91473. DOI: 10.1371/journal.pone.0091473

[23] Kurmyshkina OV, Kovchur PI, Schegoleva LV, Volkova TO. T- and NK-cell populations with regulatory phenotype and markers of apoptosis in circulating lymphocytes of patients with CIN3 or microcarcinoma of the cervix: Evidence for potential mechanisms of immune suppression. Infectious Agents and Cancer. 2017;**12**:56. DOI: 10.1186/s13027-017-0166-1.

[24] Carow K, Read C, Häfner N, Runnebaum IB, Corner A, Dürst MA. Comparative study of digital PCR and real-time qPCR for the detection and quantification of HPV mRNA in sentinel lymph nodes of cervical cancer patients. BMC Research Notes. 2017;**10**(1):532. DOI: 10.1186/s13104-017-2846-8

[25] Li Y, Wilson HL, Kiss-Toth E, Regulating STING. In health and disease. Journal of Inflammation (Lond). 2017;**14**:11. DOI: 10.1186/s12950-017-0159-2

[26] Falkenberg VR, Whistler T, Murray JR, Unger ER, Rajeevan MS. Identification of Phosphoglycerate kinase 1 (PGK1) as a reference gene for quantitative gene expression measurements in human blood RNA. BMC Research Notes. 2011;**4**:324. DOI: 10.1186/1756-0500-4-324

[27] Leitão Mda C, Coimbra EC, de Lima Rde C, Guimarães Mde L, Heráclio Sde A, Silva Neto Jda C, de Freitas AC. Quantifying mRNA and microRNA with qPCR in cervical carcinogenesis: A validation of reference genes to ensure accurate data. PLoS One. 2014;**9**(11):e111021. DOI: 10.1371/journal.pone.0111021

[28] Ng KW, Marshall EA, Bell JC, Lam WL. cGAS-STING and cancer: Dichotomous roles in tumor immunity and development. Trends in Immunology. 2017:**S1471-4906**(17):30151-30155. DOI: 10.1016/j.it.2017.07.013

[29] Wang YY, Jin R, Zhou GP, Xu HG. Mechanisms of transcriptional activation of the stimulator of interferon genes by transcription factors CREB and c-Myc. Oncotarget. 2016;**7**(51):85049-85057. DOI: 10.18632/oncotarget.13183

[30] Tang CH, Zundell JA, Ranatunga S, Lin C, Nefedova Y, Del Valle JR, Hu CC. Agonist-mediated activation of STING induces apoptosis in malignant B cells. Cancer Research. 2016;**76**(8):2137-2152. DOI: 10.1158/0008-5472.CAN-15-1885

[31] Gram AM, Sun C, Landman SL, Oosenbrug T, Koppejan HJ, Kwakkenbos MJ, Hoeben RC, Paludan SR, Ressing ME. Human B cells fail to secrete type I interferons upon

cytoplasmic DNA exposure. Molecular Immunology. 2017;**91**:225-237. DOI: 10.1016/j.molimm.2017.08.025

[32] Alvarez KLF, Beldi M, Sarmanho F, Rossetti RAM, Silveira CRF, Mota GR, Andreoli MA, Caruso EDC, Kamillos MF, Souza AM, Mastrocalla H, Clavijo-Salomon MA, Barbuto JAM, Lorenzi NP, Longatto-Filho A, Baracat E, Lopez RVM, Villa LL, Tacla M, Lepique AP. Local and systemic immunomodulatory mechanisms triggered by human papillomavirus transformed cells: A potential role for G-CSF and neutrophils. Scientific Reports. 2017;**7**(1):9002. DOI: 10.1038/s41598-017-09079-3

[33] Li Y, Huang G, Zhang S. Associations between intratumoral and peritumoral M2 macrophage counts and cervical squamous cell carcinoma invasion patterns. International Journal of Gynaecology and Obstetrics. 2017. DOI: 10.1002/ijgo.12320

[34] Heeren AM, Punt S, Bleeker MC, Gaarenstroom KN, van der Velden J, Kenter GG, de Gruijl TD, Jordanova ES. Prognostic effect of different PD-L1 expression patterns in squamous cell carcinoma and adenocarcinoma of the cervix. Modern Pathology. 2016;**29**(7):753-763. DOI: 10.1038/modpathol.2016.64

[35] Swangphon P, Pientong C, Sunthamala N, Bumrungthai S, Azuma M, Kleebkaow P, Tangsiriwatthana T, Sangkomkamhang U, Kongyingyoes B, Ekalaksananan T. Correlation of circulating CD64+/CD163+ monocyte ratio and stroma/peri-tumoral CD163+ monocyte density with human papillomavirus infected cervical lesion severity. Cancer Microenvironment. 2017. DOI: 10.1007/s12307-017-0200-2

[36] Chen Z, Pang N, Du R, Zhu Y, Fan L, Cai D, Ding Y, Ding J. Elevated expression of programmed Death-1 and programmed death Ligand-1 negatively regulates immune response against cervical cancer cells. Mediators of Inflammation. 2016;**2016**:6891482. DOI: 10.1155/2016/6891482

[37] Lopes AMM, Michelin MA, Murta EFC. Monocyte-derived dendritic cells from patients with cervical intraepithelial lesions. Oncology Letters. 2017;**13**(3):1456-1462. DOI: 10.3892/ol.2017.5595

[38] Verma V, Kim Y, Lee MC, Lee JT, Cho S, Park IK, Min JJ, Lee JJ, Lee SE, Rhee JH. Activated dendritic cells delivered in tissue compatible biomatrices induce in-situ anti-tumor CTL responses leading to tumor regression. Oncotarget. 2016;**7**(26):39894-39906. DOI: 10.18632/oncotarget.9529

[39] Zheng Y, Hu B, Xie S, Chen X, Hu Y, Chen W, Li S, Hu B. Dendritic cells infected by Ad-sh-SOCS1 enhance cytokine-induced killer (CIK) cell immunotherapeutic efficacy in cervical cancer models. Cytotherapy. 2017;**19**(5):617-628. DOI: 10.1016/j.jcyt.2017.01.008

[40] van Meir H, Nout RA, Welters MJ, Loof NM, de Kam ML, van Ham JJ, Samuels S, Kenter GG, Cohen AF, Melief CJ, Burggraaf J, van Poelgeest MI, van der Burg SH. Impact of (chemo)radiotherapy on immune cell composition and function in cervical cancer patients. Oncoimmunology. 2016;**6**(2):e1267095. DOI: 10.1080/2162402X.2016.1267095

[41] Martín-Antonio B, Suñe G, Perez-Amill L, Castella M, Urbano-Ispizua A. Natural killer cells: Angels and devils for immunotherapy. International Journal of Molecular Sciences. 2017;**18**(9):E1868. DOI: 10.3390/ijms18091868

[42] Veluchamy JP, Heeren AM, Spanholtz J, van Eendenburg JD, Heideman DA, Kenter GG, Verheul HM, van der Vliet HJ, Jordanova ES, de Gruijl TD. High-efficiency lysis of cervical cancer by allogeneic NK cells derived from umbilical cord progenitors is independent of HLA status. Cancer Immunology, Immunotherapy. 2017;**66**(1):51-61. DOI: 10.1007/s00262-016-1919-1

[43] Ferns DM, Heeren AM, Samuels S, Bleeker MCG, de Gruijl TD, Kenter GG, Jordanova ES. Classical and non-classical HLA class I aberrations in primary cervical squamous- and adenocarcinomas and paired lymph node metastases. Journal for ImmunoTherapy of Cancer. 2016;**4**:78. DOI: 10.1186/s40425-016-0184-3

[44] Chang WC, Li CH, Chu LH, Huang PS, Sheu BC, Huang SC. Regulatory T cells suppress natural killer cell immunity in patients with human cervical carcinoma. International Journal of Gynecological Cancer. 2016;**26**(1):156-162. DOI: 10.1097/IGC.0000000000000578

[45] Melsen JE, Lugthart G, Lankester AC, Schilham MW. Human circulating and tissue-resident CD56(bright) natural killer cell populations. Frontiers in Immunology. 2016;**7**:262. DOI: 10.3389/fimmu.2016.00262

[46] Wagner JA, Rosario M, Romee R, Berrien-Elliott MM, Schneider SE, Leong JW, Sullivan RP, Jewell BA, Becker-Hapak M, Schappe T, Abdel-Latif S, Ireland AR, Jaishankar D, King JA, Vij R, Clement D, Goodridge J, Malmberg KJ, Wong HC, Fehniger TA. CD56bright NK cells exhibit potent antitumor responses following IL-15 priming. The Journal of Clinical Investigation. 2017;**127**(11):4042-4058. DOI: 10.1172/JCI90387

[47] Gross CC, Schulte-Mecklenbeck A, Wiendl H, Marcenaro E, Kerlero de Rosbo N, Uccelli A, Laroni A. Regulatory functions of natural killer cells in multiple sclerosis. Frontiers in Immunology. 2016;**7**:606. DOI: 10.3389/fimmu.2016.00606

[48] Carrega P, Bonaccorsi I, Di Carlo E, Morandi B, Paul P, Rizzello V, Cipollone G, Navarra G, Mingari MC, Moretta L, Ferlazzo G. CD56(bright)perforin(low) noncytotoxic human NK cells are abundant in both healthy and neoplastic solid tissues and recirculate to secondary lymphoid organs via afferent lymph. Journal of Immunology. 2014;**192**(8):3805-3815. DOI: 10.4049/jimmunol.1301889

[49] Wulff S, Pries R, Börngen K, Trenkle T, Wollenberg B. Decreased levels of circulating regulatory NK cells in patients with head and neck cancer throughout all tumor stages. Anticancer Research. 2009;**29**(8):3053-3057

[50] Koo KC, Shim DH, Yang CM, Lee SB, Kim SM, Shin TY, Kim KH, Yoon HG, Rha KH, Lee JM, Hong SJ. Reduction of the CD16(−)CD56bright NK cell subset precedes NK cell dysfunction in prostate cancer. PLoS One. 2013;**8**(11):e78049. DOI: 10.1371/journal.pone.0078049

[51] Bauernhofer T, Kuss I, Henderson B, Baum AS, Whiteside TL. Preferential apoptosis of CD56dim natural killer cell subset in patients with cancer. European Journal of Immunology. 2003;**33**(1):119-124

[52] Nieto-Velázquez NG, Torres-Ramos YD, Muñoz-Sánchez JL, Espinosa-Godoy L, Gómez-Cortés S, Moreno J, Moreno-Eutimio MA. Altered expression of natural cytotoxicity receptors and NKG2D on peripheral blood NK cell subsets in breast cancer patients. Translational Oncology. 2016;**9**(5):384-391. DOI: 10.1016/j.tranon.2016.07.003

[53] Nair S, Dhodapkar MV, Natural Killer T. Cells in cancer immunotherapy. Frontiers in Immunology. 2017;**8**:1178. DOI: 10.3389/fimmu.2017.01178

[54] Wu D, Wu P, Qiu F, Wei Q, Huang J. Human γδT-cell subsets and their involvement in tumor immunity. Cellular & Molecular Immunology. 2017;**14**(3):245-253. DOI: 10.1038/cmi.2016.55

[55] Lawand M, Déchanet-Merville J, Dieu-Nosjean MC. Key features of gamma-delta T-cell subsets in human diseases and their immunotherapeutic implications. Frontiers in Immunology. 2017;**8**:761. DOI: 10.3389/fimmu.2017.00761

[56] Miura S, Kawana K, Schust DJ, Fujii T, Yokoyama T, Iwasawa Y, Nagamatsu T, Adachi K, Tomio A, Tomio K, Kojima S, Yasugi T, Kozuma S, Taketani Y. CD1d, a sentinel molecule bridging innate and adaptive immunity, is downregulated by the human papillomavirus (HPV) E5 protein: A possible mechanism for immune evasion by HPV. Journal of Virology. 2010;**84**(22):11614-11623. DOI: 10.1128/JVI.01053-10

[57] Hu T, Yang P, Zhu H, Chen X, Xie X, Yang M, Liu S, Wang H. Accumulation of invariant NKT cells with increased IFN-γ production in persistent high-risk HPV-infected high-grade cervical intraepithelial neoplasia. Diagnostic Pathology. 2015;**10**:20. DOI: 10.1186/s13000-015-0254-8

[58] Pita-Lopez ML, Ortiz-Lazareno PC, Navarro-Meza M, Santoyo-Telles F, Peralta-Zaragoza O. CD28-, CD45RA(null/dim) and natural killer-like CD8+ T cells are increased in peripheral blood of women with low-grade cervical lesions. Cancer Cell International 2014;**14**(1):97. DOI: 10.1186/s12935-014-0097-5

[59] Gosmann C, Mattarollo SR, Bridge JA, Frazer IH, Blumenthal A. IL-17 suppresses immune effector functions in human papillomavirus-associated epithelial hyperplasia. Journal of Immunology. 2014;**193**(5):2248-2257. DOI: 10.4049/jimmunol.1400216

[60] Lertworapreecha M, Patumraj S, Niruthisard S, Hansasuta P, Bhattarakosol P. Cytotoxic function of gamma delta (gamma/delta) T cells against pamidronate-treated cervical cancer cells. Indian Journal of Experimental Biology. 2013;**51**(8):597-605

[61] Fujii SI, Shimizu K. Exploiting antitumor immunotherapeutic novel strategies by deciphering the cross talk between invariant NKT cells and dendritic cells. Frontiers in Immunology. 2017;**8**:886. DOI: 10.3389/fimmu.2017.00886

[62] Van Acker HH, Capsomidis A, Smits EL, Van Tendeloo VF. CD56 in the immune system: More than a marker for cytotoxicity? Frontiers in Immunology. 2017;**8**:892. DOI: 10.3389/fimmu.2017.00892

[63] Lambert C, Genin C. CD3 bright lymphocyte population reveal gammadelta T cells. Cytometry Part B, Clinical Cytometry. 2004;**61**(1):45-53. DOI: 10.1002/cyto.b.20005

[64] Paget C, Chow MT, Gherardin NA, Beavis PA, Uldrich AP, Duret H, Hassane M, Souza-Fonseca-Guimaraes F, Mogilenko DA, Staumont-Sallé D, Escalante NK, Hill GR, Neeson P, Ritchie DS, Dombrowicz D, Mallevaey T, Trottein F, Belz GT, Godfrey DI, Smyth MJ. CD3bright signals on γδ T cells identify IL-17A-producing Vγ6Vδ1+ T cells. Immunology and Cell Biology. 2015;**93**(2):198-212. DOI: 10.1038/icb.2014.94

[65] Guo C, Shen X, Fu B, Liu Y, Chen Y, Ni F, Ye Y, Sun R, Li J, Tian Z, Wei H. CD3(bright) CD56(+) T cells associate with pegylated interferon-alpha treatment nonresponse in chronic hepatitis B patients. Scientific Reports. 2016;**6**:25567. DOI: 10.1038/srep25567

[66] Okoye IS, Houghton M, Tyrrell L, Barakat K, Elahi S. Coinhibitory receptor expression and immune checkpoint blockade: Maintaining a balance in CD8+ T cell responses to chronic viral infections and cancer. Frontiers in Immunology. 2017;**8**:1215. DOI: 10.3389/fimmu.2017.01215

[67] Li Y, Zhang J, Han S, Qian Q, Chen Q, Liu L, Zhang Y. B7-H3 promotes the proliferation, migration and invasiveness of cervical cancer cells and is an indicator of poor prognosis. Oncology Reports. 2017;**38**(2):1043-1050. DOI: 10.3892/or.2017.5730

[68] Han S, Li Y, Zhang J, Liu L, Chen Q, Qian Q, Li S, Zhang Y. Roles of immune inhibitory molecule B7-H4 in cervical cancer. Oncology Reports. 2017;**37**(4):2308-2316. DOI: 10.3892/or.2017.5481

[69] Yang W, YP L, Yang YZ, Kang JR, Jin YD, Wang HW. Expressions of programmed death (PD)-1 and PD-1 ligand (PD-L1) in cervical intraepithelial neoplasia and cervical squamous cell carcinomas are of prognostic value and associated with human papillomavirus status. The Journal of Obstetrics and Gynaecology Research. 2017;**43**(10):1602-1612. DOI: 10.1111/jog.13411

[70] Reddy OL, Shintaku PI, Moatamed NA. Programmed death-ligand 1 (PD-L1) is expressed in a significant number of the uterine cervical carcinomas. Diagnostic Pathology. 2017;**12**(1):45. DOI: 10.1186/s13000-017-0631-6

[71] Balsat C, Blacher S, Herfs M, Van de Velde M, Signolle N, Sauthier P, Pottier C, Gofflot S, De Cuypere M, Delvenne P, Goffin F, Noel A, Kridelka F. A specific immune and lymphatic profile characterizes the pre-metastatic state of the sentinel lymph node 10.1080/2162402X.2016.1265718

[72] Liu C, Lu J, Tian H, Du W, Zhao L, Feng J, Yuan D, Li Z. Increased expression of PD-L1 by the human papillomavirus 16 E7 oncoprotein inhibits anticancer immunity. Molecular Medicine Reports. 2017;**15**(3):1063-1070. DOI: 10.3892/mmr.2017.6102

[73] Budczies J, Bockmayr M, Denkert C, Klauschen F, Gröschel S, Darb-Esfahani S, Pfarr N, Leichsenring J, Onozato ML, Lennerz JK, Dietel M, Fröhling S, Schirmacher P, Iafrate AJ, Weichert W, Stenzinger A. Pan-cancer analysis of copy number changes in programmed death-ligand 1 (PD-L1, CD274) – associations with gene expression, mutational load, and survival. Genes, Chromosomes & Cancer. 2016;**55**(8):626-639. DOI: 10.1002/gcc.22365

[74] The Cancer Genome Atlas Research Network. Integrated genomic and molecular charac-terization of cervical cancer. Nature. 2017;**543**(7645):378-384. DOI: 10.1038/nature21386

[75] Ma Q, Zhao M, Wei X, Zhao J, Yang T, Zhang Q, Wang K, Yang X. Expressions of immune negative regulator FoxP3+Treg and PD-L1 protein in the immune microenvironment of cervical lesion. Zhongguo Yi Xue Ke Xue Yuan Xue Bao. 2017;**39**(1):128-132. DOI: 10.3881/j.issn.1000-503X.2017.01.021

[76] Mora-García ML, Ávila-Ibarra LR, García-Rocha R, Weiss-Steider B, Hernández-Montes J, Don-López CA, Gutiérrez-Serrano V, Titla-Vilchis IJ, Fuentes-Castañeda MC, Monroy-Mora A, Jave-Suárez LF, Chacón-Salinas R, Vallejo-Castillo L, Pérez-Tapia SM, Monroy-García A. Cervical cancer cells suppress effector functions of cytotoxic T cells through the adenosin-ergic pathway. Cellular Immunology. 2017;**320**:46-55. DOI: 10.1016/j.cellimm.2017.09.002

[77] Molling JW, de Gruijl TD, Glim J, Moreno M, Rozendaal L, Meijer CJ, van den Eertwegh AJ, Scheper RJ, von Blomberg ME, Bontkes HJ. CD4(+)CD25hi regulatory T-cell fre-quency correlates with persistence of human papillomavirus type 16 and T helper cell responses in patients with cervical intraepithelial neoplasia. International Journal of Cancer. 2007;**121**(8):1749-1755. DOI: 10.1002/ijc.22894

[78] Visser J, Nijman HW, Hoogenboom BN, Jager P, van Baarle D, Schuuring E, Abdulahad W, Miedema F, van der Zee AG, Daemen T. Frequencies and role of regulatory T cells in patients with (pre)malignant cervical neoplasia. Clinical and Experimental Immunology. 2007;**150**(2):199-209. DOI: 10.1111/j.1365-2249.2007.03468.x

[79] Chen Z, Ding J, Pang N, Du R, Meng W, Zhu Y, Zhang Y, Ma C, Ding Y. The Th17/Treg balance and the expression of related cytokines in uygur cervical cancer patients. Diagnostic Pathology. 2013;**8**:61. DOI: 10.1186/1746-1596-8-61

[80] de Lourdes Mora-García M, García-Rocha R, Morales-Ramírez O, Montesinos JJ, Weiss-Steider B, Hernández-Montes J, Ávila-Ibarra LR, Don-López CA, Velasco-Velázquez MA, Gutiérrez-Serrano V, Monroy-García A. Mesenchymal stromal cells derived from cervi-cal cancer produce high amounts of adenosine to suppress cytotoxic T lymphocyte func-tions. Journal of Translational Medicine. 2016;**14**(1):302. DOI: 10.1186/s12967-016-1057-8

[81] Tang A, Dadaglio G, Oberkampf M, Di Carlo S, Peduto L, Laubreton D, Desrues B, Sun CM, Montagutelli X, Leclerc C. B cells promote tumor progression in a mouse model of HPV-mediated cervical cancer. International Journal of Cancer. 2016;**139**(6):1358-1371. DOI: 10.1002/ijc.30169

[82] Schwartz M, Zhang Y, Rosenblatt JD. B cell regulation of the anti-tumor response and role in carcinogenesis. Journal for ImmunoTherapy of Cancer. 2016;**4**:40. DOI: 10.1186/s40425-016-0145-x

[83] Shen M, Sun Q, Wang J, Pan W, Ren X. Positive and negative functions of B lymphocytes in tumors. Oncotarget. 2016;**7**(34):55828-55839. DOI: 10.18632/oncotarget.10094

5

Screening for Ovarian Cancer

Poonam Jani and Rema Iyer

Abstract

Ovarian cancer is often diagnosed at an advanced stage and is associated with poor survival. Screening aims at detection of early stage disease with a view of improving overall survival. Incidence of ovarian cancer is about 1–2% in the low-risk and 10–40% in the high-risk population. Transvaginal ultrasound (TVS) and serum CA125 levels have been used for early detection. Annual screening with TVS and serum CA125 levels (using a cut-off value) has not demonstrated detection of ovarian cancer at an early stage. Multimodal screening (MMS) using sequential CA125 levels (with interpretation of risk using Risk of Ovarian Cancer Algorithm—ROCA) and ultrasound as the second-line test have been shown to have improved sensitivity when compared to annual ultrasound in the detection of ovarian cancer. However, no impact on survival has been demonstrated, and therefore, screening cannot be recommended in the general or high-risk population. There is evidence now to suggest that high-grade serous cancers originate from the fallopian tube where precursor lesions have been identified. Newer screening strategies are likely to shift the focus to detecting these precursor lesions with novel techniques such as exfoliative cytology, circulating tumour DNA and use of microbubbles in ultrasound imaging.

Keywords: screening, transvaginal ultrasound, CA125, ovarian cancer, multimodal screening

1. Introduction

Ovarian cancer is the seventh most common cancer in women worldwide, accounting for 4% of cancers in women. Incidence of ovarian cancer is increasing, especially in Europe and Northern America, being the fifth most common cancer in European women [1]. Even though the life time risk of developing ovarian cancer is 1–2% in the general population, since it is often diagnosed at a later stage, ovarian cancer has the highest mortality rate associated with gynaecological cancers in the developed world [2]. Therefore, there is a need to introduce a screening programme for early detection of this disease.

Screening for any disease is aimed at detection of premalignant conditions or early stage disease. Cervical cancer screening is a successful programme as the progression from premalignant to malignant disease is well understood. However, until recently, precursor lesions were not recognised for ovarian cancer. Now, there is evidence to suggest that some of the high-grade serous cancers start as premalignant lesions in the fimbrial end of the fallopian tube as serous tubal intraepithelial carcinoma (STIC) [3]. Strategies to detect these premalignant lesions are likely to change the approach to ovarian cancer screening.

2. Role of pelvic ultrasound in ovarian cancer screening

Ultrasound has been used as a screening tool to detect early malignant lesions in the ovary and fallopian tube. Features such as presence of septa, papillary projections and solid areas are used to distinguish possible malignant lesions from benign ones. The use of colour flow Doppler to detect altered blood flow as a result of neo-vascularisation has also been explored in diagnosing ovarian neoplasms.

Transvaginal ultrasonography (TVS) has long been considered a useful modality for estimating morphological factors of carcinogenesis. Non-invasiveness and ease of implementation are amongst its benefits for screening, and women generally find TVS an acceptable modality for detection [4]. Factors often used for the assessment of ovarian masses include morphology and volume analysis, but more advanced methods such as Doppler and neuronal network analyses are being investigated for their efficacy.

There are many challenges to overcome in the utilisation of TVS as a screening modality. Variation in operator competence is one such challenge. The United Kingdom Collaborative Trial for Ovarian Cancer Screening (UKCTOCS) trial overcame this challenge by providing standardised training regimes to all sonographers. Although this could be a viable solution, there will always be variation in competence based on operator experience. For example, more experienced sonographers may be better at detecting borderline cysts than less experienced sonographers. The lack of standardised terms to describe ovarian sonographic features is another issue. The International Ovarian Tumour Analysis (IOTA) Group have created a set of recommendations to address this by setting definitions for morphological features such as 'septum, solid, smooth, irregular', and so on. [5].

Patient acceptability of screening modality is also an essential factor to consider. In a recent study, 72.7% of women (n = 651) reported no discomfort during TVS, 23.3% of women reported some pain or discomfort and 3.5% documented moderate to severe pain during the TVS procedure. Increasing pain was attributed to history of hysterectomy and a prolonged scanning time. Interestingly, those who experienced pain were noted less likely to return for a subsequent scan 1 year later [4].

Visualisation of the ovary is a further quality assurance factor to overcome in ovarian cancer screening. Decreasing follicular activity and ovarian shrinkage in postmenopausal women makes visualisation problematic. In a study involving TVS of 43,867 women (median age 60.6 years), factors affecting visualisation of ovaries in postmenopausal women included previous hysterectomy, unilateral oophorectomy, tubal ligation, increasing age and obesity. Interestingly, factors that increased visualisation of the ovaries included a history of infertility and increasing age at menopause [6].

One of the biggest challenges in ovarian screening lies in differentiating between benign and malignant macroscopic changes. Ovarian morphology varies greatly from patient to patient, and thus benign lesions can give rise to false positive results, leading to unnecessary interventions. Unilocular cysts and those with simple septations are often benign and self-resolving. Features increasing the risk of malignancy include identification of neo-angiogenesis, multiple loculations, presence of papillary structures and solid foci [7–9]. False positives can be reduced with serial ultrasonography [10] as many ovarian lesions resolve without intervention. Benign lesions such as cysts and non-malignant solid lesions are also prevalent in the older population. In a study involving histological and ultrasound characterisation of ovarian cysts from autopsy material from 52 postmenopausal women who had died from causes other than gynaecological cancers, 56% were found to have histologically benign ovarian masses. This evidence suggests that many women will have benign lesions and so ultrasound testing could potentiate unnecessary over-investigating and surgical interventions [11]. The malignant potential of inclusion cysts are yet to be determined, however, it has been proven that TVS is a valid system for detecting malignancy after initial assessment at 1 year. In a study assessing the malignant potential of inclusion cysts, of the 1234 patients carrying ovarian inclusion cysts and 22,914 patients with normal ovaries, 432 women were diagnosed with ovarian cancer, respectively. Overall, the study showed the wider potential of application of TVS as a screening modality [12].

A well-defined criteria or reliable method of quantification needs to be introduced in order to differentiate between benign and malignant cysts. The University of Kentucky has developed a morphological index (MI) score looking at ovarian volume and macroscopic features. In their study, malignancy correlated to an increase in MI score with serial imaging, whereas benign tumours correlated to a decreased or stable MI score [13]. There is scope, therefore, for more accurate quantification of malignant potential, using risk predictors and TVS-led assessment.

New strategies to aid in accurate detection of malignant tumours include neuronal networks and pattern recognition models [14]. These developments are still in their infancy; however, a multicentre study demonstrated that borderline tumours, struma ovarii, papillary cystadenofibromas and myomas proved most difficult to reliably differentiate using ultrasound even with logistic regression models [15].

Magnetic resonance imaging (MRI) is a further imaging modality to consider for screening, due to its detailed visualisation of the pelvis. As an option for screening, however, implications of cost, duration of test, contra-indications for the wider population including placement of metal work, all pose great hurdles to acceptability.

3. Tumour markers

Tumour markers are substances, mostly proteins produced by the tumour cells, which can be detected in the blood and other bodily secretions of the affected individual. These markers can be produced by normal tissue as well but their levels are usually significantly elevated during a malignant process. Tumour markers are used for the early detection, to guide management and to assess treatment response in cancer.

CA125 is the most commonly used tumour marker for the detection of ovarian cancer. In 1981, Bast et al. developed OC125, a murine monoclonal antibody, which was found to react with ovarian carcinoma cells [16]. An immunoassay was then developed to detect the antigen CA125 in the serum of patients affected by non-mucinous ovarian cancer. CA125 levels were found to be elevated in 82% of women affected by non-mucinous epithelial ovarian cancer, and it was useful in monitoring the treatment response [17].

Elevated CA125 levels are seen in 50% of stage I and >90% of stage II–IV serous ovarian cancers [18]. However, the levels are usually not elevated with mucinous and borderline ovarian tumours. CA125 is also not very specific to ovarian cancer as the levels are increased in other malignancies such that of the gastrointestinal tract, breast and lung; and in benign gynaecological (e.g. endometriosis, fibroids, adenomyosis, benign masses and pregnancy) [18] and non-gynaecological conditions (e.g. heart failure, pancreatitis, hepatitis) [19].

A cut-off value of 35 U/ml is accepted as the upper limit of normal [17]. This cut-off value is acceptable in postmenopausal women, whereas, in premenopausal women, the cut-off value tends to be significantly higher at 50 U/ml [20]. Other factors have also been found to affect the CA125 level. A study on CA125 levels in healthy postmenopausal women observed varying levels with race (highest in Caucasian and lowest in African women), lower levels with previous hysterectomy, regular smoking and caffeine intake, and, higher levels with a previous (non-ovarian) cancer diagnosis. Age of the individual, age at menarche and menopause and previous ovarian cysts were also predictive of baseline levels in postmenopausal women [21].

The CA125 level can be elevated for up to 5 years prior to the diagnosis of ovarian cancer. This finding has been crucial for its application in screening asymptomatic women [22]. Given its low sensitivity and specificity, interpretation of CA125 level using a cut-off value has not been very useful in screening. However, sequential measurements of CA125 as a first-line test and transvaginal ultrasound as a second-line test in multimodal screening have been found to significantly improve its sensitivity and specificity [23].

Human epididymis protein 4 or HE4 is another tumour marker which is elevated in ovarian cancer but not with benign ovarian masses. It can therefore be used to distinguish between the two [24]. In a study using an algorithm combining both HE4 and CA125, 93.8% of epithelial ovarian cancers were accurately classified as high risk [25]. Other markers that have been tested include prolactin, transthyretin, CA72-4 and CA15-3. Combining these markers with CA125 has not shown to improve its efficacy in screening for ovarian cancer [26].

4. Screening population

There are two populations of women who are at risk of developing ovarian cancer—the general population whose life time risk is around 1–2% and the high-risk population (strong family history/gene mutations) whose risk can range from 10 to 46%. Most of the ovarian cancers are sporadic of which 90% occur in postmenopausal women, and for this reason, screening trials in the general population have been aimed at this cohort. In the high-risk population, however, even premenopausal women are at increased risk and are therefore included in screening studies.

5. Genetic predisposition to ovarian cancer

Approximately, 5–10% of ovarian cancers are attributed to genetic mutations. Mutations in the BRCA1 and BRCA 2 genes increase the risk of developing both breast and ovarian cancer. The life time risk of developing ovarian cancer (up to the age of 70 years) is 40% (95% CI, 35–46%) for carriers of BRCA1 mutation and 18% (95% CI, 13–23%) for BRCA2 mutation carriers [27]. A strong family history of breast and ovarian cancers could be an indicator of the presence of mutations in BRCA genes given their high penetrance [28]. The age of onset of ovarian cancer tends to be younger in BRCA carriers when compared to the general population. Median age at diagnosis is 63 years in the general population [29], 51.2 years for BRCA 1 and 57.5 years for BRCA2 mutation carriers [30].

Lynch syndrome or hereditary nonpolyposis colorectal cancer (HNPCC) is a syndrome secondary to mutations in the mismatch repair genes (MMR)—MLH1, MSH2, MSH6 and PMS2, which not only increases the risk of developing colorectal cancer but also ovarian and endometrial cancer in female carriers. The estimated cumulative risks of ovarian cancer by age 70 years for women with Lynch Syndrome is around 10% (range 6–14%) [31].

Traditionally, testing for gene mutations has been undertaken in individuals with a strong family history of ovarian cancer. Earlier studies looking at family history alone have shown that women with a first degree relative with ovarian cancer have a 4–5% life time risk of developing ovarian cancer. With two affected close relatives, the risk increases to around 10% and can become higher with even more relatives affected by ovarian cancer [32].

More recently there has been a different approach to screening for gene mutations. A randomised controlled trial looking at testing of the population regardless of family history in the Ashkenazi Jewish population reported a slightly higher incidence of BRCA mutations in the population screening group when compared with the family history group [33]. Such studies suggest that unselected testing of the population identifies 50% more carriers of genetic mutations than the traditional approach to screening based on family history alone.

Other than genetic factors, risk of ovarian cancer has also been found to increase with nulliparity, early menarche and late menopause, hormone replacement therapy and endometriosis. Factors suppressing ovulation such as use of the oral contraceptive pill, multiparity, longer periods of lactation have been associated with a decreased risk [34].

6. Symptom-based screening

Symptoms of ovarian cancer occur insidiously, with many patients presenting with non-gynaecological symptoms such as indigestion, abdominal bloating and early satiety, leading to a cascade of trial therapies and investigations until a diagnosis is reached. Hence, there may be a time lapse from initial presentation to actual diagnosis of ovarian cancer. The National Institute for Health and Care Excellence (NICE) in the UK advises primary care physicians to conduct preliminary testing if a woman reports persistent or frequent symptoms of abdominal distension, early satiety and/or appetite loss, pelvic/abdominal pain or increased urinary urgency and/or frequency [35]. This has been followed-up by a nationwide campaign, encouraging patients to present if any of the aforementioned symptoms occur.

In an effort to trigger early detection in patients presenting non-specifically, Goff et al. developed a symptom index (SI) [36]. The presence of any one of six symptoms was considered a positive result, including bloating, increased abdominal size, pelvic or abdominal pain, difficulty eating and/or early satiety. In the detection of ovarian cancer, the specificity of the SI was higher in women over 50 (90%) when compared to women under 50 (86.7%) years of age [37]. The SI also had a better sensitivity for advanced stage disease (79.5%) when compared to early stage disease (56.7%). Similar data was noted in a further study, when considering the SI as an isolated screening tool [38]. Acceptability of symptom-based screening was assessed in a subsequent prospective study. Encouragingly, of the 1261 women involved, symptom-based screening yielded a mean acceptability score of 4.8/5 and 4.7/5 for TVS and CA125 utilisation, respectively [36]. A multivariate approach involving SI, CA125 and HE4 biomarkers has also been studied for suitability [38]. Use of all three variates combined yielded an overall sensitivity of 83.8% and specificity of 98.5%. The authors concluded that these combined tests could be beneficial as first-line screening tool to aid selection for second-line imaging.

Despite these results, the question still remains as to whether detection using a symptom-based approach increases survival rates. Overall, there has been conflicting data regarding the correlation between symptom onset, referral and diagnostic delays, stage at presentation and overall survival rates in ovarian cancer patients. Several studies have demonstrated no such association [39]. Moreover, a recent Australian study discovered no correlation between time of symptom onset and FIGO stage III and IV disease, and concluded that longer time to diagnosis does not affect survival in women, even with advanced stage ovarian cancer [40]. A large qualitative study noted no difference between duration of symptom onset or time to diagnosis amongst patients with early to more advanced disease. Interestingly, women with advanced disease were more likely to report disregarding their symptoms [41]. Overall, current evidence suggests that the most successful direction of symptom-based detection of ovarian cancer is with a multivariate approach, but further research is required to ascertain its applicability.

7. Trials in ovarian cancer screening

Ultrasound and serum CA125 testing are two main modalities that have been used in ovarian cancer screening. Ultrasound alone has been used in some of the studies. In some other studies, multimodal screening with a combination of serum CA125 and ultrasound have been used. Following are some of the larger trials in the general population.

7.1. The University of Kentucky Ovarian Cancer Screening (UKOCS) trial

This trial was set up in 1987 to assess the efficacy of annual transvaginal ultrasonography (TVS) to detect ovarian cancer in asymptomatic women. All asymptomatic women: (1) 50 years or older and (2) 25 years or older with a family history of ovarian cancer in a first- or second-degree relative were eligible to participate in the trial. The control group for this study consisted of those women diagnosed with epithelial ovarian cancer entered in the University of Kentucky Tumor registry or statewide Kentucky Cancer registry between 1995 and 2001, who had not participated in screening [42].

A total of 37,293 women were screened over a period of 24 years between 1987 and 2011 with TVS. Women with an abnormal ultrasound at screening underwent repeat ultrasound in 4–6 weeks. If this scan was also abnormal, then further characterisation of the ovarian mass was performed with tumour indexing, colour Doppler and serum CA125 levels. Women underwent surgery if the second screen was also abnormal. However, if this screen was normal, then the scan was repeated in 6 months. As a result of screening, 47 invasive epithelial ovarian cancers and 15 epithelial ovarian tumours of low malignant potential were detected. An improved survival rate was noted in the screened group when compared to controls. The 5-year survival rate for all women with invasive epithelial ovarian cancer detected by screening as well as interval cancers was 74.8 ± 6.6% compared with 53.7 ± 2.3% for unscreened women with ovarian cancer from the same institution who had undergone treatment using the same protocol (p < 0.001) [43].

7.2. The Shizuoka Cohort Study of Ovarian Cancer Screening (SCSOCS) trial

A total of 82,487 asymptomatic postmenopausal women were enrolled into this study between 1985 and 1999 across 212 hospitals in Shizouka, Japan. They were randomised into an intervention group (n = 41,688) or a control group (n = 40,799) and were followed up for a mean period of 9.2 years. The women in the intervention group were screened with a pelvic ultrasound scan (USS) and a serum CA 125 test. If the USS was normal and if the CA125 was <35 U/ml, then they returned to yearly follow-up. If the scan suggested malignant disease and/or if the CA 125 was elevated, then the women were referred for surgery. However, if the scan was abnormal but suggestive of benign disease, it was repeated every 3–6 months. Also, if the CA125 was above a certain threshold with a normal scan, the women had a repeat scan in 6 months. There was no statistical difference between the number of ovarian cancers detected in the screening arm when compared to the control arm (27 vs. 32). However, there were a higher proportion of stage 1 ovarian cancers in the screened group when compared to the control group (63% vs. 38%) [44].

7.3. The Prostate Lung Colorectal and Ovarian (PLCO) Cancer Screening Randomised Controlled Trial

A total of 78,216 postmenopausal women aged 55–74 years were enrolled into this trial across 10 centres in the US. They were randomised to either annual screening (n = 39,105) or usual medical care (n = 39,111). Main outcome measure was mortality from ovarian/tubal/primary peritoneal cancers. The women in the screening arm had annual transvaginal ultrasound scan and CA125 (using a 35 kU/L cut-off) for 3 years and CA125 alone for a further 2 years. Women with an abnormal screening result were managed by their physicians. The follow-up period was 13 years in total. A total of 212 women were diagnosed with ovarian cancer in the screening arm when compared to 176 in the no screening (usual care) arm. In the screening arm, there were 118 deaths when compared to 100 deaths in the usual care arm as a result of ovarian cancer (mortality RR, 1.18; 95% CI, 0.82–1.71). This trial concluded that screening with CA125 and transvaginal ultrasound did not reduce mortality from ovarian cancer [45].

7.4. Ovarian Cancer Screening Trials in the UK

In 1993, Jacobs et al. screened 22,000 asymptomatic postmenopausal women with serum CA125 using a cut-off value of 30 kU/L. A transvaginal ultrasound was performed if the CA125 level was ≥30 kU/L. Women were referred for a gynaecological opinion if the ovarian volume was ≥ 8.8 ml. Out of the 41 women who had a positive screening result, 11 had ovarian cancer. Of the 21,959 women with a negative screening result, eight subsequently developed ovarian cancer. This protocol achieved a specificity of 99.9% and a positive predictive value of 26.8% and an apparent sensitivity of 78.6% and 57.9% at the first year and second year of follow-up, respectively [23].

Jacobs et al. then conducted a randomised controlled trial to assess the feasibility of a multi-modal approach using serum CA125 level and transvaginal ultrasound to screen for ovarian cancer [46]. A total of 21,935 postmenopausal women aged ≥45 years were randomised to either a screening group (n = 10,958) or a control group (n = 10,977). In the screening group, women were offered three annual screens using serum CA125 level as the first screening test. If the CA125 level was ≥30 kU/L, a transvaginal ultrasound scan was performed as a second test. If the ovarian volume was ≥8.8 ml on ultrasound, the women were referred for a gynaeco-logical opinion. Twenty-nine women with a positive screening test had surgical intervention out of which six were found to have ovarian cancer and the remaining 23 had a false posi-tive result. Therefore, the positive predictive value of screening was 20.7%. During the 8 year follow-up period, 10 more women in the screening group developed ovarian cancer bringing the total to 16 in the screened group. In the control group, 20 women were diagnosed with ovarian cancer. The median survival was better in the screening group when compared to the control group—72.9 months versus 41.8 months (p = 0.0112). There were nine deaths from ovarian cancer in the screened group when compared to 18 in the control group, which was not statistically significant (relative risk 2.0, 95% CI, 0.78–5.13; p = 0.083).

7.4.1. Risk of Ovarian Cancer Algorithm (ROCA)

The two UK studies discussed earlier used a cut-off value of CA125 of 30 kU/L for screening. Analysis of the serial serum CA125 data in women who subsequently developed ovarian cancer revealed a significant rise in the CA125 level after a 'change point'. In the unaffected women, however, the CA125 maintained a flat profile, fluctuating around the individual's baseline levels. The ROCA takes into account an individual woman's age, serial CA125 profile and estimates her risk of developing ovarian cancer based on known cases of ovarian cancer compared with the flat-profile model of known controls [47]. The ROCA calculates and updates the risk based on the most recent CA125 level. The risk is categorised as elevated, intermediate and normal. Women with an elevated risk are referred for an ultrasound, intermediate risk for repeat CA125 within a few months and normal risk for an annual CA125 test [48]. The ROCA has been used in subsequent screening trials.

7.4.2. The United Kingdom Collaborative Trial of Ovarian Cancer Screening (UKCTOCS)

Between 2001 and 2005, 202,638 women were randomly assigned to a control arm (n = 101,359) and an intervention arm (n = 101,279). The intervention arm was further subdivided into a multimodal screening (MMS) arm with annual CA125 screening (interpreted using the ROC algorithm) followed by ultrasound as a second-line test (n = 50,640) or annual screening with ultrasound (USS) alone (n = 50,639). Randomisation into the control arm and the two-intervention arm was carried out in a 2:1:1 ratio. The main aim of the trial was to determine the impact of screening on mortality from ovarian cancer [49].

Women in the MMS arm had their serum CA125 tested at recruitment and their risk was interpreted using the ROC algorithm. They went on to have (1) ultrasound scan if their risk was elevated or (2) repeat CA125 in 12 weeks if their risk was intermediate and (3) annual CA125 screening if the risk was low.

Women in the USS arm had transvaginal ultrasound at recruitment. They had repeat scans if the initial scan was abnormal. Women with persistent abnormalities were referred for clinical evaluation and had surgery if indicated. This trial was conducted across 13 centres in the UK.

Analysis of the prevalence screen results revealed that the MMS strategy was superior to ultrasound alone for detection of ovarian cancer (sensitivity of 89.4% and specificity of 99.8% for multimodal screening group compared to sensitivity of 84.9% and specificity of 98.2% for ultrasound only group) [50].

During the follow-up period, a total of 1282 women were diagnosed with ovarian cancer (median follow-up—11.1 years). A total of 652 women in the screening arm were diagnosed with ovarian cancer, which included 338 women in the MMS group and 314 women in the USS group when compared to 630 in the no screening group. A total of 148 women in the MMS group, 154 women in the USS group (n = 302) and 347 women in the no screening died from ovarian cancer. There was no significant reduction in mortality from ovarian cancer demonstrated in the primary analysis. However, after exclusion of the prevalent cases, further analysis of the mortality data revealed a significant reduction in mortality in the MMS group when compared to the no screening group. An overall average reduction in mortality of 20% was observed in the MMS group, with a reduction of 8% in years 0–7 and 28% in years 7–14. However, the authors concluded that further follow-up was required to ascertain the benefits of screening [51].

7.5. Screening in the high-risk population

Screening studies in the high-risk population also adopted the following two strategies: (1) annual screening with transvaginal ultrasound and CA125 and (2) multimodal screening with 3–4 monthly measurement of serum CA125 as the first and transvaginal ultrasound as the second-line test based on the CA125 levels.

In a Dutch multicentre observational study, 880 BRCA1 or BRCA2 carriers who had annual screening with CA125 and transvaginal scan were followed-up between 1993 and 2005. There were 10 incident cancers diagnosed. Five out of these ten cancers were in women who had previously had a normal screening within the last 3–10 months preceding the diagnosis. Eight out of the ten incident cancers were stage III–IV. In this study, despite annual screening, a large majority of the cancers were interval cancers that were diagnosed at an advanced stage. This study concluded that annual screening with TVS and CA125 neither helped in early diagnosis nor reduced mortality in high-risk women from ovarian cancer [52].

In the UK, Stirling et al. conducted a study involving 1110 high-risk women who were screened in three cancer genetic centres with annual CA125 and transvaginal ultrasound, between 1991 and 2004 [53]. Thirteen ovarian cancers were detected (including one borderline tumour). Three of these were detected during the first screen and seven during annual follow-up. The remaining three were interval cancers out of which one was an incidental finding following prophylactic surgery 2 months after a normal screen and the remaining two presented with symptoms, 4 and 12 months after a normal screening, respectively. This study also concluded that annual screening with CA125 and TVS was not effective in early diagnosis of ovarian cancer to have an impact on prognosis. In addition, the false positive rate was high in pre-menopausal women leading to unnecessary surgical intervention.

7.5.1. United Kingdom Familial Ovarian Cancer Screening Study (UK FOCSS)

Between 2002 and 2008, 3563 high-risk women (≥10% estimated lifetime risk) aged 35 years or above were recruited into this multicentred study across 37 centres in the UK. The trial had two phases—1 and 2.

In Phase 1, women underwent screening with annual transvaginal ultrasound scan and serum CA125 measurement. For CA125, a cut-off of 35 IU/ml for premenopausal women and 30 IU/ml for postmenopausal women was used.

A total of 27 primary ovarian/fallopian tube/peritoneal cancers were diagnosed during the course of screening and a further 10 cancers developed after 365 days following the last screen (median 539 days, range, 382–1369) in Phase 1 of the study. Nine of the primary ovarian/fallopian tube cancers were diagnosed during the prevalent screen and 13 were incident, screen-detected cancers. The positive predictive value was 25.5% (95% CI, 14.3–40.0) and negative predictive value was 99.9% (95% CI, 99.8–100) for the incident screen. Of the 13 incident cancers, only four were stage I or II. There was a delay in surgical intervention in the prevalent and screen-detected cancers (median—79 days). This study concluded that annual screening was not adequate in high-risk women for early detection of ovarian/fallopian tube cancer.

Following from the results of Phase I, women underwent more frequent screening with CA125 testing in Phase 2 (2007–2012) of the study. Serum CA125 levels were measured every 4 months, and the risk of developing ovarian cancer was estimated using the Risk of Ovarian Cancer algorithm (ROCA). Ultrasound was used as a second-line screen depending on the

ROCA estimated risk [54]. If the risk was normal, TVS was performed annually and if it was abnormal, then TVS was performed within 2 months.

There were 13 screen-detected and 6 occult (diagnosed following risk reducing salpingo-oophorectomy) primary ovarian/fallopian tube cancers in women who had been screened in the preceding year. Five out of the 13 screen-detected cancers and five out of the six occult cancers were stage I–II. Of these 19 women, 18 underwent optimal cyto-reductive surgery, with zero residual disease. This protocol had a high sensitivity of 94.7%, high negative predictive value of 100% and a positive predictive value of 10.8% for the detection of ovarian/fallopian tube cancers within 1 year of screening. The conclusion from Phase II was that ROCA-based screening could be an option for high-risk women who declined risk-reducing surgery. However, there was no conclusive evidence to suggest an impact on survival.

7.5.2. Cancer Genetics Network and Gynecologic Oncology Group study

The Cancer Genetics Network (CGN) ROCA study in Australia and the Gynecologic Oncology Group (GOG) study-GOG-0199 in the US used the same protocol to screen women at increased risk of developing ovarian/fallopian tube cancer [55]. All women received an annual transvaginal scan and CA125 testing every 3 months. The ROCA was used to estimate the risk and an interval TVS was performed for an abnormal ROCA result.

A total of 3692 women were screened in the two studies combined. There were four prevalent cancers and six incident cancers detected as a result of screening. Nine additional cancers were detected following risk reducing surgery. Three out of the six incident cases were detected at CA125 levels <35 U/ml using ROCA. The specificity for referral for ultrasound was 92% and the positive predictive value was 4.6%. This study concluded that three monthly CA125 testing with result interpretation using ROCA had a high specificity in the detection of early stage ovarian cancer with half of the incident cancers being diagnosed at CA125 levels <35 U/ml. There was a high rate of complete cytoreduction following surgery for the incident cancers diagnosed during the study period. The authors concluded that this screening regime with three monthly CA125 measurements performed better than 6–12 monthly screening using an absolute CA125 cut-off of 35 U/ml; however, larger studies were required given the small number of incident cases.

Thus, screening studies in high-risk women have demonstrated that annual screening with CA125 using a cut-off value and TVS is likely to miss the cancers that develop during the interval period. More frequent testing with CA125 with result interpretation using the ROCA helps to estimate an individual's risk based on their baseline CA125 level, aiding detection of ovarian cancer at an early stage or advanced cancer with low volume disease that can be optimally cytoreduced surgically. However, there is still paucity of evidence with regards to a mortality benefit from screening. Therefore, screening cannot be recommended as an alternative to risk reducing surgery, which remains the definitive preventative strategy in high-risk women.

7.6. Future of ovarian cancer screening

Ovarian cancer is a heterogeneous group of cancers, which includes both epithelial and non-epithelial neoplasms. Within the epithelial cancers, there are both slow growing Type 1 cancers that include mucinous, low-grade endometrioid, low-grade serous, clear cell and transitional cell carcinomas; and, the more aggressive, fast multiplying Type 2 cancers, which include high-grade serous carcinomas (HGSC), high-grade endometrioid, undifferentiated and carcinosarcomas [56]. Given their indolent nature, Type 1 tumours tend to be confined to the ovary at diagnosis, are easily detectable on ultrasound at an early stage and carry a better prognosis. Type 2 tumours, however, metastasise early in the natural history of the disease, are diagnosed at a late stage and carry a poor prognosis as a result. Traditional approach to screening using TVS and serum CA125 has not been effective in detecting these Type 2 cancers at an early stage. Detailed pathological examination of the fallopian tube from high-risk women who have undergone prophylactic salpingo-oophorectomy has revealed pre-cancer precursor lesions (serous tubal intraepithelial carcinoma or STIC) thereby, suggesting that a good majority of HGSC originate in the tube rather than in the ovary [3]. Majority of the incidental HGSCs in the low-risk population have also been shown to arise from STICs [57]. STIC lesions exhibit mutation in the TP53 gene which is likely to signal the early stages of carcinogenesis. Exfoliative cytology from the fimbrial end of the tube to detect these precursor lesions [58] and novel assays to detect TP53 mutations in circulating DNA are being explored [59, 60]. Angiogenesis is present early in the development of cancer. The use of microbubbles that are small enough to pass through capillaries is being explored to detect micro-vascularity in ovarian tumours on ultrasound [61].

A better understanding of tumourigenesis is opening up new avenues in ovarian cancer screening. Studies have shown that the target lesion is not always the ovary in 'ovarian cancer' and that STIC is the pre-malignant lesion in a good majority of HGSCs which include primary ovarian/fallopian tube/peritoneal cancers. The focus of future screening strategies will be used to detect low volume early disease either from the primary site of origin using exfoliative cytology or novel imaging modalities, or, in circulation using sensitive assays to detect low levels of tumour DNA and tumour markers.

Author details

Poonam Jani and Rema Iyer*

*Address all correspondence to: rema@doctors.org.uk

Department of Gynaecological Oncology, Women's Health Directorate, East Kent Hospitals University NHS Foundation Trust, Kent, England, United Kingdom

References

[1] Ferlay JSI, Ervik M, et al. GLOBOCAN 2012 v1.0, Cancer Incidence and Mortality Worldwide: IARC CancerBase No. 11 [Internet]. Lyon: France: International Agency for Research on Cancer; 2013

[2] Seidman JD, Horkayne-Szakaly I, Haiba M, Boice CR, Kurman RJ, Ronnett BM. The histologic type and stage distribution of ovarian carcinomas of surface epithelial origin. International Journal of Gynecological Pathology. 2004;**23**(1):41-44

[3] Crum CP, Drapkin R, Miron A, Ince TA, Muto M, Kindelberger DW, et al. The distal fallopian tube: A new model for pelvic serous carcinogenesis. Current Opinion in Obstetrics and Gynecology. 2007;**19**(1):3-9

[4] Gentry-Maharaj A, Sharma A, Burnell M, Ryan A, Amso NN, Seif MW, et al. Acceptance of transvaginal sonography by postmenopausal women participating in the United Kingdom Collaborative Trial of Ovarian Cancer Screening. Ultrasound in Obstetrics & Gynecology. 2013;**41**(1):73-79

[5] Timmerman D, Valentin L, Bourne TH, Collins WP, Verrelst H, Vergote I. Terms, definitions and measurements to describe the sonographic features of adnexal tumors: A consensus opinion from the International Ovarian Tumor Analysis (IOTA) group. Ultrasound in Obstetrics and Gynecology. 2000;**16**(5):500-505

[6] Sharma A, Burnell M, Gentry-Maharaj A, Campbell S, Amso NN, Seif MW, et al. Factors affecting visualization of postmenopausal ovaries: Descriptive study from the multi-center United Kingdom Collaborative Trial of Ovarian Cancer Screening (UKCTOCS). Ultrasound in Obstetrics & Gynecology. 2013;**42**(4):472-477

[7] Timmerman D, Ameye L, Fischerova D, Epstein E, Melis GB, Guerriero S, et al. Simple ultrasound rules to distinguish between benign and malignant adnexal masses before surgery: Prospective validation by IOTA group. BMJ. 2010;**341**:c6839

[8] Ferrazzi E, Zanetta G, Dordoni D, Berlanda N, Mezzopane R, Lissoni G. Transvaginal ultrasonographic characterization of ovarian masses: Comparison of five scoring systems in a multicenter study. Ultrasound in Obstetrics and Gynecology. 1997;**10**(3):192-197

[9] Timmerman D, Testa AC, Bourne T, Ameye L, Jurkovic D, Van Holsbeke C, et al. Simple ultrasound-based rules for the diagnosis of ovarian cancer. Ultrasound in Obstetrics and Gynecology. 2008;**31**(6):681-690

[10] Pavlik EJ, Ueland FR, Miller RW, Ubellacker JM, DeSimone CP, Elder J, et al. Frequency and disposition of ovarian abnormalities followed with serial transvaginal ultrasonography. Obstetrics & Gynecology. 2013;**122**(2, PART 1):210-217

[11] Valentin L, Skoog L, Epstein E. Frequency and type of adnexal lesions in autopsy material from postmenopausal women: Ultrasound study with histological correlation. Ultrasound in. Obstetrics and Gynecology. 2003;**22**(3):284-289

[12] Sharma A, Gentry-Maharaj A, Burnell M, Fourkala EO, Campbell S, Amso N, et al. Assessing the malignant potential of ovarian inclusion cysts in postmenopausal women within the UK Collaborative Trial of Ovarian Cancer Screening (UKCTOCS): A prospective cohort study. BJOG: An International Journal of Obstetrics & Gynaecology. 2012;**119**(2):207-219

[13] Elder JW, Pavlik EJ, Long A, Miller RW, DeSimone CP, Hoff JT, et al. Serial ultrasonographic evaluation of ovarian abnormalities with a morphology index. Gynecologic Oncology. 2014;**135**(1):8-12

[14] Timmerman D, Verrelst H, Bourne T, De Moor B, Collins W, Vergote I, et al. Artificial neural network models for the preoperative discrimination between malignant and benign adnexal masses. Ultrasound in Obstetrics and Gynecology. 1999;**13**(1):17-25

[15] Valentin L, Ameye L, Jurkovic D, Metzger U, Lécuru F, Van Huffel S, et al. Which extra-uterine pelvic masses are difficult to correctly classify as benign or malignant on the basis of ultrasound findings and is there a way of making a correct diagnosis? Ultrasound in Obstetrics & Gynecology. 2006;**27**(4):438-444

[16] Bast RC, Feeney M, Lazarus H, Nadler LM, Colvin RB, Knapp RC. Reactivity of a monoclonal antibody with human ovarian carcinoma. Journal of Clinical Investigation. 1981;**68**(5):1331-1337

[17] Bast RCJ, Klug TL, John ES, Jenison E, Niloff JM, Lazarus H, et al. A radioimmunoassay using a monoclonal antibody to monitor the course of epithelial ovarian cancer. New England Journal of Medicine. 1983;**309**(15):883-887

[18] Jacobs I, Bast JRC. The CA 125 tumour-associated antigen: A review of the literature. Human Reproduction. 1989;**4**(1):1-12

[19] Buamah P. Benign conditions associated with raised serum CA-125 concentration. Journal of Surgical Oncology. 2000;**75**(4):264-265

[20] Skates SJ, Mai P, Horick NK, Piedmonte M, Drescher CW, Isaacs C, et al. Large prospective study of ovarian cancer screening in high-risk women: CA125 cut-point defined by menopausal status. Cancer Prevention Research. 2011;**4**(9):1401-1408

[21] Pauler DK, Menon U, McIntosh M, Symecko HL, Skates SJ, Jacobs IJ. Factors influencing serum CA125II levels in healthy postmenopausal women. Cancer Epidemiology Biomarkers & Prevention. 2001;**10**(5):489-493

[22] Zurawski VR, Orjaseter H, Andersen A, Jellum E. Elevated serum CA 125 levels prior to diagnosis of ovarian neoplasia: Relevance for early detection of ovarian cancer. International Journal of Cancer. 1988;**42**(5):677-680

[23] Jacobs I, Davies AP, Bridges J, Stabile I, Fay T, Lower A, et al. Prevalence screening for ovarian cancer in postmenopausal women by CA 125 measurement and ultrasonography. British Medical Journal. 1993;**306**(6884):1030-1034

[24] Montagnana M, Lippi G, Ruzzenente O, Bresciani V, Danese E, Scevarolli S, et al. The utility of serum human epididymis protein 4 (HE4) in patients with a pelvic mass. Journal of Clinical Laboratory Analysis. 2009;**23**(5):331-335

[25] Moore RG, McMeekin DS, Brown AK, DiSilvestro P, Miller MC, Allard WJ, et al. A novel multiple marker bioassay utilizing HE4 and CA125 for the prediction of ovarian cancer in patients with a pelvic mass. Gynecologic Oncology. 2009;**112**(1):40-46

[26] Skates SJ, Horick N, Yu Y, F-J X, Berchuck A, Havrilesky LJ, et al. Preoperative sensitivity and specificity for early-stage ovarian cancer when combining cancer antigen CA-125II, CA 15-3, CA 72-4, and macrophage colony-stimulating factor using mixtures of multivariate normal distributions. Journal of Clinical Oncology. 2004;**22**(20):4059-4066

[27] Chen S, Parmigiani G. Meta-analysis of BRCA1 and BRCA2 penetrance. Journal of Clinical Oncology. 2007;**25**(11):1329-1333

[28] Berry DA, Giovanni P, Sanchez J, Schildkraut J, Winer E. Probability of carrying a mutation of breast-ovarian cancer gene BRCA1 based on family history. Journal of the National Cancer Research Institute. 1997;**89**(3):227-237

[29] Ovarian Cancer Reserach Fund Alliance. https://ocrfa.org/patients/about-ovarian-cancer/statistics/

[30] Risch HA, McLaughlin JR, Cole D, Rosen B, Bradley L, Kwan E, et al. Prevalence and penetrance of germline BRCA1 and BRCA2 mutations in a population series of 649 women with ovarian cancer. American Journal of Human Genetics. 2001;**68**(3):700-710

[31] Bonadona VBB, Olschwang S, Grandjouan S, Huiart L, Longy M, Guimbaud R, Buecher B, Bignon Y, Caron O, Colas C, Noguès C, Lejeune-Dumoulin S, Olivier-Faivre L, Polycarpe-Osaer F, Nguyen TD, Desseigne F, Saurin J, Berthet P, Leroux D, Duffour J, Manouvrier S, Frébourg T, Sobol H, Lasset C, Bonaïti-Pellié C. Cancer risks associated with germline mutations in mlh1, msh2, and msh6 genes in lynch syndrome. Journal of the American Medical Association. 2011;**305**(22):2304-2310

[32] Stratton JF, Pharoah P, Smith SK, Easton D, Ponder BAJ. A systematic review and meta-analysis of family history and risk of ovarian cancer. BJOG: An International Journal of Obstetrics & Gynaecology. 1998;**105**(5):493-499

[33] Manchanda R, Loggenberg K, Sanderson S, Burnell M, Wardle J, Gessler S, et al. Population testing for cancer predisposing BRCA1/BRCA2 mutations in the Ashkenazi-Jewish Community: A randomized controlled trial. Journal of the National Cancer Research Institute. 2015;**107**(1):1-11

[34] Jelovac D, Armstrong DK. Recent progress in the diagnosis and treatment of ovarian cancer. CA: A Cancer Journal for Clinicians. 2011;**61**(3):183-203

[35] NICE. Suspected cancer: Recognition and referral. 2015. www.nice.org.uk/guidance/ng12

[36] Goff BA, Lowe KA, Kane JC, Robertson MD, Gaul MA, Andersen MR. Symptom triggered screening for ovarian cancer: A pilot study of feasibility and acceptability. Gynecologic Oncology. 2012;**124**(2):230-235

[37] Goff BA, Mandel LS, Drescher CW, Urban N, Gough S, Schurman KM, et al. Development of an ovarian cancer symptom index. Cancer. 2007;**109**(2):221-227

[38] Andersen MR, Goff BA, Lowe KA, Scholler N, Bergan L, Drescher CW, et al. Use of a symptom index, CA125, and HE4 to predict ovarian cancer. Gynecologic Oncology. 2010;**116**(3):378-383

[39] Neal RD, Allgar VL, Ali N, Leese B, Heywood P, Proctor G, et al. Stage, survival and delays in lung, colorectal, prostate and ovarian cancer: Comparison between diagnostic routes. British Journal of General Practice. 2007;**57**(536):212-219

[40] Nagle CM, Francis JE, Nelson AE, Zorbas H, Luxford K, Fazio AD, et al. Reducing time to diagnosis does not improve outcomes for women with symptomatic ovarian cancer:

A report from the Australian ovarian cancer study group. Journal of Clinical Oncology. 2011;**29**(16):2253-2258

[41] Goff BA, Mandel L, Muntz HG, Melancon CH. Ovarian carcinoma diagnosis. Cancer. 2000;**89**(10):2068-2075

[42] van Nagell JR, PD DP, Ueland FR, CP DS, Cooper AL, JM MD, Pavlik EJ, Kryscio RJ. Ovarian cancer screening with annual transvaginal sonography. Cancer. 2007;**109**(9):1887-1896

[43] van Nagell JRJ, Miller RW, DeSimone CP, Ueland FR, Podzielinski I, Goodrich ST, et al. Long-term survival of women with epithelial ovarian cancer detected by ultrasonographic screening. Obstetrics & Gynecology. 2011;**118**(6):1212-1221

[44] Kobayashi H, Yamada Y, Sado T, Sakata M, Yoshida S, Kawaguchi R, et al. A randomized study of screening for ovarian cancer: A multicenter study in Japan. International Journal of Gynecological Cancer. 2008;**18**(3):414-420

[45] Buys SS, Partridge E, Black A. Effect of screening on ovarian cancer mortality: The prostate, lung, colorectal and ovarian (plco) cancer screening randomized controlled trial. Journal of the American Medical AssociationJAMA. 2011;**305**(22):2295-2303

[46] Jacobs IJ, Skates SJ, MacDonald N, Menon U, Rosenthal AN, Davies AP, et al. Screening for ovarian cancer: A pilot randomised controlled trial. The Lancet. 1999;**353**(9160):1207-1210

[47] Skates SJ, Menon U, MacDonald N, Rosenthal AN, Oram DH, Knapp RC, et al. Calculation of the risk of ovarian cancer from serial CA-125 values for preclinical detection in postmenopausal women. Journal of Clinical Oncology. 2003;**21**(10 suppl):206-210

[48] Menon U, Skates SJ, Lewis S, Rosenthal AN, Rufford B, Sibley K, et al. Prospective study using the risk of ovarian cancer algorithm to screen for ovarian cancer. Journal of Clinical Oncology. 2005;**23**(31):7919-7926

[49] Menon U, Gentry-Maharaj A, Ryan A, Sharma A, Burnell M, Hallett R, et al. Recruitment to multicentre trials—Lessons from UKCTOCS: Descriptive study. BMJ. 2008;**337**:a2079

[50] Menon U, Gentry-Maharaj A, Hallett R, Ryan A, Burnell M, Sharma A, et al. Sensitivity and specificity of multimodal and ultrasound screening for ovarian cancer, and stage distribution of detected cancers: Results of the prevalence screen of the UK Collaborative Trial of Ovarian Cancer Screening (UKCTOCS). Lancet Oncology. 2009;**10**(4):327-340

[51] Jacobs IJ, Menon U, Ryan A, Gentry-Maharaj A, Burnell M, Kalsi JK, et al. Ovarian cancer screening and mortality in the UK Collaborative Trial of Ovarian Cancer Screening (UKCTOCS): A randomised controlled trial. The Lancet. 2016;**387**(10022):945-956

[52] Hermsen BBJ, Olivier RI, Verheijen RHM, Beurden Mv, de Hullu JA, Massuger LF, et al. No efficacy of annual gynaecological screening in BRCA1/2 mutation carriers; an observational follow-up study. British Journal of Cancer. 2007;**96**:1335-1342

[53] Stirling D, Evans DGR, Pichert G, Shenton A, Kirk EN, Rimmer S, et al. Screening for familial ovarian cancer: Failure of current protocols to detect ovarian cancer at an early stage according to the International Federation of Gynecology and Obstetrics System. Journal of Clinical Oncology. 2005;**23**(24):5588-5596

[54] Rosenthal AN, Fraser LSM, Philpott S, Manchanda R, Burnell M, Badman P, et al. Evidence of stage shift in women diagnosed with ovarian cancer during phase II of the United Kingdom Familial Ovarian Cancer Screening Study. Journal of Clinical Oncology. 2017;**35**(13):1411-1420

[55] Skates SJ, Greene MH, Buys SS, Mai PL, Brown PH, Piedmonte M, et al. Early detection of ovarian cancer using the risk of ovarian cancer algorithm with frequent CA125 testing in women at increased familial risk—combined results from two screening trials. Clinical Cancer Research. 2017 Jul 15;**23**(14):3628-3637

[56] Kurman RJ, Shih L-M. The origin and pathogenesis of epithelial ovarian cancer—A proposed unifying theory. AmericanJournal of Surgical Pathology. 2010;**34**(3):433-443

[57] Gilks CB, Irving J, Köbel M, Lee C, Singh N, Wilkinson N, et al. Incidental nonuterine high-grade serous carcinomas arise in the fallopian tube in most cases: Further evidence for the tubal origin of high-grade serous carcinomas. The American Journal of Surgical Pathology. 2015;**39**(3):357-364

[58] Rodriguez EF, Lum D, Guido R, Austin RM. Cytologic findings in experimental in vivo fallopian tube brush specimens. Acta Cytologica. 2013;**57**(6):611-618

[59] Forshew T, Murtaza M, Parkinson C, Gale D, Tsui DWY, Kaper F, et al. Noninvasive identification and monitoring of cancer mutations by targeted deep sequencing of plasma DNA. Science Translational Medicine. 2012;**4**(136):136ra68-ra68

[60] Kinde I, Bettegowda C, Wang Y, Wu J, Agrawal N, Shih I-M, et al. Evaluation of DNA from the papanicolaou test to detect ovarian and endometrial cancers. Science Translational Medicine. 2013;**5**(167):167ra4-ra4

[61] Willmann JK, Bonomo L, Testa AC, Rinaldi P, Rindi G, Valluru KS, et al. Ultrasound molecular imaging with BR55 in patients with breast and ovarian lesions: First-in-human results. Journal of Clinical Oncology. 2017;**35**(19):2133-2140. DOI: 10.1200/JCO. 2016.70.8594

6

Microenvironment in Vagina as a Key-Player on Cervical Cancer: Interaction of Polymorphic Genetic Variants and Vaginal Microbiome as Co-Factors

Andreia Matos, Alda Pereira da Silva, Rui Medeiros,
Manuel Bicho and Maria Clara Bicho

Abstract

Current knowledge point to persistence of risk factors for the development of cervical intraepithelial neoplasia. The infection with a high-risk oncogenic Human Papillomavirus (HPV) subtypes, most commonly 16 and 18, is a necessary, although not sufficient, condition for development of invasive cervical cancer (ICC) and its precancerous precursor, cervical intra-epithelial neoplasia (CIN). It has been suggested that CIN disease severity and the diversity of vaginal microbiota are associated and this may determine viral persistence and disease behaviour. Our work focuses on the genetic variability associated to the modulation of genotoxicity induced by vaginal microbiota diversity. Relatively little is known about the mechanisms associated with clearance or persistence of HPV infection, therefore we hypothesized that may be under the influence of the genetic background.

Keywords: factors of persistence, genetic variation, microbiome, onco-microbiota, cervical cancer

1. Introduction

The vaginal microenvironment plays an important role in reproductive health. Human microbiome research has shown commensal bacteria to be a major factor in both wellness and disease pathogenesis. Interest in the microbiome has recently expanded beyond the gut to include a multitude of other organ systems for which the microbiome may have health implications. Here, we review the role of the vaginal microbiome in health and disease, with a particular focus on gynecologic malignancies, specifically cervical cancer. Further research is required to understand the molecular mechanisms involved in the complex role that bacterial communities can play in the development of cancer.

Cervical cancer is one of the most preventable cancers. However, its progression and above all, the progress towards prevention is often frustrating. Moreover, and despite the continuously growing body of knowledge, the role of factors that affect the human papillomavirus (HPV) persistence are not yet fully understood.

Indeed, the oncogenic HPVs are a necessary cause of cervical cancer; however, they are not a sufficient cause, being other cofactors implicated in the increase of risk. We have also to consider external factors to the host, such as smoking habits, nutritional and behavioural factors (number of partners and their characteristics, age at onset of sexual activity), hormonal therapies-sexual steroids (oral contraceptives and post-menopausal substitution therapy), herpes simplex infections, *Chlamydia trachomatis* or other sexually transmitted infectious diseases and also nonspecific inflammatory diseases. Genetic and immunological factors and other endogenous co-factors may induce initiation and progression associated with genotoxicity, mutagenicity and irreversible cell proliferation [1, 2].

Dysbiosis results from the disruption of equilibrium of the microbiome. Given that the vaginal microbiome composition has been shown to play a role in the HPV infection and the rate of HPV clearance, the vaginal microbiome structure may be associated with the development of cervical cancer secondary to a persistent HPV infection.

Nevertheless, recent and concise data show that composition of the early-life microbiota is critical in the development of the immune system, and how deviations from homeostasis can induce disease later in life [3].

Our group has been presenting data that reflects mainly the influence of genetic, epigenetic and environmental including the vaginal microbiota-derived factors in the natural history of HPV associated lesions leading to cervical cancer as a multifactorial disease process.

In this scenario, the microbiota and its genome (microbiome) fulfils part of the natural history of cervical cancer. In the last years, it has been characterized HPV-genotypes profile, and bacterial vaginosis (BV) leading to its association with the prevalence of HSIL and progression to invasive cervical cancer (ICC) in adult women.

Despite the risk factors status knowledge, we may consider the need of a more proactive behaviour, namely, a strategy for improving the local fora with topic therapy. In this chapter, we will focus in the role of genetic susceptibility associated to the development of cervical cancer. Furthermore, we will discuss opportunities for interventions that modify the microbiome for therapeutic purpose.

2. Factors of persistence

2.1. Vaginal microbiota, HPV and co-infections

More than ever, the association of a disrupted microbiota and the increasing incidence of chronic human diseases have been addressed [4]. Locally, the microbiota affects the functions and regulates the immunity of epithelial barrier. Therefore, the vaginal microbiome plays an essential role not only in health and dysbiosis, but also in modulation of immune response and, possible, in the carcinogenic process. Additionally, the persistence of risk factors, namely, HPV and other co-infections, may be associated to the disruption of these barriers [5].

The carcinogenic process in cervical cancer results in systemic and persistent damages, with important changes in immune checkpoints of the involved microenvironment [6]. From the key-players involved in this process, the microbiota influences, locally, physiological functions from the maintenance of barrier homeostasis to the regulation of metabolism, hematopoiesis, inflammation, immunity and other functions systematically [4, 7]. This barrier is supported by immune cells, for example, B cells, which produces IgA that helps to neutralize pathogenic bacteria (**Figure 1**) [8]. When this barrier locally fails it is created a favourable environment for carcinogenesis, the dysregulation of the integrity of vaginal epithelial cells will lead to more susceptibility for infections, causing low-grade chronic inflammation that leads to disease.

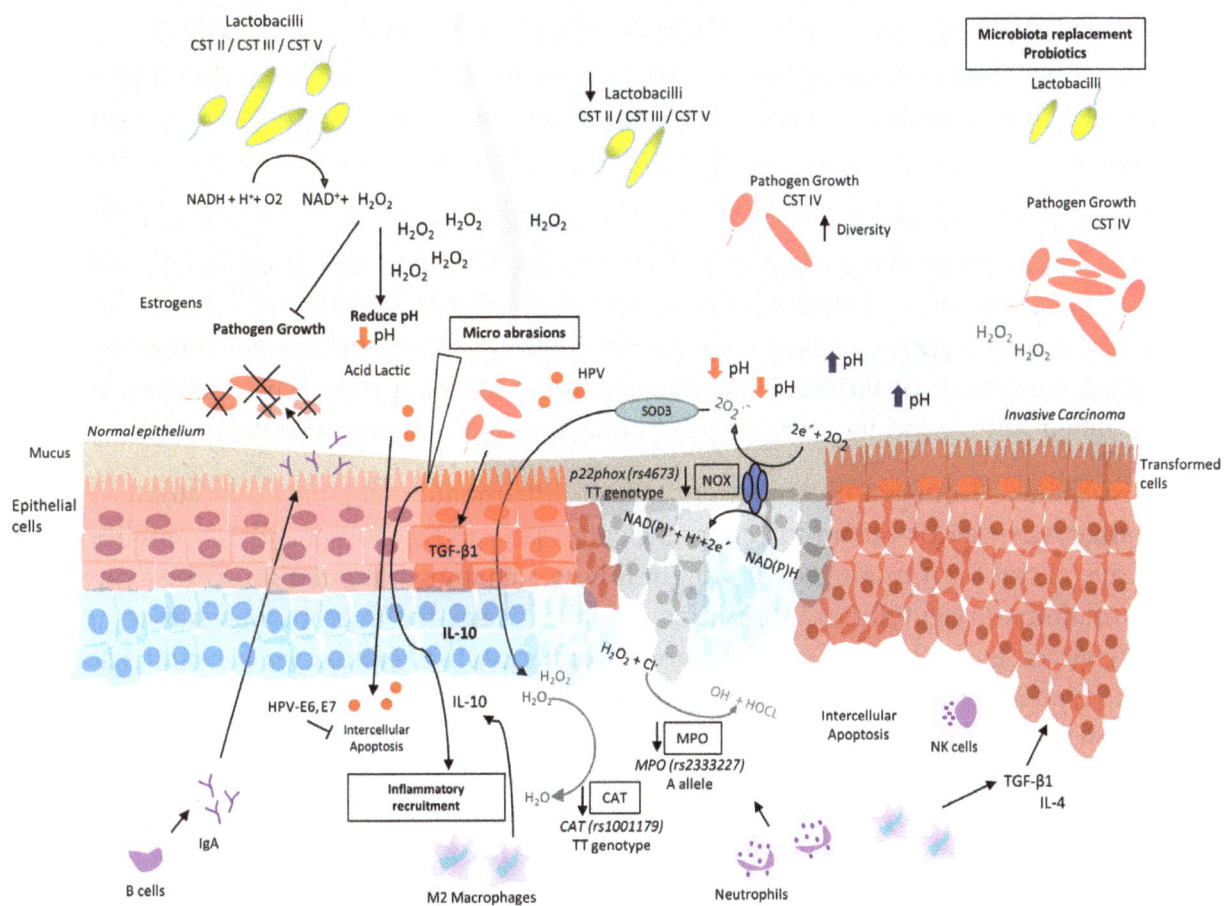

Figure 1. The presence of certain types of lactobacillus lowers pH and induces H_2O_2, which may contribute to the formation of HOCL by myeloperoxidase. CSTs IV are associated to bacterial vaginosis and the other microorganisms, to pre-cancerous lesions and cervical cancer. The types of groups of bacillus may be preponderant for maintaining the vaginal balance. Four species are most important for the balance of the vagina ecosystem: *L. gasseri* (II) *L. crispatus* (I), *L. jensenii* (V) and *L. iners* (III). The inter-individual genetic polymorphic variations should be integrated in a complex model, since a compromise vaginal microflora and inefficient genetic profile may contribute to the development of cervical cancer; CSTs, community state types; CSTs I, *Lactobacillus crispatus*; CSTs II, *Lactobacillus gasseri*; CSTs III, *Lactobacillus iners*; CSTs IV, *Lactobacillus, Sneathia amnii* and *Fusobacterium*; CSTs V, *Lactobacillus jensenii*.

The collection of microorganisms (or microbiota) populates complex ecosystems where genome is called microbiome and the implications on women health, from conception to the next generation, has been recently discussed [9]. A healthy vaginal microbiome is apparently dominated mainly by Community State Types (CST): *Lactobacillus crispatus (CSTs I)*, *Lactobacillus gasseri (CSTs II)*, *Lactobacillus iners (CSTs III)* and *Lactobacillus jensenii (CSTs V)*, which, regulate for instance, the balance of reactive oxygen species (ROS) (**Figure 1**) [7]. Although vaginal dysbiosis presents biological plausibly by influencing host's innate immune response, susceptibility to infection, and the development of cervical disease, the underlying cause is not yet well understood. Nevertheless, greater diversity in the vaginal microbiota was associated in women with HPV-positive with cervical intra-epithelial neoplasia (CIN) [10].

There is a strong relationship between infection with HPV, pre-neoplastic lesions and cervical cancer. Moreover, the prevalence of high-risk HPV genital infection (HSIL) and cervical cancer in adult women has been documented. Therefore, the determination of this specific environment correlated with demographic, behavioural and clinical parameters will contribute to a better knowledge of key-players that triggers the carcinogenic pathways in cervical cancer. Other different risk factors including early age at first intercourse, multiple sex partners and low socioeconomic status also have significant role in disease initiation [11].

The HPV infects only epithelial cells, firstly, throughout the basal layer of the epithelium, probably via microabrasions in the epithelial surface, then the viral DNA is released from the capsid and transported into the nucleus as free genetic material or extrachromosomal episomes (**Figure 1**) [12]. Environmental factors might locally influence the initiation of this invasion, among other co-factors, HPV allows potential tumour cells to escape from lactobacilli-mediated control and interfering with intracellular induction of apoptosis [7].

Recently, changes from pro-inflammatory to anti-inflammatory signals - the cytokine milieu - may affect whether or not an infection is cleared [13] and hypothetically an environment favourable or not for tumour growth, might follow a change in regulation of the expression of pro-inflammatory cytokines. After infection takes place, the microbiome changes and its diversity increases. HPV proteins E2, E6 and E7 enhance IL-10 expression secondary to macrophages type 2 presence. These latter are also enhanced in its activity by TGFβ-1 in cytokines expression and its phagocytic efficacy, which is in turn stimulated by the microbiota present. The increase of diversity in the microbiota, through its toxins (FadA from *Fusobacterium* spp.) will promote a metastasis phenotype similar to what happens in cervical cancer [13].

Moreover, polymorphic genetic variants used as surrogate markers might explain the inter-individual variations and the differential immune response causing the persistence and the progression of HPV effects. We had studied some polymorphisms that are associated with genetic susceptibility to cervical infection and increase for risk of acquiring and transmitting HPV infection. These polymorphisms are involved in several pathways, throughout the production of metabolites or other carcinogenic substances, by increasing the susceptibility of the inflamed epithelium or by changing the immune system equilibrium (**Figure 1**).

2.2. Lactobacilli enhance reactive oxygen species and the role of genetic susceptibility in the vaginal microbiome

The ROS, comprise a group of oxygen derivatives from distinct oxidation status of O_2, such as, superoxide radical anion (O_2^-), and hydroxyl free-radical (OH^-) and as well as non-radical forms, namely H_2O_2 [14]. The latter has a role as a second messenger molecule in signalling cascades that regulates gene expression and fundamental cellular processes such as proliferation, differentiation and migration [15]. Lactobacilli's H_2O_2 production in the absence of peroxidase may result in toxic concentrations of H_2O_2 and cause damage of the mucosa [16]. The presence of peroxidases guarantees the generating of hypochlorous acid (HOCL) in the vagina inducing a steady removal of excess of H_2O_2 and generation of HOCL [17].

H_2O_2-producing lactobacilli strains, use a NADH oxidase that directly generates H_2O_2 in a two-electron reduction of O_2 (**Figure 1**). Klebanoff et al. proposed that hydrogen peroxide H_2O_2, product of lactobacilli and peroxidase, in the vagina of healthy women might be responsible for the prevention of vaginosis and also might exert an antitumour effect [18]. The antimicrobial effect of H_2O_2-generating lactobacilli is efficiently enhanced in the presence of peroxidases (such as myeloperoxidase and eosinophil peroxidase) and halides [18]. This points to a role of HOCL as superior antimicrobial compound. The vaginal fluid of the majority of healthy women contains sufficiently high concentration of peroxidase to allow biologically significant HOCL synthesis in the presence of H_2O_2-generating lactobacilli [18].

Bauer proposed that peroxidase, which converts H_2O_2 into HOCL, is responsible for creating a microbicial vaginal milieu by maintaining a balanced, non-toxic [18]. The papers of Bauer had highlighted the role of lactobacilli in the vaginal flora of healthy premenopausal women pointing to the beneficial effects for the predominance of microorganisms. Lactobacilli adhere to epithelial cells and thus cause sterile prevention of cell infections with undesirable microorganisms. Lactobacilli cause low pH through production of lactate and also release bactericidal compounds (**Figure 1**) [7]. Others ROS are the highly reactive and toxic by-products of oxygen metabolism, which can damage bacterial nucleic acids, proteins and cell membranes [19].

Recent work of Kruger and Baeur 2017, confirms that the lactobacillus-derived H_2O_2 per se is not likely to be beneficial for the vaginal epithelium, because it causes nonselective lesions in nontransformed as well as transformed cells. The combination of lactobacillus and peroxidase is more favourable. Moreover, the lactobacilli in this system can be completely mimicked in vitro by H_2O_2 generated by glucose oxidase, indicating that its contribution for potential tumour prevention is fully explained by bacterial generation of H_2O_2 [17].

This idyllic scenario is considered for normal cells or untransformed cells, which have a wide antioxidant regulatory defence system that serves to prevent the oxidative stress and the development of neoplasms [20]. Nevertheless, the papillomavirus infected cells (in particular by oncogenic types HPV 16, 33, 31) are resistant to this pathway of apoptosis induction. In transformed cells caused by damages induced by HPV, cells lose control of senescence and p53 activity is abrogated [21].

The combination of the host genome and microbiome increases genetic variation and phenotypic plasticity, enabling the holobiont to increase its overall fitness [22]. Genome-wide association studies identified cervical cancer susceptibility variants across different populations [23]. Therefore, the input of these and other polymorphic variants, may reflect the interindividuality of response in women with cervical cancer. In this chapter, we will focus on some these polymorphisms involved in the modulation of ROS production.

2.2.1. NAD(P)H oxidase (NOX)

The production of O_2^- through NAD(P)H oxidase (NOX) by transformed cells or cervical cancer cells, can be specifically targeted with production of OH^- that induces apoptosis of these cells. The spontaneous dismutation of superoxide anions produce H_2O_2, at low pH, causes mutagenic effects that initiate malignant transformation (**Figure 1**). The high local concentrations of ROS through expression of SOD and catalase, it has also the potential to prevent elimination of transformed cells trough ROS/Reactive Nitrogen Species (RNS)-dependent intercellular apoptosis-inducing signalling [14].

The changes in the gut influences the vaginal microbiome, for instance the expression of NOX is modulated by, for example, the presence of *Helicobacter pylori*, which induces an indirect prooxidative mechanism through recruitment of neutrophils and by assembling of their NOX2 components to the cell membrane [1, 24].

NOX are membrane-associated oligomeric proteins that produce $O_2\cdot$ for host defence and other functions. Generation of extracellular $O_2\cdot$ through NOX is associated with oncogene activation and seems to be required for the control of cell proliferation and maintenance of the transformed state [25]. This protein consists of among other peptides by a regulatory 22-kDa α- subunit (p22phox) and a 91-kDa catalytic β-subunit (gp91phox). The p22phox protein is the NOX element responsible for the regulation of electron transfer to gp91phox [26]. The *p22phox* (*CYBA* gene) polymorphism with rs4673 (C-242 T) causes a functional non-conservative substitution from histidine-72 to a tyrosine residue that decreases its activity [27] (**Figure 1**). Our previous work unravels the association between *CYBA* polymorphism in women with ICC, having been observed a heterosis phenomenon with a protective profile in ICC [14]. This U type curve reflects, on one hand, the homozygote genotype CC leaded to increased ROS production, mainly H_2O_2 resulting from dismutation of O2·, which in turn results in excessive cell growth; on the other hand, the homozygote genotype TT lowers ROS production, mainly decreasing O2· mediated apoptosis cell capacity, resulting in a higher risk for the development of tumours in both cases [14]. Updated data from our cohort, we found that the TT genotype of *ph22phox* polymorphism was a tendency for increased risk in ICC (**Figure 1**) (OR = 3.57, 95% [0.85–13.48], P = 0.057), being age and smoking habits dependent factors.

Women with cervical cancer will have a lower induction of O2· and, consequently, compromising the dismutation by SOD3 of this apoptotic factor into H_2O_2. The continuous modification of vaginal microbiota throughout depletion of lactobacillus or infections with HPV, contribute to increase of pH, influencing the concentrations of ROS in vaginal milieu. Moreover, women with TT genotype of *p22phox* polymorphisms will have a worse response to these important modifications (**Figure 1**).

2.2.2. Catalase

The NOX and catalase (CAT) proteins work in sequence in a metabolic pathway. Transformed cells, spontaneous and enzymatic dismutated O_2^- into H_2O_2 by SOD occurs at right density to allow optimal velocity of the ROS interactions [28]. The CAT is a heme enzyme that plays a predominant role in controlling H_2O_2 and $O2\cdot$ protecting in this way cells from deleterious effects of oxidative stress. In healthy women, this protector effect rises from the conversion of H_2O_2 into H_2O and O_2 but in cervical cancer transformed cells, the ROS signalling is inhibited by a membrane associated catalase and causing control system failure that ultimately results in cell apoptosis failure [26, 29]. Notwithstanding, women with a genetic variant of CAT associated with a decrease activity will not contribute to this control system (**Figure 1**).

In humans, the CAT gene is located on chromosome 11p13 and its rs1001179 polymorphism (C-262 T) is located on the promoter region and influences transcription and consequent expression of this enzyme and hence the oxidative status of cells and its microenvironment [30]. In a case–control study, we observed a greater risk for developing ICC associated with the homozygote genotype TT of CAT polymorphism C-262 T polymorphism of the CAT gene (OR = 3.03, 95% CI 1.46–6.29, P = 0.003) [31]. Similarly to other cancers types, the T variant of this polymorphism is associated to a decreased enzyme activity, generating high levels of ROS [32–34]. The interaction of CC genotype of p22phox polymorphism and the TT genotype of CAT leads to a higher risk for ICC (OR = 3.95, 95% CI 1.07–14.52, P = 0.032) [31].

Moreover, recent reports have suggested a connection between oestrogen exposure, CAT activity and polymorphism in breast cancer [35]. These findings suggest that CAT genotype modifies the effect of hormone replacement therapy (HRT) use on breast cancer risk and that HRT may affect risk by affecting oxidative stress. This scenario, also might be important in cervical cancer, namely, women with CAT TT genotype (associated to a decreased catalase activity), will deficiently protects cells from ROS.

2.2.3. Myeloperoxidase

The oxidative stress conditions are generated by the release of ROS at the infection site by host immune cells such as neutrophils and monocytes. Additionally, resistance of oncogenic papilloma virus-expressing cells to apoptosis induction by the HOCL/hydroxyl anion pathways is likely, as papilloma virus-containing cells are also resistant to intercellular induction of apoptosis [36].

The toxic concentrations of H_2O_2 could be converted by myeloperoxidase (MPO). MPO, a lysosomal enzyme expressed in polymorphonuclear neutrophils, has the potential to kill HPV transformed cells, as a component of an intercellular induced-apoptosis pathway. The MPO was also being pointed as a key-player on controlling of vaginal microenvironment, namely, the H_2O_2-generating *Lactobacillus acidophilus*. In healthy women, this production inhibits the overgrowth of potentially pathogenic organisms; in fact, it can be toxic to other bacteria, fungi, viruses, spermatozoa, or tumour cells [37].

Supposedly, there are no resident neutrophils and macrophages on vaginal microenvironment, nevertheless the persistence of risk co-factors and ROS may lead to the recruitment of inflammatory cells. The presence of MPO on vaginal milieu is activated. Probably, the persistence of death cells recalls of neutrophils to vagina, being MPO important for the control of excess production of HOCl. In the vaginal microenvironment, the MPO catalyzes the reaction between H_2O_2 and either thiocyanate ions or a halide, such as iodide, bromide or chloride ions, yielding HOCl, which participates in the oxidative burst during the innate host defence [38]. MPO may act in synergy with other proteins. Therefore, an imbalance between oxidants/antioxidants could mean a higher chance for mutations and oncogenesis leading to diseases, including cancer—since MPO produces ROS secondary derivatives can be involved in the neoplastic transformation of cells through this pathway.

H_2O_2, and a halide form a powerful antimicrobial system in phagocytes and tissue fluids, which certain microorganisms can serve as the source of H_2O_2 for this system. The equilibrium of the production of H_2O_2 by *Lactobacilli* in the vagina appears to be a nonspecific host defence mechanism, which can be potentiated by myeloperoxidase that produces HOCl (**Figure 1**).

The production of superoxide through NADPH oxidase from cervical cancer cells, can be specifically targeted with production of OH⁻ radicals that induces selective apoptosis of these cells [16].

The polymorphism in the *MPO* gene induce a transition G463A (rs2333227), in the promotor region of the gene, where the wild-type G allele promotes the binding of transcription factors leading to a higher transcriptional activity than the A allele [39].

We found that women with the GG genotype had lower risk for cervical cancer than the women who displayed the heterozygous genotype GA (OR = 0.546, 95% CI = 0.315–0.939, P = 0.028, OR = 2.210, 95% CI [1.257–3.886], p = 0.008, respectively). The genotype that leads to a higher concentration of ROS (GG) presents itself as a protection factor in comparison to the homozygous genotype (AA) [39]. Moreover, recently, we observed that the A carriers of MPO polymorphism were about 5-fold of increased risk for cervical cancer (OR = 5.41, 95% CI [2.15–13.64], P < 0.0001) (**Figure 1**), being dependent of age (OR = 3.38, 95% CI [0.85–13.48], P = 0.085) and independent of smoking habits (OR = 3.85, 95% CI [1.33–11.11], P = 0.013). The interaction of HOCl and superoxide of transformed cells will generate apoptosis-inducing hydroxyl radicals.

We suggest that there is an association between the H_2O_2-producing strains found in the vaginal microbial flora and high activity of MPO leading to a clearance of the HPV-infected cells, the relation may also lead to the apoptosis of the transformed cells, producing O2· and OH·, acting as a protective factor for a cervical cancer [16, 17, 26].

2.2.4. Reactive nitrogen species

Nitric oxide is generated by nitric oxide synthase (NOS) and presents 3 isoforms: neuronal (NOS1), endothelial (NOS3) and inducible (NOS2). High local concentrations of ROS through expression of SOD and catalase might be associated to prevention of elimination of transformed cells trough ROS/RNS-dependent intercellular apoptosis-inducing signalling [14, 16]. Conversely the excess of NO inhibits the apoptosis induction associated to H_2O_2 and reversely NO-mediated apoptosis induction was inhibited by excess of H_2O_2 [29].

The NOS3 gene is located in the 7q35–36 region of chromosome 7 and the genetic polymorphism with a great clinical relevance is the 27 bp-VNTR 4b/a intron 4 [40]. In addition, NO produced by endothelial and epithelial cells, also modulates the regulation of vascular endothelial growth factor and is possibly associated to increase in processes of invasiveness and metastasis [41]. Preliminary results from our group, although only with a trend, identify that the A variant of NOS3 polymorphism, which is associated with higher activity of this enzyme, predisposes to ICC OR = 7.50, 95%CI [0.88–63.9], P = 0.066).

2.2.5. Catechoestrogens and cytochrome P450 (CYP1A1)

There is a clear association between the excessive and cumulative exposure to oestrogens and the development of cancer in hormone-sensitive tissues, such as the cervix. Therefore, we found that CYP1A1 and Catechol-o-methyltransferase (COMT) work in a metabolic sequence and their interaction could lead to an alternative pathway of oestrogen metabolism with production of 16-OH-estrone that is more proliferative and less apoptotic [42, 43]. The role of oestrogen and the association of CSTs favourable for balance vaginal milieu, was previously debated [44].

Aryl hydroxylase (AhR) the transcription factor of CYP1A1 is also associated with immuno-suppression after activation of IL-22 pathway, and the maintenance of intraepithelial in innate lymphocytes leading to the mucosal protection from inflammation [45].

Recently, a very interesting work unlighted the mechanism, where the Lactobacillus-derived H_2O_2 suppress host kynurenine metabolism, by inhibiting the expression of the metabolizing enzyme, indoleamine 2,3-dioxygenase (IDO1), in the intestine [46]. Moreover, maintaining elevated kynurenine levels during Lactobacillus supplementation diminished the treatment benefits.

3. Treatment and prevention: microbiota-derived factors

Finally, as suggested by other authors, it may be possible to expand the use of probiotics in the treatment of gynecologic cancers. The study of the role of probiotic bacteria for the prevention of colon and cervical cancer has led to the conclusion the tumour preventive effects of probiotic bacteria might be due to their control of the microbial flora, establishment of beneficial metabolic effects and stimulation of the immune system [37, 47]. Therefore, we can act in the prevention, specifically, the relapses.

Genetic analysis based on single nucleotide polymorphisms identified genetic variants associated with tumour rejection in mice, which could potentially affect ROS production and NK cell activity. That results also supports that B cells play a detrimental role in antitumour immunity and suggest that targeting B cells could enhance the antitumour response and improve the efficacy of therapeutic cancer vaccines [8].

The conventional photon radiotherapy for cervical cancer irradiates parts of the healthy tissue. This treatment perturbs the vaginal microbiome and disrupt the epithelial barrier function, permitting translocation of pathogenic bacteria and causing an inflammatory response [48]. The role of probiotic bacteria for the prevention of colon cancer has led to conclusion of the tumour preventive potential by the microbes. Additionally, the genetic polymorphism might be related to genetic susceptibility to infections and so, the implementations of probiotics may reinforce the immune system. A better understanding of this line will allow for the development of therapies that can manipulate the microbiome to reinstate homeostasis.

The application of probiotic strains *Lactobacillus rhamnosus* GR-1 and *Lactobacillus reuteri* RC-14 concomitantly with specific anti-infective agents provides more reliable cytological diagnostics, reduces the number of false positive and false negative findings on cervical malignancy and normalizes vaginal microflora in higher percentage of patients with vaginal infections compared with therapy including anti-infective agents only [49].

The use of probiotics, such as L. acidophilus, concomitant with the subsequent use of antibiotics, helps to restore the natural bacteria in the digestive tract that eventually are killed by antibiotics.

Recently, due to changes in the sexual behaviour of the general population, especially in developed countries, there has been an increase in the incidence of HPV infection in other parts of the body, including oropharynx and anus, among others.

In summary, a personalized clinical / therapeutic approach is suggested to avoid unnecessary treatments, based on previous history (onset of sexual activity, number of partners, anovulatory, parity, nutrition, alcohol, tobacco, genetics-immunity, etc.), in vaginal pH, Lactobacillus, in the diagnosis of HPV, viral load, mRNA, HSV, CMV, HSIL, AGC, CINI and CINII / III. *Chlamydia trachomatis, Mycoplasma, Ureaplasma, Neisseria gonorrhoeae*) and in the immunohistochemical study (p16 and Ki-67) of dysplasia [50, 51].

4. Conclusions

The HPV is not a sufficient cause for developing of cervical cancer, therefore other factors may be involved in this susceptibility, namely the microenvironment in vagina and inter-individual genetic polymorphic variations. These variables must be integrated in a complex model that integrates other co-factors, such as, smoking, diet and oral contraceptives. According to this review based on recent data, it seems that a deficiency of an antioxidant mechanism associated to a compromise vaginal microflora and inefficient genetic profile may contribute to the development of cervical cancer. We hypothesis that the genetic background and dysbiosis may contribute to increase risk for gynecologic advanced cancer.

Therefore, the equilibrium of gut/vaginal microbiota and adequate supplementation for a homeostasis of oxidant and antioxidant species may contribute to the regression of the persistence of factors associated with cervical cancer.

Acknowledgements

The authors would like to acknowledge the Instituto de Investigação Científica Bento da Rocha Cabral and Sociedade Portuguesa de Papillomavírus for support.

Conflict of interest

The authors declare that they have no competing interests.

Author details

Andreia Matos[1,2]*, Alda Pereira da Silva[1], Rui Medeiros[3,4,5], Manuel Bicho[1,2] and Maria Clara Bicho[1,2,6]

*Address all correspondence to: andreiamatos@medicina.ulisboa.pt

1 Genetics Laboratory and Environmental Health of Faculty of Medicine of University of Lisbon, Lisbon, Portugal

2 Instituto de Investigação Científica Bento da Rocha Cabral, Lisbon, Portugal

3 Faculty of Medicine, University of Porto, Portugal

4 Research Department, Portuguese League Against Cancer, CEBIMED, Portugal

5 Faculty of Health Sciences of the Fernando Pessoa University, Porto, Portugal

6 Dermatology Research Unit, Instituto de Medicina Molecular, Lisboa, Portugal

References

[1] Villain P, Gonzalez P, Almonte M, Franceschi S, Dillner J, Anttila A, et al. European code against cancer 4th edition: Infections and cancer. Cancer Epidemiology. 2015;**39**(Suppl 1): S120-S138

[2] Bui TC, Thai TN, Tran LT-H, Shete SS, Ramondetta LM, Basen-Engquist KM. Association between vaginal douching and genital human papillomavirus infection among women in the United States. The Journal of Infectious Diseases. 2016;**214**(9):1370-1375

[3] Tamburini S, Shen N, Wu HC, Clemente JC. The microbiome in early life: Implications for health outcomes. Nature Medicine. 2016;**22**(7):713-722

[4] Blaser MJ. The theory of disappearing microbiota and the epidemics of chronic diseases. Nature Reviews. Immunology. 2017;**17**(8):461-463

[5] de Abreu AL, Malaguti N, Souza RP, Uchimura NS, Ferreira EC, Pereira MW, et al. Association of human papillomavirus, Neisseria gonorrhoeae and chlamydia trachomatis co-infections on the risk of high-grade squamous intraepithelial cervical lesion. American Journal of Cancer Research 2016;**6**(6):1371-1383

[6] Heong V, Ngoi N, Tan DSP. Update on immune checkpoint inhibitors in gynecological cancers. Journal of Gynecologic Oncology. 2017;**28**(2):e20

[7] Mitra A, MacIntyre DA, Marchesi JR, Lee YS, Bennett PR, Kyrgiou M. The vaginal microbiota, human papillomavirus infection and cervical intraepithelial neoplasia: What do we know and where are we going next? Microbiome. 2016;**4**(1):58

[8] Tang A, Dadaglio G, Oberkampf M, Di Carlo S, Peduto L, Laubreton D, et al. B cells promote tumor progression in a mouse model of HPV-mediated cervical cancer. International Journal of Cancer. 2016;**139**(6):1358-1371

[9] Younes JA, Lievens E, Hummelen R, van der Westen R, Reid G, Petrova MI. Women and their microbes: The unexpected friendship. Trends in Microbiology. 2017

[10] Mitra A, MacIntyre DA, Lee YS, Smith A, Marchesi JR, Lehne B, et al. Cervical intraepithelial neoplasia disease progression is associated with increased vaginal microbiome diversity. Scientific Reports. 2015;**5**(16865)

[11] Matos A, Moutinho J, Pinto D, Medeiros R. The influence of smoking and other cofactors on the time to onset to cervical cancer in a southern European population. European Journal of Cancer Prevention. 2005;**14**(5):485-491

[12] Schiffman M, Wentzensen N. Human papillomavirus infection and the multistage carcinogenesis of cervical cancer. Cancer Epidemiology, Biomarkers & Prevention. 2013;**22**(4):553-560

[13] Audirac-Chalifour A, Torres-Poveda K, Bahena-Roman M, Tellez-Sosa J, Martinez-Barnetche J, Cortina-Ceballos B, et al. Cervical microbiome and cytokine profile at various stages of cervical cancer: A pilot study. PLoS One. 2016;**11**(4):e0153274

[14] Costa A, Scholer-Dahirel A, Mechta-Grigoriou F. The role of reactive oxygen species and metabolism on cancer cells and their microenvironment. Seminars in Cancer Biology. 2014;**25**:23-32

[15] Sies H, Berndt C, Jones DP. Oxidative stress. Annual Review of Biochemistry. 2017;**86**(1):715-748

[16] Bauer G. Signaling and proapoptotic functions of transformed cell-derived reactive oxygen species. Prostaglandins, Leukotrienes, and Essential Fatty Acids. 2002;**66**(1):41-56

[17] Kruger H, Bauer G. Lactobacilli enhance reactive oxygen species-dependent apoptosis-inducing signaling. Redox Biology. 2017;**11**:715-724

[18] Klebanoff SJ, Hillier SL, Eschenbach DA, Waltersdorph AM. Control of the microbial flora of the vagina by H_2O_2-generating lactobacilli. The Journal of Infectious Diseases. 1991;**164**(1):94-100

[19] Netea MG, Joosten LAB, van der Meer JWM, Kullberg B-J, van de Veerdonk FL. Immune defence against Candida fungal infections. Nature Reviews. Immunology. 2015;**15**(10):630-642

[20] Zhou D, Shao L, Spitz DR. Reactive oxygen species in normal and tumor stem cells. Advances in Cancer Research. 2014;**122**:1-67

[21] Stiasny A, Freier CP, Kuhn C, Schulze S, Mayr D, Alexiou C, et al. The involvement of E6, p53, p16, MDM2 and Gal-3 in the clinical outcome of patients with cervical cancer. Oncology Letters. 2017;**14**(4):4467-4476

[22] Bordenstein SR, Theis KR. Host biology in light of the microbiome: Ten principles of Holobionts and Hologenomes. PLoS Biology. 2015;**13**(8):e1002226

[23] Martinez-Nava GA, Fernandez-Nino JA, Madrid-Marina V, Torres-Poveda K. Cervical cancer genetic susceptibility: A systematic review and meta-analyses of recent evidence. PLoS One. 2016;**11**(7):e0157344

[24] Suerbaum S, Michetti P. Helicobacter pylori infection. The New England Journal of Medicine. 2002;**347**(15):1175-1186

[25] Skonieczna M, Hejmo T, Poterala-Hejmo A, Cieslar-Pobuda A, Buldak RJ. NADPH oxidases: Insights into selected functions and mechanisms of action in cancer and stem cells. Oxidative Medicine and Cellular Longevity. 2017;**2017**:9420539

[26] Bechtel W, Bauer G. Catalase protects tumor cells from apoptosis induction by intercellular ROS signaling. Anticancer Research. 2009;**29**(11):4541-4557

[27] Najafi M, Alipoor B, Shabani M, Amirfarhangi A, Ghasemi H. Association between rs4673 (C/T) and rs13306294 (A/G) haplotypes of NAD(P)H oxidase p22phox gene and severity of stenosis in coronary arteries. Gene. 2012;**499**(1):213-217

[28] Mittal M, Siddiqui MR, Tran K, Reddy SP, Malik AB. Reactive oxygen species in inflammation and tissue injury. Antioxidants & Redox Signaling. 2014;**20**(7):1126-1167

[29] Bechtel W, Bauer G. Modulation of intercellular ROS signaling of human tumor cells. Anticancer Research. 2009;**29**(11):4559-4570

[30] Khodayari S, Salehi Z, Fakhrieh Asl S, Aminian K, Mirzaei Gisomi N, Torabi Dalivandan S. Catalase gene C-262T polymorphism: Importance in ulcerative colitis. Journal of Gastroenterology and Hepatology. 2013;**28**(5):819-822

[31] Castaldo SA, da Silva AP, Matos A, Inacio A, Bicho M, Medeiros R, et al. The role of CYBA (p22phox) and catalase genetic polymorphisms and their possible epistatic interaction in cervical cancer. Tumour Biology. 2015;**36**(2):909-914

[32] Liu K, Liu X, Wang M, Wang X, Kang H, Lin S, et al. Two common functional catalase gene polymorphisms (rs1001179 and rs794316) and cancer susceptibility: Evidence from 14,942 cancer cases and 43,285 controls. Oncotarget. 2016;**7**(39):62954-62965

[33] Funke S, Risch A, Nieters A, Hoffmeister M, Stegmaier C, Seiler CM, et al. Genetic polymorphisms in genes related to oxidative stress (GSTP1, GSTM1, GSTT1, CAT, MnSOD, MPO, eNOS) and survival of rectal cancer patients after radiotherapy. Journal of Cancer Epidemiology. 2009;**2009**:302047

[34] Fabre EE, Raynaud-Simon A, Golmard J-L, Hebert M, Dulcire X, Succari M, et al. Gene polymorphisms of oxidative stress enzymes: Prediction of elderly renutrition. The American Journal of Clinical Nutrition. 2008;**87**(5):1504-1512

[35] Quick SK, Shields PG, Nie J, Platek ME, McCann SE, Hutson AD, et al. Effect modification by catalase genotype suggests a role for oxidative stress in the association of hormone replacement therapy with postmenopausal breast cancer risk. Cancer Epidemiology, Biomarkers & Prevention. 2008;**17**(5):1082-1087

[36] zur Hausen H. Viruses in human cancers. Science. 1991;**254**(5035):1167-1173

[37] Tachedjian G, Aldunate M, Bradshaw CS, Cone RA. The role of lactic acid production by probiotic lactobacillus species in vaginal health. Research in Microbiology. 2017

[38] Klebanoff SJ. Myeloperoxidase: Friend and foe. Journal of Leukocyte Biology. 2005;**77**(5): 598-625

[39] Castelao C, da Silva AP, Matos A, Inacio A, Bicho M, Medeiros R, et al. Association of myeloperoxidase polymorphism (G463A) with cervix cancer. Molecular and Cellular Biochemistry. 2015;**404**(1-2):1-4

[40] Ezzidi I, Mtiraoui N, Mohamed MBH, Mahjoub T, Kacem M, Almawi WY. Endothelial nitric oxide synthase Glu298Asp, 4b/a, and T-786C polymorphisms in type 2 diabetic retinopathy. Clinical Endocrinology. 2008;**68**(4):542-546

[41] Gao X, Wang J, Wang W, Wang M, Zhang J. eNOS genetic polymorphisms and cancer risk: A meta-analysis and a case–control study of breast cancer. Alkhiary W, editor. Medicine (Baltimore). 2015;**94**(26):e972

[42] Bicho MC, Pereira da Silva A, Matos A, Silva RM, Bicho MD. Sex steroid hormones influence the risk for cervical cancer: Modulation by haptoglobin genetic polymorphism. Cancer Genetics and Cytogenetics. 2009;**191**(2):85-89

[43] Matos A, Castelao C, Pereira da Silva A, Alho I, Bicho M, Medeiros R, et al. Epistatic interaction of CYP1A1 and COMT polymorphisms in cervical cancer. Oxidative Medicine and Cellular Longevity. 2016;**2016**(2769804)

[44] Brotman RM, Ravel J, Bavoil PM, Gravitt PE, Ghanem KG. Microbiome, sex hormones, and immune responses in the reproductive tract: Challenges for vaccine development against sexually transmitted infections. Vaccine. 2014;**32**(14):1543-1552

[45] Cella M, Colonna M. Aryl hydrocarbon receptor: Linking environment to immunity. Seminars in Immunology. 2015;**27**(5):310-314

[46] Marin IA, Goertz JE, Ren T, Rich SS, Onengut-Gumuscu S, Farber E, et al. Microbiota alteration is associated with the development of stress-induced despair behavior. Scientific Reports. 2017;**7**:43859

[47] Brady LJ, Gallaher DD, Busta FF. The role of probiotic cultures in the prevention of colon cancer. The Journal of Nutrition. 2000;**130**(2S Suppl):410S-414S

[48] Chase D, Goulder A, Zenhausern F, Monk B, Herbst-Kralovetz M. The vaginal and gastrointestinal microbiomes in gynecologic cancers: A review of applications in etiology, symptoms and treatment. Gynecologic Oncology. 2017;**138**(1):190-200

[49] Perisic Z, Perisic N, Golocorbin Kon S, Vesovic D, Jovanovic AM, Mikov M. The influence of probiotics on the cervical malignancy diagnostics quality. Vojnosanitetski Pregled. 2011;**68**(11):956-960

[50] Cuschieri K, Wentzensen N. Human papillomavirus mRNA and p16 detection as biomarkers for the improved diagnosis of cervical neoplasia. Cancer Epidemiology, Biomarkers & Prevention. 2008;**17**(10):2536-2545

[51] Bicho MC. Biomarkers of cervical carcinogenesis associated with genital HPV infection. Acta Médica Portuguesa. 2013;**26**(2):79-80

7

Ethnic Differences in Susceptibility to the Effects of Platinum-Based Chemotherapy

Andrey Khrunin, Alexey Moisseev,
Vera Gorbunova and Svetlana Limborska

Abstract

There is substantial interindividual variability in the efficacy and tolerability of anticancer drugs. Such differences can be greater between individuals of different ethnicities. The clinical studies demonstrate that individuals from Asia (East Asia) are more susceptible to the effects of platinum-containing chemotherapies than their Western counterparts. To determine whether population-related genomics (i.e., frequencies of DNA polymorphisms) contribute to differences in patient outcomes, polymorphisms in 109 genes involved mainly in xenobiotic metabolism, DNA repair, the cell cycle, and apoptosis were tested in Russian (Caucasians) and Yakut (North Asians) ovarian cancer patients receiving cisplatin-based chemotherapy. Totally, 232 polymorphisms were genotyped in individual DNA samples using conventional PCR and arrayed primer extension technology. Single nucleotide polymorphisms (SNPs) in more than 30 genes were found to be associated with one or more of clinical end points (i.e., tumor response, progression-free survival, overall survival, and side effects). However, all associations between SNPs and clinical outcomes were specific for each of ethnic group studied. These findings let us to propose the existence of distinctive ethnic-related characteristics in molecular mechanisms determining the sensitivity of patients to platinum drug effects.

Keywords: cisplatin, DNA polymorphisms, ethnic diversity, chemotherapy, ovarian cancer

1. Introduction

There is substantial interindividual variability in the efficacy and tolerability of pharmaceuticals, including anticancer drugs. Such differences can be greater between individuals of different ethnicities [1]. Currently, pharmacoethnicity, or ethnic diversity in drug effectiveness and/or toxicity, is an increasingly recognized factor for accounting interindividual variations in drug response [2]. Although the reasons underlying ethnic diversity in drug response are likely multifactorial [3], the results of numerous population studies suggest that they may be attributed, at least in part, to the interpopulation differences in frequencies of DNA polymorphisms – inherited variations at the DNA sequence level [4–6]. In terms of F_{ST}, the most commonly used measure of population differentiation; the proportion of such differences is 5–13% of total genetic diversity depending on the type of polymorphic markers chosen [6]. The opponents of ethnic-/race-based explorations in pharmacogenomics often consider these portions of variation as non-essential in the context of considerably larger proportions of within population variation which represents the average difference between members of the same population and accounts for 87–95% of total variance [7, 8]. Nevertheless, significant differences in the population prevalence of functionally impaired allelic variants of genes may create a potential for ethnic differences in responses to drugs that are detoxified (transported or targeted) by the proteins that are encoded by those genes [9–11]. A prominent example how population-based genetic differences can affect the drug response is the significantly greater risk for Stevens-Johnson syndrome and toxic epidermal necrolysis among East/Southeast Asian carbamazepine users, particularly Han-Chinese, Thais, and Malaysians, that has been associated with *HLA-B*1502* allele [12]. The relationship was not evident in non-Asian patients as well as in Japanese and Koreans due to infrequency of the allele in these populations. Another example is the lower average warfarin requirements of Asians linked to the higher frequency of AA genotype at SNP rs9923231 upstream of *VKORC1* gene among them [13]. Finally, considering potential pharmacoethnicity of anticancer drugs, one of the most illustrative examples, although not associated with germline variations, is the higher response rate to EGFR inhibitors (e.g., gefitinib) of Asian (East Asian) lung cancer patients compared to Caucasians that correlates to higher frequencies of activating *EGFR* mutations in East Asians [14].

Keeping all that in mind, we carried out a comparative study aimed to explore the genetic bases of differences between Asian and Caucasian cancer patients in their sensitivity to the effects of platinum-containing chemotherapy. Platinum-based drugs are among the most widely used cytotoxic agents for the treatment of many types of cancer [15]. The first information about lesser tolerance of Asian patients to standard, approved for Europeans, doses of platinum-containing regimens came from Japanese physicians [16]. In both individual small studies and some common arm trials conducted in Japan and by Southwest Oncology Group, the higher frequency of toxicity, particularly hematologic toxicity, was registered in Asian patients than non-Asians (mostly Caucasians) [1, 17]. Moreover, it was also found that the incidence of toxicity was still higher among Asians even after appropriate dose reduction [1]. Although some comparative pharmacogenetic studies have been conducted, the reasons underlying the higher sensitivity/toxicity of Asians to the systemic platinum-containing therapy are not yet well understood [18–20]. To assess the effect of population genomics on difference in patient response, we comparatively explored the results of cisplatin-based chemotherapy in Russian (Caucasians) and Yakut (North Asians) ovarian cancer patients. Principal component analysis, performed by us using genotype data of a common set of 125,000 genome-wide SNPs, demonstrated significant differences between gene pools of Asian and non-Asian populations (**Figure 1**).

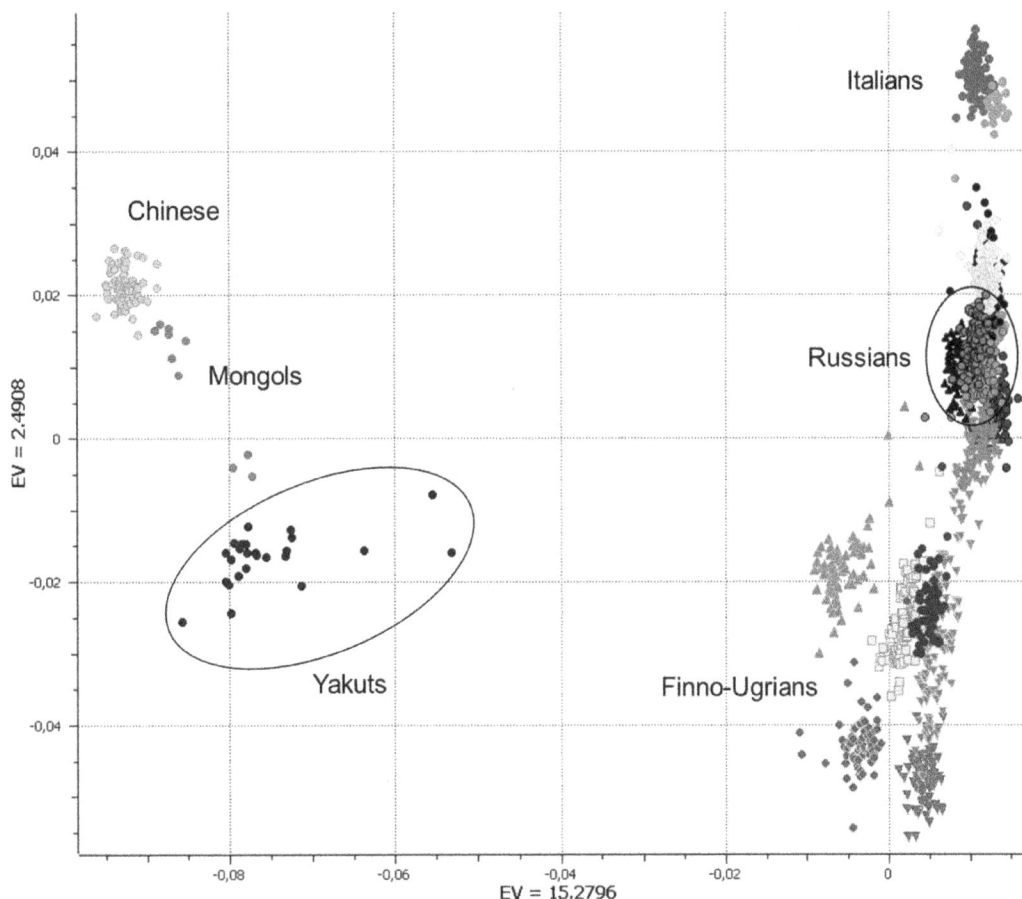

Figure 1. Genetic structure of Eurasian populations (based on 125,000 autosomal SNPs). The first two PCs are shown. Each individual is represented by a sign and the label corresponding to their self-identified population origin.

The estimates, obtained using the same set of polymorphic markers, showed that a portion of variation accounted for population-related differences, F_{ST}, in allele frequency between Russians and Yakuts was as high as 0.08, creating the potential for searching a causative polymorphism(s) with corresponding prevalence in population frequency. In the current study such candidates were searched among 232 polymorphisms from 109 genes involved mainly in xenobiotic metabolism, DNA repair, the cell cycle, and apoptosis.

2. Materials and methods

2.1. Patients

Ovarian cancer patients were identified and treated between 2003 and 2007 years at the N. N. Blokhin Cancer Research Centre and the Yakutsk Republic Cancer Clinic. Once identified, patients were invited to participate and were enrolled after they signed an informed consent. Detailed procedures of patient enrolment and data collection have been described previously [21, 22]. Briefly, unrelated Russian and Yakut women with morphologically confirmed epithelial ovarian carcinoma, who had received no previous chemotherapy or radiation therapy, were recruited. The upper age limit was 65 years. Exclusion criteria were serious concomitant diseases (diabetes, uncontrolled hypertension, myocardial infarction within the last 6 months, etc.), and clinically significant hearing impairment (grade 2 or higher). To ascertain ethnicity, women completed a questionnaire about their ancestry; only self-described Russian and Yakut patients with no history of interethnic marriages in the past two generations were recruited. Before the initiation of chemotherapy, venous blood samples were obtained for genetic testing. The chemotherapy regimen was intravenous cisplatin (100 mg/m^2) plus cyclophosphamide (600 mg/m^2) on day 1, every 3 weeks, for a maximum of 6 cycles. Intraperitoneal chemotherapy and radiotherapy were not allowed. Toxicity of the treatment was described according to standard National Cancer Institute Common Toxicity Criteria version 2.0 [23]. All patients were assessed for the maximal grades of nephrotoxicity, ototoxicity, neurotoxicity, emesis, neutropenia, anemia, and thrombocytopenia.

The tumor response was assessed every 2 cycles. After the completion of chemotherapy, the patients were followed-up for disease relapse and survival. Patients with progressive disease were treated with second-line chemotherapy, mostly taxane based. The study protocol and informed consent form were approved by the Ethics Committee of the N. N. Blokhin Cancer Research Centre.

2.2. Genotyping

DNA was isolated from the venous blood samples (leukocytes) using a conventional approach including proteinase K treatment with subsequent phenol-chloroform extraction [24]. Some polymorphisms (**Table 1**) were genotyped using a polymerase chain reaction restriction fragment length polymorphism (RFLP)-based technique or determined directly through evaluation of their PCR product lengths.

Other polymorphisms were genotyped using a microarray "DNA repair single nucleotide polymorphism detection test" (version 2, Asper Biotech, Tartu, Estonia). The microarray genotypes 228 SNPs in 106 genes involved in[1] DNA repair, cell cycle control, apoptosis, and xenobiotic metabolism. Most of manually genotyped loci were also in the list of the microarray's polymorphisms and served as controls of genotyping efficiency. To check into account the potential mistakes in genotyping with the microarray [25], all polymorphisms, which were associated with any clinical endpoints, were additionally tested using the RFLP method.

2.3. Statistical analysis

A permutation exact test, a two-sided Fisher exact test, and a χ^2 test were used to determine the relationship between the variables and alleles/genotypes tested. Correlations between survival and genotype or genetic polymorphism were assessed using the Kaplan-Meier product limit method and the log-rank test. The significance of associations was set at $P < 0.05$ [26]. The statistical analyses were performed using the Statistica software (version 6.0, StatSoft, Inc., Tulsa, OK, USA) or the IBM SPSS Statistics software package (version 19, SPSS, Inc., IBM Company, IBM Corporation, Armonk, NY, USA), GraphPadInStat (version 3.00, GraphPad Software, San Diego, CA, USA), and the PowerMarker software (version 3.0) [27].

---

[1]Alternative variant – "genes which are involved in".

Polymorphism	#rs ID	Genotypes (No. patients)*			P
GSTA1 – 69 C/T	rs3957357	CC (43/60)	CT (49/22)	TT (12/5)	0.0007
GSTM1 gene deletion		0/0 (47/28)	+/0** (57/59)	NA	0.0754
GSTM3 AGG deletion	rs1799735	AGG/AGG (83/75)	AGG/– (16/12)	–/– (5/0)	0.1054
GSTM3 Val^{224}Ile	rs7483	Val/Val (39/30)	Val/Ile (57/37)	Ile/Ile (8/20)	<0.0001
GSTP1 Ile^{105}Val	rs1695	Ile/Ile (41/67)	Ile/Val (53/17)	Val/Val (10/3)	<0.0001
GSTP1 Ala^{114}Val	rs1138272	Ala/Ala (80/84)	Ala/Val (24/3)	—***	0.0001
GSTT1 gene deletion		0/0 (18/22)	+/0** (86/65)	NA	0.2123
ERCC1 19007 T/C	rs11615	TT (43/53)	TC (46/29)	CC (15/5)	0.0146
ERCC1 8092 C/A	rs3212986	CC (61/52)	CA (37/31)	AA (6/4)	0.9351
ERCC2 Asp^{312}Asn	rs1799793	Asp/Asp (34/66)	Asp/Asn (50/19)	Asn/Asn (20/2)	<0.0001
ERCC2 Lys^{751}Gln	rs13181	Lys/Lys (28/67)	Lys/Gln (54/18)	Gln/Gln (22/2)	<0.0001
XRCC1 Arg^{194}Trp	rs1799782	Arg/Arg (94/69)	Arg/Trp (10/18)	—	0.0398
XRCC1 Arg^{280}His	rs25489	Arg/Arg (95/80)	Arg/His (9/6)	His/His (0/1)	0.5007
XRCC1 Arg^{399}Gln	rs25487	Arg/Arg (49/40)	Arg/Gln (45/39)	Gln/Gln (10/8)	0.9752
TP53 Arg^{72}Pro	rs1042522	Arg/Arg (52/47)	Arg/Pro (40/35)	Pro/Pro (12/5)	0.3733
CYP2E1 96bp insertion		–/– (100/74)	–/ins (4/13)	—	0.0097
CYP2E1 – 1053 C/T	rs2031920	CC (102/68)	CT (2/18)	—	<0.0001
CYP2E1 7632 T/A	rs6413432	TT (91/67)	TA (12/20)	AA (1/0)	0.0753
CYP2E1 9896 C/G	rs2070676	CC (82/78)	CG (20/9)	GG (2/0)	0.0908

*The first value in parentheses means the number of patients with corresponding genotype in Russian group, the second one – in Yakut group.

**The genotype was defined as positive if at least one copy of gene was present.

***The corresponding genotype was not occurred in populations.

NA – not available (not determined with the genotyping method used).

Table 1. Genotype frequencies in Russian and Yakut patients.

3. Results and discussion

During 2003–2007 years, 104 Russian patients and 87 Yakut patients were enrolled in the study. The median age of patients was 52 and 51 years, respectively. The majority of patients in both groups had stage III disease (72 and 53 women, respectively). Stages I, II, and IV were detected in 14, 6, and 10 Russian patients and 1, 8, and 25 Yakut patients. A total of 21 Russian patients and 11 Yakut patients were receiving adjuvant chemotherapy and were not eligible for evaluation of tumor response (i.e., they had no residual disease after surgery). Overall response rates, comprising complete and partial responders, were 85% in the Russian group and 58% in the Yakut group.

The median progression-free survival (PFS) in the Russian group was 12 months, and the median overall survival (OS) was 55 months. In the Yakut group, both intervals were shorter —8 and 29 months, respectively. However, being adjusted for disease stage, the values became similar to those for the Russian group.

More contrast results were obtained in analysis of occurrence of adverse events. To assess the association between genotype and the toxicity of the treatment used, patients were classified as having good or poor tolerance to treatment (grades 3–4 of neutropenia, grades 2–4 of anemia, grades 2–4 of neuropathy, grades 3–4 of emesis, all grade of thrombocytopenia, nephrotoxicity, and ototoxicity were considered as clinically significant toxicities). Comparison of the frequencies of side effects registered in Russian and Yakut patients confirmed higher toxicity of platinum-based regimens for patients of Asian origin than for Europeans. Particularly, Yakut patients suffered more frequently than Russians from nephrotoxicity and severe emesis (P = 0.027 and P = 0.061, respectively), which both were known to be the most common adverse events observed in regimens using cisplatin [28].

Genetic testing of the patients from our groups was performed in two stages. At first, we explored the associations between outcomes of a cisplatin-cyclophosphamide regimen in Russian and Yakut ovarian cancer patients and some most common polymorphisms in several genes [21, 22], among the tested genes, were glutathione S-transferase (GST) genes (GSTA1, GSTM1, GSTM3, GSTP1 and GSTT1), DNA repair genes (ERCC1, ERCC2 and XRCC1) as well as TP53 and CYP2E1 genes (**Table 1**). GST and DNA repair genes have been described as important for cisplatin metabolism and activity [29, 30]. GSTs can directly limit the amount of reactive cisplatin species available for interaction with DNA, by catalyzing their binding to tripeptide glutathione. The resulting cisplatin-glutathione conjugates can be further easily excreted from the cell by the GS-X pump transporters [31]. DNA repair proteins remove platinum-DNA adducts, the persistence of which underpins the antitumor potential of platinum drugs. In contrast to GST and the DNA repair proteins, TP53 protein does not seem to directly affect cisplatin metabolism or transformation. At the same time, it has a crucial role in mediating cellular responses to DNA damage, initiating programmed cell death when the effective DNA repair is impossible [29, 30, 32]. There is also no evidence that cisplatin is metabolized by CYP2E1. However, CYP2E1 is a significant potential source of catalytic iron and can serve as a site for generating reactive oxygen species in the presence of cisplatin [33]. It has been proposed that this mechanism underlies cisplatin-induced nephrotoxicity and hepatotoxicity [34, 35].

One of the most significant associations found in the first part of the study was the correlation between the survival time intervals and GSTP1 Ile105Val polymorphism registered in Russian subjects (P = 0.004 and P = 0.016 for PFS and OS, respectively). Russian ovarian cancer patients with a homozygous Ile/Ile genotype had longer PFS and OS than those ones who carried Ile/Val and Val/Val genotypes. However, the association was not observed in Yakut patients. PFS and OS of Yakut women with Ile/Ile genotype did not differ from the corresponding time intervals of patients with 1 or 2 Val alleles. In the Yakut group, PFS correlated with CYP2E1 7632 T/A polymorphism (P = 0.015), being longer in patients with a homozygous TT genotype than in patients with the heterozygous TA genotype.

Analysis of genotype distribution in the population groups for toxicities revealed that occurrence of nephrotoxicity and severe emesis in Yakut patients correlated with GSTT1 and

CYP2E1 genotypes, respectively. Patients with a homozygous *GSTT1* gene deletion (*GSTT1* null) suffered more frequently from nephrotoxicity than carriers of functional *GSTT1* variants (OR = 3.31, 95% CI 1.15–9.54, P = 0.028). Patients who had a 96 bp insertion in the promoter region of the *CYP2E1* were more prone to severe emesis (OR = 4.69, 95% CI 1.31–16.77, P = 0.027). Grade 3 or 4 emesis was also associated with another *CYP2E1* polymorphism—a single nucleotide substitution (9896 C/G) in intron 7. Patients with a heterozygous CG genotype had a higher risk of severe emesis than patients with the homozygous CC genotype (OR = 16.96, 95% CI 2.01–143.16, P = 0.002). In contrast, in Russian patients, *CYP2E1* polymorphisms were not associated with any clinical outcomes and distribution of *GSTT1* genotypes correlated with severity of emesis. The risk of severe emesis was higher in Russian patients with the *GSTT1*-null genotype than in patients with a functional *GSTT1* variant (OR = 4.06, 95% CI 1.40–11.78; P = 0.014). As for the nephrotoxicity in Russian subjects, it was associated with *ERCC1* 19007 T/C or 8092 C/A polymorphisms, and cases of renal dysfunction were more prevalent among patients with the heterozygous genotypes of each locus. Other found genotype-clinical end point associations were also discordant in Russians and Yakuts (**Table 2**).

When genotype distributions in both groups were compared significant differences in population genotype frequencies were noted for 10 of 19 polymorphisms studied but only 5 of them were associated with clinical outcomes (**Tables 1** and **2**).

Evaluation of the direction/strength of the associations showed that they were not correlated with the differences in population frequencies of corresponding genotypes. For example, the absence of correlation between the *GSTP1* Ile105Val polymorphism and survival in Yakut patients was not simply due to the higher prevalence of Ile/Ile genotype among them because carriers of Ile/Ile genotype did not differ in PFS or OS from those who had genotypes with 1 or 2 Val alleles. Similar results were obtained for the *GSTA1-69* C/T polymorphism. Its CT and TT genotypes were associated with a risk of anemia in Yakuts; yet the greater frequencies of the CT and TT genotypes in Russians did not result in a higher risk of anemia. Similarly, risk genotypes of *ERCC1* 19007 T/C and ERCC2 Asp312Asn polymorphisms (i.e., heterozygous genotypes in Russians) were not rare among Yakut patients but they did not demonstrate correlations with the corresponding side effects (**Tables 1** and **2**). It seems that only in the case of *CYP2E1* 96 bp insertion polymorphism an effect of allele frequency differences could be proposed but due to small number of individuals with the insertion containing genotypes in Russians the suggestion requires verification in a larger sample.

Taken in the context of other data, the obtained results generally supported the role of ethnicity as an additional reason for differences in the outcomes of clinical trials in which the same treatment is used. At the same time, the results of genetic testing suggested that a single genotypic difference was unlikely to account for the observed ethnic variation in toxicity and survival. Moreover, they also suggested that assessing traditionally tested common polymorphisms in GST and DNA repair genes is not enough for relevant description of lesser tolerability of Asians (North/East Asians) to the effects of platinum-containing chemotherapies and further studies involving more polymorphic markers are required.

In the second part of our study, we systematically investigated the associations between patients' outcomes and SNPs in more than 100 genes using the microarray "DNA repair single nucleotide polymorphism detection test" (version 2) [36, 37]. Like similar genotyping panels, the list of genes tested comprised candidate genes involved in key pathways of cellular

Gene name	#rs ID	Clinical outcomes**															
		PFS		OS		Anemia		Neutropenia		Thrombocitopenia		Nephrotoxicity		Ototoxicity		Emesis	
		R	Y	R	Y	R	Y	R	Y	R	Y	R	Y	R	Y	R	Y
GSTA1	rs3957357						+										
GSTM1	gene deletion					+				+							
GSTM3	rs1799735					+				+							
GSTM3	rs7483																
GSTP1	rs1695	+		+													
GSTP1	rs1138272																
GSTT1	gene deletion												+			+	
ERCC1	rs11615											+					
ERCC1	rs3212986											+					
ERCC2	rs1799793									+							
ERCC2	rs13181																
XRCC1	rs1799782																
XRCC1	rs25489																
XRCC1	rs25487							+									
TP53	rs1042522							+									
CYP2E1	96bp insertion																+
CYP2E1	rs2031920																
CYP2E1	rs6413432		+														
CYP2E1	rs2070676																+

*The registered associations are indicated by "+" in the corresponding cells.
**Tumor response and ototoxicity were not included in the table as there were no associations between them and polymorphisms tested.

Table 2. The associations between polymorphisms and clinical outcomes observed in Russian (R) and Yakut (Y) patient groups (the first stage of the study)*.

response to different drugs [38, 39], including many genes that are related to the cisplatin pathway (platinum pathway) [40]. A total of 213 SNPs from 228 genotyped SNPs were new (i.e., they did not include SNPs from the first stage) and 27 SNPs were associated with one or more of the assessed clinical end points (**Table 3**).

Increasing number of polymorphisms yielded an association with tumor response. To assess the association, patients who achieved a complete remission were compared with those without it (i.e., patients with partial response, stable and progressive disease). In the Russian group, a significant difference in complete response was observed according to polymorphism in the *ADH1C* gene (A/G, rs698) (P = 0.0002). The proportion of patients who achieved a complete response was higher among carriers of homozygous genotypes AA and GG compared with patients with a heterozygous variant AG. In Yakut patients, the occurrence of complete response was correlated with an allelic status of SNP in *CDKN1B* gene (T/C, rs34330), particularly with an allele C. There were no cases of complete remission among patients who carried a homozygous genotype TT at rs34330. The SNP was also associated with PFS in Yakut subjects (P = 0.0051); patients with the genotype TT had shorter PFS than patients with CC and CT genotypes. The protein encoded by *CDKN1B* gene participates in regulation of the cell cycle by binding and inhibiting activation of cyclin E-CDK2 or cyclin D-CDK4 complexes, and thus blocking the transition of the cell into the S-phase. C > T substitution at rs34330 locus results in decreasing the levels of mRNA and CDKN1B protein [41]. Reduced level of *CDKN1B* expression has been associated with a poor outcome in various cancers [42, 43]. In contrast, the *ADH1C* SNP (rs698) has been associated with a risk of alcoholism and ethanol-related cancers [44], but our study was the first to demonstrate an association with a chemotherapy outcome (i.e., tumor response) but the mechanism is not obvious.

Genotypes of seven SNPs were associated with differences in PFS in the Russian group (**Table 3**). The most significant SNPs were rs1142345 (A/G) in *TPMT* (P = 3×10^{-8}) and rs4986998 (C/T) and rs1800566 (C/T) in *NQO1* genes (P = 2×10^{-6} and P = 9×10^{-11}, respectively). The longer PFS was seen in patients with the most frequent genotypes AA and CC. SNPs in *NQO1* demonstrated similar correlations with OS.

Thiopurine S-methyltransferase (TPMT) is a cytosolic methylating enzyme with unknown physiological role [45]. However, this enzyme is known to be able to catalyze the S-methylation of some aromatic and heterocyclic compounds, particularly thio-compounds (e.g., 6-mercaptopurine and 6-thioguanine). Discussing the associations revealed between SNPs in *TPMT* and cisplatin ototoxicity, Ross et al. [46] have hypothesized that TPMT can affect cisplatin-induced hearing impairment through inactivation of cisplatin-purine compounds that form cytotoxic DNA cross-links, and cause cell death. As might be expected from that data, those patients in our study who had the loss-of-function genotype AG at rs1142345 should demonstrate a better outcome as a result of decreased inactivation of cisplatin-purine compounds, but such a correlation was not observed. Moreover, patients with an AG genotype had even shorter PFS than those who carried the functionally normal AA genotype.

The tested SNPs in *NQO1* gene are characteristic polymorphic variants affecting functional ability of the corresponding protein — a cytosolic flavoenzyme NAD(P)H: quinone oxidoreductase 1 (NQO1). *NQO1* polymorphic status has been associated with anticancer chemotherapy

Gene name	#rs ID	Clinical outcomes																
		Response		PFS		OS		Anemia		Neutropenia		Thrombocitopenia		Nephrotoxicity		Ototoxicity		Emesis	
		R	Y	R	Y	R	Y	R	Y	R	Y	R	Y	R	Y	R	Y	R	Y
ADH1C	rs698	+																	
ALDH2	rs4646777			+															
APEX1	rs1048945																+		
CCNH	rs2266690							+											
COMT	rs4633			+															
CDKN1B	rs34330		+		+														
CYP1A1	rs4646903						+												
CYP1A2	rs2470890						+												
DRD2	rs1079597				+														
EPHX1	rs1051740							+						+					
EPHX1	rs2234922															+			
ERCC5	rs1047768									+									
ERCC5	rs17655									+									
GRPR	rs4986946			+															
GSTA4	rs405729							+											
LIG3	rs1052536									+									
MSH3	rs26279											+							
MSH6	rs1042821																	+	
MUTYH	rs3219484									+									
MUTYH	rs3219489									+									
NAT2	rs1801280							+											

Gene name	#rs ID	Clinical outcomes																	
		Response		PFS		OS		Anemia		Neutropenia		Thrombocitopenia		Nephrotoxicity		Ototoxicity		Emesis	
		R	Y	R	Y	R	Y	R	Y	R	Y	R	Y	R	Y	R	Y	R	Y
NBN	rs1063045																		+
NQO1	rs1800566			+		+													
NQO1	rs4986998			+		+													
RAD52	rs11226									+									
TPMT	rs1142345			+															

The designations are the same as in **Table 2.**

Table 3. The associations between polymorphisms and clinical outcomes observed in Russian (R) and Yakut (Y) patient groups (the second stage of the study)*.

outcome (i.e., individuals with CT and TT genotypes at rs1800566 showed reduced survival compared to CC homozygotes) [47, 48]. The same correlations were observed in our study. Taking into account the key role of NQO1 in preventing the formation of reactive semiquinone radicals and generating reactive oxygen species (ROS) via redox cycling, one can propose that the worse survival of carriers of CT and TT genotypes is at least the consequence of a chronically elevated level of ROS, which results in enhanced ROS-mediated DNA damage, increased genetic instability, and further cancer progression [47].

In addition to *CDKN1B*, SNPs in *CYP1A1* (T/C, rs4646903) and *CYP1A2* (C/T, rs2470890) were found to also be associated with survival, particularly with OS, in Yakut patients (P = 0.007 and P = 0.0072, respectively). In each case the longer OS occurred in patients with homozygous genotypes TT. In contrast to TPMT and NQO1, the role of CYP1A1 and CYP1A2 in cisplatin metabolism or toxicity is difficult to discern. At the same time, it cannot be excluded that the observed associations are related to metabolic pathways of drugs used in the second and subsequent lines of the chemotherapy (taxanes and anthracyclines).

Totally, 16 SNPs were associated with the side effects of chemotherapy. Thirteen such SNPs were revealed in the Russian group and three SNPs in Yakuts (**Table 3**). A total of 6 of 13 SNPs were associated with an incidence of severe neutropenia in Russian patients. A strong association was estimated for SNP rs1052536 in *LIG3*. Carriers of its homozygous genotype CC had more than 20-fold higher risk of grade 3 or 4 neutropenia than patients with other genotypes (OR = 23.211, 95% CI =2.976–181.02, P = 2 × 10^{-6}). However, the most significant was SNP rs3219484 in *MUTYH*. The SNP was represented by only two genotypes, and patients who carried a heterozygous genotype AG had very low (actually unobserved) risk of developing severe neutropenia (OR = 0.013, 95% CI 0.000–0.220, P = 4 × 10^{-8}). *MUTYH* encodes a DNA glycosylase involved in repair of oxidatively damaged DNA, in particular by excising adenines misincorporated opposite 7,8-dihydro-8-oxoguanines. Such mispairs are promutagenic, and if left unrepaired before the next round of replication, they can give rise to CG → AT transversion mutations [49]. The observed association may reflect the substantial contribution of oxidative stress (i.e., ROS) into cisplatin-induced cytotoxicity. On the other hand, an associative grouping of *MUTYH* SNPs together with SNPs from other DNA repair genes, particularly *RAD52* and *ERCC5*, may also indicate a role of MUTYH in the repair of cisplatin-produced DNA lesions (e.g., participation in detection of the lesions) [50].

Another side effect for which multiple associations were found in the Russian group was anemia. SNPs in *NAT2*, *GSTA4*, *CCNH*, and *EPHX1* genes were associated with the toxicity (**Table 3**). The most significant was SNP rs1801280 in *NAT2*. Cases of anemia occurred more frequently among patients with the heterozygous CT genotypes (78.4%) compared with the homozygous variants (OR = 5.945, 95% CI 2.351–15.031, P = 0.00009). This association is of particular interest because there is no information about a role of NAT2 in the metabolism or toxicity of cisplatin or cyclophosphamide (the second drug in our chemotherapy regimen) [51]. One can propose that the association found is due to linkage between the SNP with a functional SNP(s) in other gene(s). Unlike *NAT2*, three other genes (i.e., *GSTA4*, *CCNH*, and *EPHX1*) are more relevant to the effects of intracellular processing of cisplatin. The cyclin encoded by *CCNH* is a part of a TFIIH complex that is an essential component of a nucleotide excision repair pathway, widely accepted as a main player in removing platinum-DNA adducts from DNA molecules [52].

GSTA4 plays an important role for the detoxification of 4-hydroxynonenal [53], a toxic product of lipid peroxidation, increasing immensely under oxidative stress conditions (e.g., overproduction of ROS), including cisplatin treatment [54, 55]. The role of epoxide hydrolases (EPXHs) in cisplatin-induced toxicity appears to be also related to the effects of oxidative stress. However, in contrast to GSTA4, EPXHs role is inhibitory and results from the abilities of epoxide hydrolases to metabolize epoxyeicosatrienoic acids (EETs) possessing multiple functions, particularly anti-inflammatory effects. The data about relationships between EET hydrolysis and cisplatin toxicity have been mainly obtained from the studies of cisplatin nephrotoxicity [56, 57]. It has been shown that the anti-inflammatory effect of EETs substantially depends on EPHX2, a cytosolic partner of EPHX1. EPHX1 also accepts EETs, although generally to a much lesser extent than EPHX2 [58]. Therefore, a role for EPHX1 in cisplatin toxicity should not be excluded, particularly because of its high expression in kidneys. The association between the SNP rs1051740 in *EPHX1* and nephrotoxicity of the regimen used supports this suggestion.

Three SNPs in *APEX1* (rs1048945), *MSH3* (rs26279), and *MSH6* (rs1042821) were associated with ototoxicity, thrombocytopenia, and emesis in Russian patients (**Table 3**). *APEX1* gene encodes apurinic/apyrimidinic endodeoxyribonuclease 1 playing an essential role in the DNA base excision repair pathway, where it removes apurinic/apyrimidinic sites produced during the repair of bases modified by ROS, alkylating agents, or ionizing radiation [59]. High *APEX1* expression has been associated with a poor outcome for chemoradiotherapy, poor complete response rate, shorter local relapse-free interval, poorer survival, and high angiogenesis [59]. At the same time, a role for APEX1 in protection against toxicity, particularly neurotoxicity, induced by ionizing radiation, and cisplatin treatment, has also been demonstrated [60–62]. ROS and oxidative DNA damage induced by them were shown to be important components of the deleterious effects of cisplatin on neuronal cells. Taking into account the proposed role of ROS in the mechanism of cisplatin-induced hearing loss [63], a contribution of APEX1 can also be hypothesized.

The protein products of *MSH3* and *MSH6* are essential components of the DNA mismatch repair system (MMR). The presence of MMR is thought to be important in mediating cisplatin and carboplatin cytotoxicity, whereas its deficiency, by contrast, may contribute to desensitization of cancer cells to the drugs [64, 65]. In our study, SNPs in *MSH3* and *MSH6* were not associated with tumor response or survival. Nevertheless, patients with minor alleles of the SNPs rs26279 and rs1042821 were at higher risk of thrombocytopenia and emesis, respectively.

Only one gene from the list above was also present among the genes whose polymorphisms were associated with the adverse reactions in Yakut patients, namely, *EPXH1* gene. However, it was associated with a different side effect (i.e., ototoxicity). Furthermore, the corresponding polymorphisms were also different (A/G, rs2234922 and C/G, rs2260863) (**Table 3**). Higher risk of ototoxicity was observed in patients with the most frequent genotypes AA and CC (OR = 26.26, 95% CI 1.502–458.98, P = 0.0005). Although the role of EPXHs in cisplatin toxicity has been mainly associated with their effects on cisplatin-induced kidney injury, the observed link between the *EPHX1* polymorphism and cisplatin ototoxicity can be due to similarity of mechanisms underlying cisplatin-induced hearing impairment and renal dysfunction [66].

The second gene whose allelic variants were associated with a side effect of chemotherapy in Yakut patients (i.e., severe emesis) was *NBN* (G/A, rs1063045). The risk factor for the development of severe emesis in patients was their heterozygous status at the rs1063045 locus. The protein encoded by NBN gene is an important component of the system repairing DNA double-strand breaks that can be induced by different environmental and endogenous agents, including cisplatin. The existing data suggest connections between polymorphic variants of the NBN gene and the results of cisplatin-based chemotherapy [67].

Intergroup comparison of genotypes generated with the microarrays revealed substantial differences in population frequencies of alleles and genotypes for many polymorphic markers. More than half of all markers differed significantly in the occurrence of their allelic variants in Russian and Yakut patients.

The proportion of significant genotype frequency differences resembled the results obtained in the first part of the study where a smaller number of polymorphic markers was involved (**Table 2**). Furthermore, the results of the comparisons of population-related associative spectra were also the same: there were no identical correlations for any of significant polymorphisms. All associations between the polymorphic markers and clinical outcomes were specific for each of the ethnic group studied.

These findings are generally compatible with the results of the HapMap project studying of the toxicity of platinum compounds (i.e., cisplatin and carboplatin) to lymphoblastoid cell lines from three groups of racially different individuals [19]. One can propose that the failure to detect common associations/commonly associated polymorphisms in our two groups was due to distinctive ethnic-related characteristics in the molecular mechanisms determining the sensitivity of patients to platinum drugs. Hence the difference in platinum drug sensitivity might not exclusively depend on the difference in variant frequencies of given polymorphisms. Another, but not exclusive, explanation of the findings could be a limitation of the number of polymorphisms tested and a possible omission of other potentially important markers. The latest may be mainly due to the misunderstanding of molecular phenotype(s) of the particular drug(s) [68]. The more relevant is the molecular phenotype, the higher is the potential to optimize the use of a particular drug. For some drugs, such as fluorouracil, irinotecan, and mercaptopurine, some relevant variants (i.e., DPYD*2A, DPYD 2846T/A, and TYMS 2R/3R; UGT1A1*28 and UGT1A1*6; TPMT *2, TPMT *3A, and TPMT*3C) have been established but for other ones, including platinum-containing agents, they are less apparent [68, 69].

The importance of DNA repair, particularly nucleotide excision repair, for platinum cytotoxicity is widely accepted [64]. However, the overall contribution of even the most common genetic variants to predictions of response to platinum-based therapy is not yet well established [70, 71]. In principle, the situation with other "canonical" pathways affecting mainly cisplatin pharmacokinetics could be described the same way [72]. Therefore, the role of additional mechanisms that are not directly related to cisplatin cellular processing has also been proposed [73]. The results of our study overrepresented with the associations with polymorphisms in genes for different metabolic enzymes (TPMT, NQO1, EPXH1, etc.) supports the suggestion (the associations would remain significant even if they were adjusted with the Bonferroni method). The abundance of associations with genes involved in processing of

ROS or ROS-mediated lesions is of particular interest. First, it can point to the higher potential of ROS in total cisplatin-related cytotoxicity [66, 73]. Second, it has been proposed that populations from different geographic regions possess a difference in efficiency of coupling mitochondrial oxidation with phosphorylation, with more heat production and lower ROS generation in North/Northeastern Asians [74, 75]. Consequently, we can expect in Asians lower ability to utilize extra ROS and higher sensitivity to effects of platinum-based drugs. However, because of the relatively small sample sizes and limited number of markers tested, further studies are required to confirm this hypothesis.

In summary, comprehensive exploration of genotypes of polymorphisms in more than 100 genes in ovarian cancer patients from Russian and Yakut ethnic groups, receiving cisplatin-based chemotherapy, revealed pronounced differences in associative spectra between them. Taken in the context of absence of correlations between the associations and polymorphic genotype frequencies, the differences suggest a potential for distinct ethnic-related molecular mechanisms determining the sensitivity of patients to platinum drug effects. The mechanisms are thought to be associated with activity of different metabolic enzymes, including those involved in processing the reactive oxygen species. These genetic findings and differential responses to platinum-based chemotherapy between ethnic groups suggest that future genetic testing may be invaluable not only in predicting chemotherapy response but also in deciding the most appropriate chemotherapy regimen. It may be possible to identify in detail the susceptibility differences to chemotherapy sensitivity at the molecular level and harness this for therapeutic gains.

Acknowledgements

This study was supported by grants from the Programs "Fundamental Researches for Development of Biomedical Technologies" and "Molecular and Cell Biology" of the Russian Academy of Sciences and Russian Foundation for Basic Research.

Author details

Andrey Khrunin[1*], Alexey Moisseev[2], Vera Gorbunova[3] and Svetlana Limborska[1]

*Address all correspondence to: khrunin@img.ras.ru

1 Department of Molecular Bases of Human Genetics, Institute of Molecular Genetics, Russian Academy of Sciences, Moscow, Russia

2 Institute of Modern Information Technologies in Medicine, Russian Academy of Sciences, Moscow, Russia

3 Department of Chemotherapy, N.N.Blokhin Cancer Research Centre, Ministry of Healthcare of the Russian Federation, Moscow, Russia

References

[1] O'Donnell PH, Dolan ME. Cancer pharmacoethnicity: Ethnic differences in susceptibility to the effects of chemotherapy. Clinical Cancer Research. 2009;15:4806-4814. DOI: 10.1158/1078-0432.CCR-09-0344

[2] Ortega VE, Meyers DA. Pharmacogenetics: Implications of race and ethnicity on defining genetic profiles for personalized medicine. The Journal of Allergy and Clinical Immunology. 2014;133:16-26. DOI: 10.1016/j.jaci.2013.10.040

[3] Morris AM, Rhoads KF, Stain SC, Birkmeyer JD. Understanding racial disparities in cancer treatment and outcomes. Journal of the American College of Surgeons. 2010;211:105-113. DOI: 10.1016/j.jamcollsurg.2010.02.051

[4] Kidd KK, Pakstis AJ, Speed WC, Kidd JR. Understanding human DNA sequence variation. The Journal of Heredity. 2004;95:406-420

[5] Li JZ, Absher DM, Tang H, Southwick AM, Casto AM, Ramachandran S, Cann HM, Barsh GS, Feldman M, Cavalli-Sforza LL, Myers RM. Worldwide human relationships inferred from genome-wide patterns of variation. Science. 2008;319:1100-1104. DOI: 10.1126/science.1153717

[6] Barbujani G, Colonna V. Human genome diversity: Frequently asked questions. Trends in Genetics. 2010;26:285-295. DOI: 10.1016/j.tig.2010.04.002

[7] Pena SD. The fallacy of racial pharmacogenomics. Brazilian Journal of Medical and Biological Research. 2011;44:268-275

[8] Jobling MA, Rasteiro R, Wetton HJ. In the blood: The myth and reality of genetic markers of identity. Ethnic and Racial Studies. 2016;39:142-161. DOI: 10.1080/01419870.2016.1105990

[9] Xie HG, Kim RB, Wood AJ, Stein CM. Molecular basis of ethnic differences in drug disposition and response. Annual Review of Pharmacology and Toxicology. 2001;41:815-850

[10] Phan VH, Moore MM, McLachlan AJ, Piquette-Miller M, Xu H, Clarke SJ. Ethnic differences in drug metabolism and toxicity from chemotherapy. Expert Opinion on Drug Metabolism & Toxicology. 2009;5:243-257. DOI: 10.1517/17425250902800153

[11] Phan VH, Tan C, Rittau A, Xu H, McLachlan AJ, Clarke SJ. An update on ethnic differences in drug metabolism and toxicity from anti-cancer drugs. Expert Opinion on Drug Metabolism & Toxicology. 2011;7:1395-1410. DOI: 10.1517/17425255.2011.624513

[12] Tangamornsuksan W, Chaiyakunapruk N, Somkrua R, Lohitnavy M, Tassaneeyakul W. Relationship between the HLA-B*1502 allele and carbamazepine-induced Stevens-Johnson syndrome and toxic epidermal necrolysis: A systematic review and meta-analysis. JAMA Dermatology. 2013;149:1025-1032. DOI: 10.1001/jamadermatol.2013.4114

[13] Limdi NA, Wadelius M, Cavallari L, Eriksson N, Crawford DC, Lee MT, Chen CH, Motsinger-Reif A, Sagreiya H, Liu N, Wu AH, Gage BF, Jorgensen A, Pirmohamed M,

Shin JG, Suarez-Kurtz G, Kimmel SE, Johnson JA, Klein TE, Wagner MJ, International Warfarin Pharmacogenetics Consortium. Warfarin pharmacogenetics: A single VKORC1 polymorphism is predictive of dose across 3 racial groups. Blood. 2010;**115**:3827-3834. DOI: 10.1182/blood-2009-12-255992

[14] Ma BB, Hui EP, Mok TS. Population-based differences in treatment outcome following anticancer drug therapies. The Lancet Oncology. 2010;**11**:75-84. DOI: 10.1016/S1470-2045(09)70160-3

[15] Ho GY, Woodward N, Coward JI. Cisplatin versus carboplatin: Comparative review of therapeutic management in solid malignancies. Critical Reviews in Oncology/Hematology. 2016;**102**:37-46. DOI: 10.1016/j.critrevonc.2016.03.014

[16] Watanabe A, Taniguchi M, Sasaki S. Induction chemotherapy with docetaxel, cisplatin, fluorouracil and l-leucovorin for locally advanced head and neck cancers: A modified regimen for Japanese patients. Anti-Cancer Drugs. 2003;**14**:801-807

[17] Soo RA, Kawaguchi T, Loh M, Ou SH, Shieh MP, Cho BC, Mok TS, Soong R. Differences in outcome and toxicity between Asian and caucasian patients with lung cancer treated with systemic therapy. Future Oncology. 2012;**8**:451-462. DOI: 10.2217/fon.12.25

[18] Gandara DR, Kawaguchi T, Crowley J, Moon J, Furuse K, Kawahara M, Teramukai S, Ohe Y, Kubota K, Williamson SK, Gautschi O, Lenz HJ, McLeod HL, Lara PN Jr, Coltman CA Jr, Fukuoka M, Saijo N, Fukushima M, Mack PC. Japanese-US common-arm analysis of paclitaxel plus carboplatin in advanced non-small-cell lung cancer: A model for assessing population-related pharmacogenomics. Journal of Clinical Oncology. 2009;**27**:3540-3546. DOI: 10.1200/JCO.2008.20.8793

[19] O'Donnell PH, Gamazon E, Zhang W, Stark AL, Kistner-Griffin EO, Stephanie Huang R, Eileen Dolan M. Population differences in platinum toxicity as a means to identify novel genetic susceptibility variants. Pharmacogenetics and Genomics. 2010;**20**:327-337. DOI: 10.1097/FPC.0b013e3283396c4e

[20] Wheeler HE, Gamazon ER, Stark AL, O'Donnell PH, Gorsic LK, Huang RS, Cox NJ, Dolan ME. Genome-wide meta-analysis identifies variants associated with platinating agent susceptibility across populations. The Pharmacogenomics Journal. 2013;**13**:35-43. DOI: 10.1038/tpj.2011.38

[21] Khrunin AV, Moisseev A, Gorbunova V, Limborska S. Genetic polymorphisms and the efficacy and toxicity of cisplatin-based chemotherapy in ovarian cancer patients. The Pharmacogenomics Journal. 2010;**10**:54-61. DOI: 10.1038/tpj.2009.45

[22] Khrunin A, Ivanova F, Moisseev A, Khokhrin D, Sleptsova Y, Gorbunova V, Limborska S. Pharmacogenomics of cisplatin-based chemotherapy in ovarian cancer patients of different ethnic origins. Pharmacogenomics. 2012;**13**:171-178. DOI: 10.2217/pgs.11.140

[23] National Cancer Institute. Common Toxicity Criteria, version 2.0. April 30, 1999. Available from: https://ctep.cancer.gov/protocoldevelopment/electronic_applications/ctc.htm [Accessed: 2017-04-06]

[24] Milligan BG. Total DNA isolation. In: Hoelzel AR, editor. Molecular Genetic Analysis of Populations. London: Oxford University Press; 1998. pp. 29-60

[25] Kweekel DM, Antonini NF, Nortier JW, Punt CJ, Gelderblom H, Guchelaar HJ. Explorative study to identify novel candidate genes related to oxaliplatin efficacy and toxicity using a DNA repair array. British Journal of Cancer. 2009;101:357-362. DOI: 10.1038/sj.bjc.6605134

[26] Perneger TV. What's wrong with Bonferroni adjustments. BMJ. 1998;316:1236-1238

[27] Liu K, Muse SV. PowerMarker: An integrated analysis environment for genetic marker analysis. Bioinformatics. 2005;21:2128-2129

[28] Ardizzoni A, Boni L, Tiseo M, Fossella FV, Schiller JH, Paesmans M, Radosavljevic D, Paccagnella A, Zatloukal P, Mazzanti P, Bisset D, Rosell R. Cisplatin- versus carboplatin-based chemotherapy in first-line treatment of advanced non – small-cell lung cancer: An individual patient data meta-analysis. Journal of the National Cancer Institute. 2007;99:847-857

[29] Siddik ZH. Cisplatin: Mode of cytotoxic action and molecular basis of resistance. Oncogene. 2003;22:7265-7279

[30] Jung Y, Lippard SJ. Direct cellular responses to platinum-induced DNA damage. Chemical Reviews. 2007;107:1387-1407

[31] Hall MD, Okabe M, Shen DW, Liang XJ, Gottesman MM. The role of cellular accumulation in determining sensitivity to platinum-based chemotherapy. Annual Review of Pharmacology and Toxicology. 2008;48:495-535

[32] Sullivan A, Syed N, Gasco M, Bergamaschi D, Trigiante G, Attard M, et al. Polymorphism in wild-type p53 modulates response to chemotherapy in vitro and in vivo. Oncogene. 2004;23:3328-3337

[33] Liu H, Baliga M, Baliga R. Effect of cytochrome P450 2E1 inhibitors on cisplatin-induced cytotoxicity to renal proximal tubular epithelial cells. Anticancer Research. 2002;22:863-868

[34] Liu H, Baliga R. Cytochrome P450 2E1 null mice provide novel protection against cisplatin-induced nephrotoxicity and apoptosis. Kidney International. 2003;63:1687-1696

[35] Lu Y, Cederbaum AI. Cisplatin-induced hepatotoxicity is enhanced by elevated expression of cytochrome P450 2E1. Toxicological Sciences. 2006;89:515-523

[36] Khokhrin DV, Khrunin AV, Ivanova FG, Moiseev AA, Gorbunova VA, Limborskaia SA. Pharmacogenomics of cisplatin-based chemotherapy in ovarian cancer patients from Yakutia. Molekuliarnaia Genetika, Mikrobiologiia i Virusologiia. 2013;(4):6-9

[37] Khrunin AV, Khokhrin DV, Moisseev AA, Gorbunova VA, Limborska SA. Pharmacogenomic assessment of cisplatin-based chemotherapy outcomes in ovarian cancer. Pharmacogenomics. 2014;15:329-337. DOI: 10.2217/pgs.13.237

[38] Dai Z, Papp AC, Wang D, Hampel H, Wolfgang S. Genotyping panel for assessing response to cancer chemotherapy. BMC Medical Genomics. 2008;1:24. DOI: 10.1186/1755-8794-1-24

[39] Sissung TM, English BC, Venzon D, Figg WD, Deeken JF. Clinical pharmacology and pharmacogenetics in a genomics era: The DMET platform. Pharmacogenomics. 2010; **11**:89-103. DOI: 10.2217/pgs.09.154

[40] Platinum pathway. Available from: http://www.pharmgkb.org/pathway/PA150642262 [assessed 2017-03-27]

[41] Landa I, Montero-Conde C, Malanga D, De Gisi S, Pita G, Leandro-García LJ, Inglada-Pérez L, Letón R, De Marco C, Rodríguez-Antona C, Viglietto G, Robledo M. Allelic variant at −79 (C/T) in CDKN1B (p27Kip1) confers an increased risk of thyroid cancer and alters mRNA levels. Endocrine-Related Cancer. 2010;**17**:317-328. DOI: 10.1677/ ERC-09-0016

[42] DE Almeida MR, Pérez-Sayáns M, Suárez-Peñaranda JM, Somoza-Martín JM, García-García A. p27Kip1 expression as a prognostic marker for squamous cell carcinoma of the head and neck. Oncology Letters. 2015;**10**:2675-2682

[43] Lin TC, Tsai LH, Chou MC, Chen CY, Lee H. Association of cytoplasmic p27 expression with an unfavorable response to cisplatin-based chemotherapy and poor outcomes in non-small cell lung cancer. Tumour Biology. 2016;**37**:4017-4023. DOI: 10.1007/ s13277-015-4272-7

[44] Xue Y, Wang M, Zhong D, et al. ADH1C Ile350Val polymorphism and cancer risk: Evidence from 35 case-control studies. PLoS One. 2012;**7**:e37227. DOI: 10.1371/journal. pone.0037227

[45] Fotoohi AK, Coulthard SA, Albertioni F. Thiopurines: Factors influencing toxicity and response. Biochemical Pharmacology. 2010;**79**:1211-1220. DOI: 10.1016/j.bcp.2010.01.006

[46] Ross CJ, Katzov-Eckert H, Dubé MP, Brooks B, Rassekh SR, Barhdadi A, Feroz-Zada Y, Visscher H, Brown AM, Rieder MJ, Rogers PC, Phillips MS, Carleton BC, Hayden MR, CPNDS Consortium. Genetic variants in TPMT and COMT are associated with hearing loss in children receiving cisplatin chemotherapy. Nature Genetics. 2009;**41**:1345-1349. DOI: 10.1038/ng.478

[47] Fagerholm R, Hofstetter B, Tommiska J, et al. NAD(P)H:Quinone oxidoreductase 1 NQO1*2 genotype (P187S) is a strong prognostic and predictive factor in breast cancer. Nature Genetics. 2008;**40**:844-853. DOI: 10.1038/ng.155

[48] Kolesar JM, Dahlberg SE, Marsh S, et al. The NQO1*2/*2 polymorphism is associated with poor overall survival in patients following resection of stages II and IIIa non-small cell lung cancer. Oncology Reports. 2011;**25**:1765-1772. DOI: 10.3892/or.2011.1249

[49] Markkanen E, Dorn J, Hübscher U. MUTYH DNA glycosylase: The rationale for removing undamaged bases from the DNA. Frontiers in Genetics. 2013;**4**:18. DOI: 10.3389/ fgene.2013.00018

[50] Jansson K, Alao JP, Viktorsson K, Warringer J, Lewensohn R, Sunnerhagen P. A role for Myh1 in DNA repair after treatment with strand-breaking and crosslinking chemotherapeutic agents. Environmental and Molecular Mutagenesis. 2013;**54**:327-337. DOI: 10.1002/em.21784

[51] Elkiran T, Harputluoglu H, Yasar U, Babaoglu MO, Dincel AK, Altundag K, Ozisik Y, Guler N, Bozkurt A. Differential alteration of drug-metabolizing enzyme activities after cyclophosphamide/adriamycin administration in breast cancer patients. Methods and Findings in Experimental and Clinical Pharmacology. 2007;**29**:27-32

[52] Zhovmer A, Oksenych V, Coin F. Two sides of the same coin: TFIIH complexes in transcription and DNA repair. ScientificWorldJournal. 2010;**10**:633-643. DOI: 10.1100/tsw.2010.46

[53] Balogh LM, Atkins WM. Interactions of glutathione transferases with 4-hydroxynonenal. Drug Metabolism Reviews. 2011;**43**:165-178. DOI: 10.3109/03602532.2011.558092

[54] Lee JE, Nakagawa T, Kim TS, Endo T, Shiga A, Iguchi F, Lee SH, Ito J. Role of reactive radicals in degeneration of the auditory system of mice following cisplatin treatment. Acta Oto-Laryngologica. 2004;**124**:1131-1135

[55] Li W, Yan MH, Liu Y, Liu Z, Wang Z, Chen C, Zhang J, Sun YS. Ginsenoside Rg5 ameliorates Cisplatin-induced nephrotoxicity in mice through inhibition of inflammation, oxidative stress, and apoptosis. Nutrients. 2016;**8**:E566. DOI: 10.3390/nu8090566

[56] Parrish AR, Chen G, Burghardt RC, Watanabe T, Morisseau C, Hammock BD. Attenuation of cisplatin nephrotoxicity by inhibition of soluble epoxide hydrolase. Cell Biology and Toxicology. 2009;**25**:217-225. DOI: 10.1007/s10565-008-9071-0

[57] Liu Y, Webb HK, Fukushima H, et al. Attenuation of cisplatin-induced renal injury by inhibition of soluble epoxide hydrolase involves nuclear factor κB signaling. The Journal of Pharmacology and Experimental Therapeutics. 2012;**341**:725-734. DOI: 10.1124/jpet.111.191247

[58] Decker M, Arand M, Cronin A. Mammalian epoxide hydrolases in xenobiotic metabolism and signalling. Archives of Toxicology. 2009;**83**:297-318. DOI: 10.1007/s00204-009-0416-0

[59] Fishel ML, Kelley MR. The DNA base excision repair protein Ape1/Ref-1 as a therapeutic and chemopreventive target. Molecular Aspects of Medicine. 2007;**28**:375-395

[60] Vasko MR, Guo C, Thompson EL, Kelley MR. The repair function of the multifunctional DNA repair/redox protein APE1 is neuroprotective after ionizing radiation. DNA Repair (Amst). 2011;**10**:942-952. DOI: 10.1016/j.dnarep.2011.06.004

[61] Jiang Y, Guo C, Vasko MR, Kelley MR. Implications of apurinic/apyrimidinic endonuclease in reactive oxygen signaling response after cisplatin treatment of dorsal root ganglion neurons. Cancer Research. 2008;**68**:6425-6434. DOI: 10.1158/0008-5472.CAN-08-1173

[62] Kim HS, Guo C, Thompson EL, Jiang Y, Kelley MR, Vasko MR, Lee SH. APE1, the DNA base excision repair protein, regulates the removal of platinum adducts in sensory neuronal cultures by NER. Mutation Research. 2015;**779**:96-104. DOI: 10.1016/j.mrfmmm.2015.06.010

[63] Mukherjea D, Rybak LP. Pharmacogenomics of cisplatin-induced ototoxicity. Pharmacogenomics. 2011;**12**:1039-1050. DOI: 10.2217/pgs.11.48

[64] Martin LP, Hamilton TC, Schilder RJ. Platinum resistance: The role of DNA repair pathways. Clinical Cancer Research. 2008;**14**:1291-1295. DOI: 10.1158/1078-0432.CCR-07-2238

[65] Topping RP, Wilkinson JC, Scarpinato KD. Mismatch repair protein deficiency compromises cisplatin-induced apoptotic signaling. The Journal of Biological Chemistry. 2009; **284**:14029-14039. DOI: 10.1074/jbc.M809303200

[66] Deavall DG, Martin EA, Horner JM, Roberts R. Drug-induced oxidative stress and toxicity. Journal of Toxicology. 2012;**2012**:645460. DOI: 10.1155/2012/645460

[67] Xu JL, Hu LM, Huang MD, Zhao W, Yin YM, Hu ZB, Ma HX, Shen HB, Shu YQ. Genetic variants of NBS1 predict clinical outcome of platinum-based chemotherapy in advanced non-small cell lung cancer in Chinese. Asian Pacific Journal of Cancer Prevention. 2012; **13**:851-856

[68] Loh M, Chua D, Yao Y, Soo RA, Garrett K, Zeps N, Platell C, Minamoto T, Kawakami K, Iacopetta B, Soong R. Can population differences in chemotherapy outcomes be inferred from differences in pharmacogenetic frequencies? The Pharmacogenomics Journal. 2013; **13**:423-429. DOI: 10.1038/tpj.2012.26

[69] Patel JN. Cancer pharmacogenomics: Implications on ethnic diversity and drug response. Pharmacogenetics and Genomics. 2015;**25**:223-230. DOI: 10.1097/FPC.0000000000000134

[70] Bowden NA. Nucleotide excision repair: Why is it not used to predict response to platinum-based chemotherapy? Cancer Letters. 2014;**346**:163-171. DOI: 10.1016/j.canlet. 2014.01.005

[71] Macerelli M, Ganzinelli M, Gouedard C, Broggini M, Garassino MC, Linardou H, Damia G, Wiesmüller L. Can the response to a platinum-based therapy be predicted by the DNA repair status in non-small cell lung cancer? Cancer Treatment Reviews. 2016;**48**:8-19. DOI: 10.1016/j.ctrv.2016.05.004

[72] Campbell JM, Bateman E, MDjP, Bowen JM, Keefe DM, Stephenson MD. Fluoropyrimidine and platinum toxicity pharmacogenetics: An umbrella review of systematic reviews and meta-analyses. Pharmacogenomics. 2016;**17**:435-451. DOI: 10.2217/pgs.15.180

[73] Macciò A, Madeddu C. Cisplatin: An old drug with a newfound efficacy – From mechanisms of action to cytotoxicity. Expert Opinion on Pharmacotherapy. 2013;**14**:1839-1857. DOI: 10.1517/14656566.2013.813934

[74] Mishmar D, Ruiz-Pesini E, Golik P, Macaulay V, Clark AG, Hosseini S, Brandon M, Easley K, Chen E, Brown MD, Sukernik RI, Olckers A, Wallace DC. Natural selection shaped regional mtDNA variation in humans. Proceedings of the National Academy of Sciences of the United States of America. 2003;**100**:171-176

[75] Ruiz-Pesini E, Mishmar D, Brandon M, Procaccio V, Wallace DC. Effects of purifying and adaptive selection on regional variation in human mtDNA. Science. 2004;**303**:223-226

8

Ovarian Cancer Overview: Molecular Biology and Its Potential Clinical Application

Joana Assis, Deolinda Pereira,
Augusto Nogueira and Rui Medeiros

Abstract

Over the previous two decades, there has been a shift in the ovarian cancer paradigm to consider it as a multiplicity of disease types rather than a single disease, requiring specialized medical management from molecular diagnosis through to treatment. Despite the achieved improvements in diagnosis, surgery, and systemic treatment, ovarian cancer remains the leading cause of death from gynecological tumors in western countries. The study of ovarian cancer at a molecular level could reveal potential biomarkers of disease diagnosis and progression, as well as possible therapeutic targets in areas such as angiogenesis and homologous recombination deficiencies. Although this area of research is proving invaluable concerning newer therapeutic approaches, platinum-based chemotherapy continues to be the core of the first-line treatment. Genomic screening focusing on the identification of prognostic and predictive markers is considered one of the leading areas for future ovarian cancer research.

Keywords: ovarian cancer, epithelial ovarian cancer, clinics, molecular biology, diagnosis, treatment, prognostic biomarkers, predictive biomarkers

1. Introduction

Ovarian cancer (OC) represents almost 4% of all cancer diagnoses among women worldwide. It is the eighth most common cause of death by cancer, resulting in 152,000 deaths (4.3% of all cancer deaths) [1, 2]. Besides its low incidence, OC is associated with a high mortality rate attributable, in part, to the frequent diagnosis at an advanced stage. The late diagnosis of OC is due to several factors including symptomatology absence and/or nonspecificity to the inexistence of an effective screening method and to the aggressive biology of this tumor with the ability to disseminate.

The geographic variability in OC incidence is considerable, being frankly higher in developed countries with rates surpassing 7.5/100,000 women. The highest continental rate is registered in Europe, where 65,584 new OC cases were observed. In opposite, the lowest continental values were registered in African regions, with incidence rates below 5/100,000 women [1]. Concerning mortality, for women with less than 75 years, the average risk of dying from OC is twice as high in more than less-developed regions. Inclusively, for developed countries, OC stands as the fifth most lethal cancer among women [1]. In Europe, in 2012, 42,749 deaths were observed, which corresponds to more than 25% of all worldwide OC deaths [3, 4]. Among the gynecological tumors, OC is the leading cause of death even being only the third most common, preceded by cervical and endometrial cancers [2–4].

Nevertheless, the numerous attempts to characterize the ovarian carcinogenesis and etiology, age is considered as a major determinant for OC development: there is an increased disease risk after the menopause, being 63 the median age at diagnosis [5].

Beyond age, an important risk factor for OC is the familiar history. Although the germline mutations in genes that predispose to OC are relatively rare in the general population, they are responsible for approximately 10–20% of all cases [6, 7]. The critical genes involved in hereditary OC are *BRCA1* and *BRCA2*, associated with hereditary breast/ovarian cancer syndrome. The risk of spontaneous OC development, throughout life, is around 1.7%, while the heritage of germline mutations that alter *BRCA1* gene function confers a cumulative risk from 40 to 60%, mainly to serous carcinoma. The presence of pathogenic mutations in *BRCA2* gene lowers the risk for about a half (10–30%). OC hereditary women tend to develop the disease nearly 10 years earlier than women with sporadic OC [8–10].

Moreover, reproductive and endocrine factors seem to be important, whereby the nulliparity, early menarche (<12 years), late menopause (>52 years), endometriosis, polycystic ovary syndrome, and the recent exposure to hormone replacement treatment might be associated with a higher risk to develop OC [11–14]. Therefore, some behaviors and lifestyles were associated with a decrease in OC incidence, namely breastfeeding, multiparity, and the oral contraceptives use [11, 13]. Surgical procedures such as tubal ligation, hysterectomy with salpingectomy, and oophorectomy correlate with a lower incidence of this tumor but are mainly reserved for women with higher disease risk, after the completion of familiar planning.

Standard treatment of epithelial ovarian cancer (EOC) is based on cytoreductive surgery, followed by platinum-based first-line chemotherapy. This neoplasia is considered chemosensitive, yielding 40–60% of complete responses rates for advanced disease stages. Despite the apparent efficacy of treatment, up to 75% of patients will relapse and become candidates for second-line chemotherapy. As a result, the high percentage of late-stage diagnosis and the occurrence of tumor recurrence limit the treatment efficacy, and the overall 5-year survival rate remains only around 45%.

In the clinical practice, several pathological factors are considered prognostic for EOC patients, and many efforts are made to identify those that will improve patient's stratification and be useful tools for therapeutic decisions. Current research is focusing on the identification of both prognostic and predictive biomarkers that would help to optimize EOC treatment strategies and to improve the cost-effective incorporation of emerging biological agents.

2. Clinics and diagnosis

Upon the detection of an adnexal mass suspected of malignancy, the diagnostic approach should be based on a careful clinical history that should include the overall physical examination, as well as gynecological, rectal, and abdominal evaluation. After the clinical evaluation, additional diagnostic and biochemical tests should be requested, judiciously and objectively, to aid in the differential diagnosis of a pelvic mass. Among the complementary diagnostic tests, transvaginal ultrasonography (TVU) and CA125 tumor marker determination are mandatory [8, 12, 15]. Other markers are also used in the diagnostic investigation for suspected EOC cases, such as CEA and CA19.9.

In the suspicion of ovarian neoplasia, abdominal-pelvic computed tomography (CT) should be requested to confirm and characterize the presence of lesions, to evaluate the tumor extension, to identify unresectable disease, and to exclude nonovarian metastatic disease. Nevertheless, the EOC diagnosis is surgical as only the anatomopathological exam confirms the definitive diagnosis. Diagnostic radiologically guided aspiration/biopsy or laparoscopy should be requested, whenever neoadjuvant chemotherapy is being considered [8, 16].

Late disease diagnosis explains, in part, the high mortality rate of these patients [12, 17]. Over the past 25 years, there has been little improvement in the survival rate, being around 37% in the early 1970 and 44% in 2000, despite the advances in the medical treatment [18]. However, the currently available tests lack adequate sensitivity and specificity, promoting a noneffective screening strategy. Prospective studies have shown that the combined use of serum CA125 and TVU improved the specificity of the tests and allowed the detection of a number of OC cases in the preclinical phase (this is discussed in detail in another chapter).

3. Histopathology

Ovarian tumors are classified according to the World Health Organization (WHO) proposal for gynecological tumors. Ovarian cancer has high cellular heterogeneity, and most of the primary ovarian tumors can be integrated into three major groups, namely epithelial, sex cord and ovarian stroma, and germ cell tumors [2].

Although the ovarian epithelial surface represents only a small fraction of all ovarian cell types, EOC is the most common, corresponding to almost 60% of all ovarian tumors [19, 20]. According to the criteria proposed by the WHO in 2014, EOC can be divided into seven histological subcategories, namely serous, mucinous, endometrioid, clear cell, Brenner, seromucinous, and undifferentiated [2]. All the mentioned histological subtypes, except for the undifferentiated type, are further subdivided into benign, borderline, and malignant neoplasia, depending on the optical microscopy characteristics.

Sex cord and stroma tumors arise from the ovarian connective tissue, often responsible for hormone secretion. These tumors encompass a vast group of tumors, for which the subgroup of "pure" ovarian stromal tumor is the most frequent (9% of all OC), usually with benign behavior. Also in this group of tumors, granulosa cell tumors are associated with aggressive behavior and represent 1% of all OC. Regarding the germ subgroup, a mature cystic teratoma is very common (32% of all OC), although the remaining germ cell tumors, both benign and malignant, are rare, representing 3–5% of all OC cases [2, 21].

4. Staging

Ovarian cancer staging is surgical, being performed according to the International Federation of Gynecology and Obstetrics (FIGO) criteria [22]. CT or magnetic resonance imaging scans, although of limited impact for OC early diagnosis, allow to establish a surgery plan and to determine tumor irresectability criteria for 70–90% of all patients. The ability to detect peritoneal implants in both exams depends upon their location, size, and the presence of ascites. However, CT is the imaging modality of choice for OC staging, since it is indispensable for the preoperative evaluation to optimize maximal cytoreduction surgery or to help in the decision of neoadjuvant chemotherapy.

Ovarian cancer dissemination can occur through all known propagation routes, i.e., lymphatic, hematogenic, transcavitary, and contiguous. The transcavitary course is undoubtedly the most clinically relevant and, in the vast majority of cases, has an impact on the patient prognosis [23, 24]. The dissemination to the peritoneal cavity is an early phenomenon in the natural history of the disease, since the malignant cells follow the peritoneal fluid, flow concerning intra-abdominal pressure variations. Ovarian cells are characterized as anchorage-dependent cells, meaning that they could only survive when adherent to the extracellular matrix or in contact with neighbor cells. However, when OC cells exfoliate into the peritoneal cavity, they can avoid anoikis (apoptosis process triggered by the loss of binding to the extracellular matrix) and survive even when isolated. Cancer cells in this state can survive and disseminate into the peritoneum, depositing accordingly to the passive flow distribution of peritoneal fluid, predominantly into the paracolic gutters, diaphragmatic surfaces, liver capsule, intestine surface, and omentum. The adhesion of malignant cells to the peritoneum precedes the local invasion and the secondary metastasis, namely to the pleural cavity by the transdiaphragmatic pores (Stage IV) [25]. The transcavitary route seems to be related to the OC cells predilection for the abdominal cavity (homing) rather than the deposition in other organs such as liver, lungs, brain, or bone (rarely in these latter two locations). The dissemination by contiguity is also important and of particular interest for organs like fallopian tubes, uterus, contralateral appendix and bladder, rectum, and pouch of Douglas. The iatrogenic route by contiguity, for example, to the abdominal wall is less frequent. Lymphatic dissemination is frequently observed when the disease is confined to the ovary, being found in almost 15% of FIGO I–II cases [26]. In fact, for a proper FIGO staging, lymphadenectomy is required, and the removal of bulky lymph nodes should be performed to achieve complete macroscopic resection. Although the systematic lymphadenectomy in advanced OC surgical management is still discussed, it has an impact in early disease stages not only to define FIGO staging but also to establish the need for adjuvant treatment, with a significant impact in survival [27, 28]. Blood dissemination is less frequent and usually occurs in advanced disease stages [23, 24].

5. Prognostic factors

A considerable number of clinical-pathological factors have been implicated in OC prognosis. Disease stage, tumor size, histological subtype, differentiation degree, and residual tumor after surgery are considered as the classic prognostic factors. More specifically, the extent of residual disease after surgery is regarded as a major prognostic factor, shown to influence the chemotherapy response and survival [29–33]. Inclusively, a recent meta-analysis has shown that residual tumor is a more powerful prognostic determinant than FIGO stage [31]. The correct histological classification of EOC is also crucial, since it is an independent prognostic factor and provides a guideline for therapeutic management [8, 27]. Performance status (PS) and age are also important factors having an impact on the prognosis and, ultimately, in the decision of medical treatment [27].

Numerous studies have been conducted to assess the clinical significance of molecular alterations in OC. However, so far, the obtained results do not allow a prognostic biomarker to be universally accepted, although the determination of *BRCA* germline mutations has been recently approved as a predictive biomarker for OC. Recently, the development and the application of new genomic technologies have allowed the description of molecular signatures integrated into prognostic and predictive models. In particular, the Cancer Genome Atlas Project (TCGA) has been critical in adding to our knowledge, as it has been used to confirm the importance of *BRCA* genes to serous OC patients survival, as well as being able to help to describe a transcriptional signature with prognostic relevance [34] (this will be investigated further in a separate chapter).

6. Treatment

6.1. First-line treatment

The therapeutic strategy for EOC is based on cytoreductive surgery and staging, followed by adjuvant chemotherapy with the duplet platinum/taxane [8, 20]. As mentioned above, the extent of surgery is a determinant for survival and response to chemotherapy, since these parameters vary significantly depending on the success (optimal or suboptimal) of the surgical procedure [33]. Systemic therapy with cytotoxic agents plays a fundamental role in the treatment of this neoplasia. Chemotherapy is generally recommended in the EOC, including early stages with histopathological criteria of poor prognosis (FIGOIA/IB G3, FIGO IC, FIGO II, or clear cell histology at any stage). However, stage IA or IB G1 or G2 tumor patients, if adequately staged (i.e., with peritoneal washings, assessment of the contralateral ovary and fallopian tube, pelvic and para-aortic node assessment and omentectomy), have a better prognosis and can be treated with surgery alone without the need for adjuvant chemotherapy [35–37] (**Figure 1**).

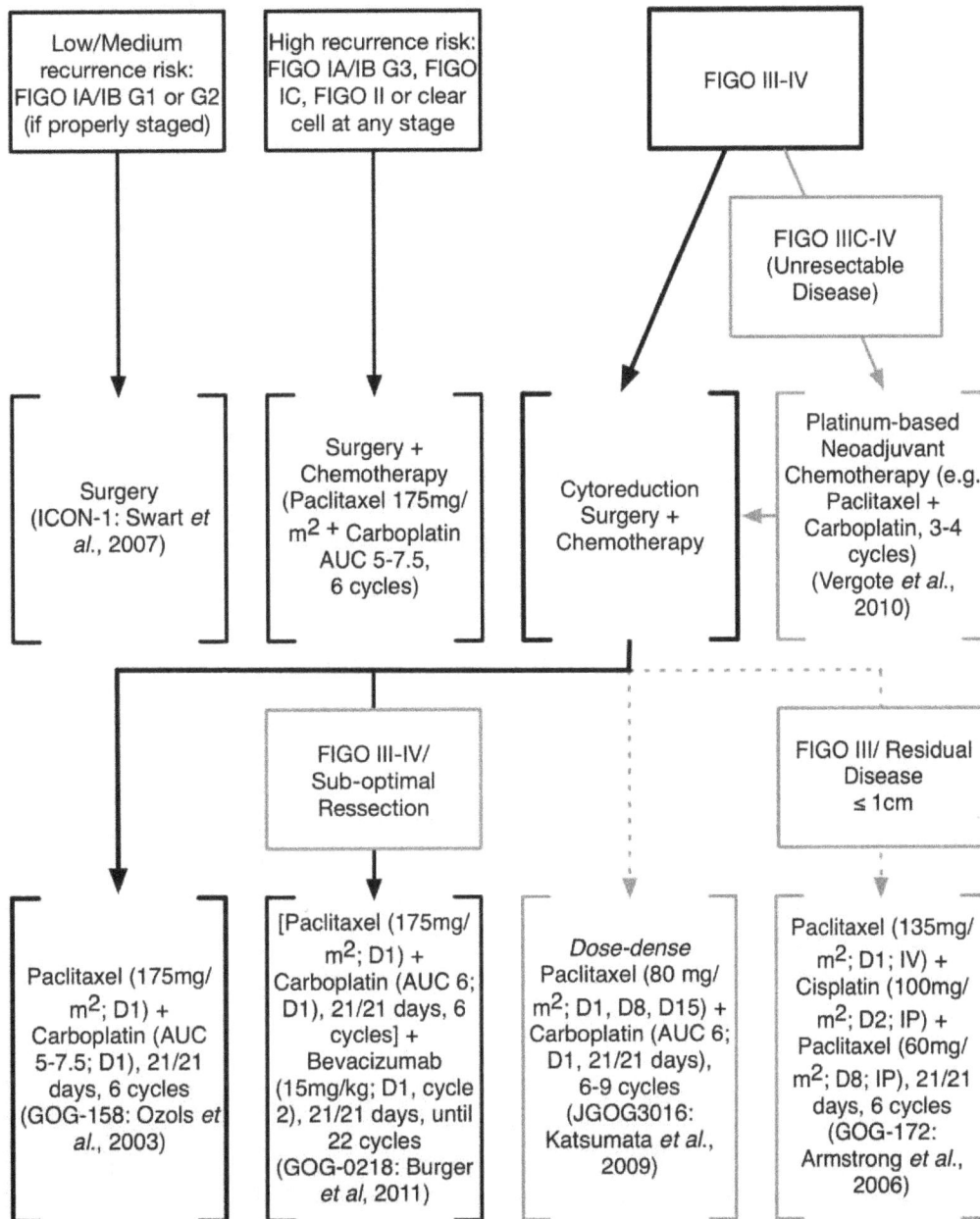

Figure 1. EOC first-line treatment algorithm according to the clinical trial that determines their approval.

The last decades have brought significant advances in the medical treatment of EOC. The association of paclitaxel with platinum has been shown to prolong both progression-free survival (PFS) and overall survival (OAS) of advanced stage patients when compared to the previous nontaxane treatment regimens. Globally, the inclusion of paclitaxel in the adjuvant chemotherapy scheme resulted in a 30% reduction in the risk of death [38–40]. Thus, the intravenous combination of paclitaxel (175 mg/m²) and carboplatin (AUC 5–7.5), every 3 weeks, for six cycles, was established as the standard primary adjuvant chemotherapy for advanced stage disease, after cytoreductive surgery (**Figure 1**) [8, 38, 39, 41–43].

This treatment regimen has been the standard for more than 15 years, and the clinical trials conducted in the last decades for the introduction of a third agent, as in the ICON-5/GOG182 clinical trial, have not shown any improvement in the survival [44]. For patients that develop allergy or toxicity to paclitaxel, namely hypersensitivity or neurotoxicity, the combination of docetaxel/carboplatin or pegylated liposomal doxorubicin (PLD)/carboplatin can be considered as an alternative [42, 45]. The cisplatin/paclitaxel duplet is equally valid but associated with increased toxicity and less convenience in the administration, being currently reserved for patients who have developed hypersensitivity to carboplatin [8, 41].

The inclusion of bevacizumab, an anti-VEGF (Vascular Endothelial Growth Factor) monoclonal antibody, is recommended for advanced OC patients with poor prognostic characteristics (Stage IV or suboptimal resection). This targeted therapy should be administered concomitantly with paclitaxel/carboplatin (after the first cycle) and be maintained after the six cycles of chemotherapy. Regarding the dose and duration of maintenance, the results are not clear, although a similar benefit is obtained with the administration of 7.5 mg/kg and 15 mg/kg for 12 and 15 months, respectively [46, 47]. Although not licensed in the United States of America and not consistently used in Europe, bevacizumab was approved by the European Medicines Agency (EMA) at a dose of 15 mg/kg for 22 cycles (15 months) [8, 46].

To improve the efficacy of the primary treatment, several clinical trials have evaluated the addition of a third cytotoxic agent (such as epirubicin, topotecan, gemcitabine, or PLD) to the first-line regimen, but none have demonstrated a benefit for triplets [8]. In addition, the Japanese JGOG-3016 trial evaluated the impact of a dose-dense therapeutic regimen (paclitaxel, weekly, 80 mg/m^2) on the chemotherapy effectiveness for OC patients. The results were promising for the benefits in PFS and OAS although associated with higher toxicity, especially myelotoxicity. Although it was a trial with potential impact on the clinical practice, because of the pharmacogenetic differences between the Japanese and Caucasian populations, further study was required to confirm these results. The European MITO-7 study did not confirm these findings in Caucasian patients, showing no benefit in the PFS and OAS with the weekly carboplatin (AUC 2) and paclitaxel (60 mg/m^2) regimen [48]. In the absence of new data, paclitaxel dose-dense administration can only be considered as an option [8].

Clinical data demonstrate that, despite the high response rate to the first-line treatment, a significant proportion of OC patients will develop disease recurrence, which in most cases is confined to the abdominal cavity. Based on this particular feature, intraperitoneal chemotherapy administration was associated with an improvement in PFS and OAS in phase III randomized studies (GOG 104, 114 and 172), in combination with intravenous chemotherapy [49, 50]. However, this strategy is not widely used in clinical practice due to its high toxicity [8]. Chemotherapy administered directly in the abdominal cavity might also be performed in the surgical setting using hyperthermal intraperitoneal chemotherapy (HIPEC). The justification for the use of the last therapeutic approach is based on studies that demonstrated that high temperatures help to overcome the resistance to cisplatin, as a result of increased penetration and cellular accumulation of this drug when administrated intraperitoneally in association with hyperthermia [51]. Although it represents a promising strategy, the use of HIPEC remains controversial.

Numerous studies have shown that neoadjuvant chemotherapy is feasible in advanced disease (Stage IIIC–IV), for which the disease is considered unresectable or when optimal primary cytoreduction is not possible due to the disease extension and/or comorbidities that increase the surgical risk [30, 52]. Neoadjuvant chemotherapy is associated with some advantages, including tumor size and disease extension reduction, improvement of optimal cytoreduction rate, less extensive surgery with lower morbidity/mortality, improvement of patients' PS before surgery, and evaluation of tumor chemosensitivity. The chemotherapy scheme to be applied should be based on platinum (often a paclitaxel/carboplatin combination), and it is not recommended to perform more than 3–4 cycles to avoid the emergence of resistant clones [8, 30]. Consequently, the use of primary chemotherapy with interval surgery has become widely accepted, whereas the role of secondary interval debulking surgery after primary surgery (suboptimal cytoreduction and three cycles of chemotherapy) is less clear, as improved survival was reported by the European Organization for Research and Treatment of Cancer (EORTC) trial [32] but not confirmed by the Gynecological Oncology Group (GOG) [53]. Also, the "second look" diagnostic laparoscopy or laparotomy to evaluate the intraperitoneal condition is obsolete and should not be considered an option [8].

6.2. Recurrent disease treatment

The maximal surgery resection strategy combined with adjuvant chemotherapy achieves complete clinical remission in about 75% of EOC patients. However, after 12–18 months, approximately 75% of these patients will develop recurrent disease and be subjected to further treatment. The OC recurrence is defined according to the progression-free interval (PFI) after the end of the initial treatment (**Figure 2**) [8, 21, 41, 54–56].

The prognosis and the likelihood of response to second-line therapy (and subsequent lines) are dependent on the PFI after the last cycle of the previous chemotherapy line. This categorization defines "platinum-refractory," when disease progresses during therapy or within 4 weeks after the last cycle; "platinum-resistant," whose progression occurs within 6 months after platinum therapy completion; "partially platinum-sensitive," for disease which progression occurs between the 6 and 12 months; and "platinum-sensitive," whose progression occurs in a period superior to 12 months [57]. The biological behavior of tumors in these groups is quite variable, with distinct response rates and variable symptoms with different treatment needs. If relapse occurs 6 months after the completion of first-line chemotherapy, a platinum-based regimen should be performed, since the disease is considered platinum sensitive. For patients with platinum-sensitive relapses, there are several therapeutic strategies available which, since this phenomenon can occur repeatedly, allows the selection of different therapeutic combinations [8]. However, the time to subsequent relapse will be progressively shorter until the tumor becomes virtually resistant to these agents [21].

The platinum re-administration is associated with a response rate around 30%, similar to the improvement seen in the PFI. Available treatment options for OC platinum-sensitive relapse are ideally based on the association of platinum with paclitaxel, gemcitabine (with or without bevacizumab), or with PLD [58–62] (**Figure 2**). The therapeutic scheme selection should consider the toxicity profile of each regimen, the residual toxicities of the previous regimens, and the patients' preferences.

First line treatment | 0 | 6M | 12M | 18M

Platinum Refractory	Platinum Resistant	Partially Platinum Sensitive	Platinum Sensitive

Likelihood of response to platinum re-administration

(0%)   (< 10%)   (30%)   (60%)

Recommended treatment

Monoterapy without Platinum		Platinum-based Chemotherapy	
Bevacizumab + [*1] weekly Paclitaxel (AURELIA: Pujade-Lauraine *et al.*, 2014)	Paclitaxel (21/21 dias)	Carboplatin + Paclitaxel (ICON 4/AGO-OVAR 22: Parmar *et al.*, 2003)	Cisplatin + Gemcitabine (Rose *et al.*, 2003)
Bevacizumab + [*1] Pegylated Lipossomal Doxorubicin (AURELIA: Pujade-Lauraine *et al.*, 2014)	Paclitaxel (Regime *dose-sense*) (Markman *et al.*, 2006)	Carboplatin + Docetaxel (Kushner *et al.*, 2007; Strauss *et al.*, 2007)	Carboplatin + Gemcitabine (AGO-OVAR 2.5: Pfisterer *et al.*, 2006)
Bevacizumab + [*1] Topotecan (AURELIA: Pujade-Lauraine *et al.*, 2014)	Docetaxel (Rose *et al.*, 2003)	Carboplatin + Pegylated Lipossomal Doxorubicin (CALYPSO: Pujade-Lauraine *et al.*, 2010)	Carboplatin + [*3] Gemcitabine + Bevacizumab (OCEANS:Aghajanian *et al.*,2012)
Topotecan (Markman *et al.*, 2004; Gordon *et al.*, 2004; Sehouli *et al.*, 2011)	Etoposide (Rose *et al.*, 1998)	Olaparib [*2] (Lederman *et al.*, 2014)	Clinical Trial
Gemcitabine (Mutch *et al.*, 2007; Fernandina *et al.*, 2008)	Pegylated Lipossomal Doxorubicin (Mutch *et al.*, 2007; Ferrandina *et al.*, 2008)		
Clinical Trial			

Other Potentially Active Drugs	Partially Platinum-sensitive

- Hormonotherapy:
  Megestrol Acetate
  Tamoxifen (Markman *et al.*, 1996)
  Aromatase Inhibitors
- Ciclophosphamide
- Vinorelbine
- Capecitabine (Wolf *et al.*, 2006)
- Melphalan
- Irinotecan
- Ifosfamide (Markman *et al.*, 1992)
- Altretamine (Alberts *et al.*, 2004)
- Nab-Paclitaxel (Tenerielo *et al.*, 2009)
- Pemetrexed (Miller *et al.*, 2009)
- Oxaliplatin
- Hyperthermic Intraperitonial Chemotherapy (HIPEC)
- Radiotherapy (Palliative)
- Clinical Trial
	Trabectidine + Pegylated Lipossomal Doxorubicin (OVA 301: Monk *et al.*, 2008)
	
	Clinical Trial

[*1] Patients previously submitted up to two therapeutical lines
[*2] *BRCA* germline mutated patients
[*3] Patients not previously submitted to Bevacizumab

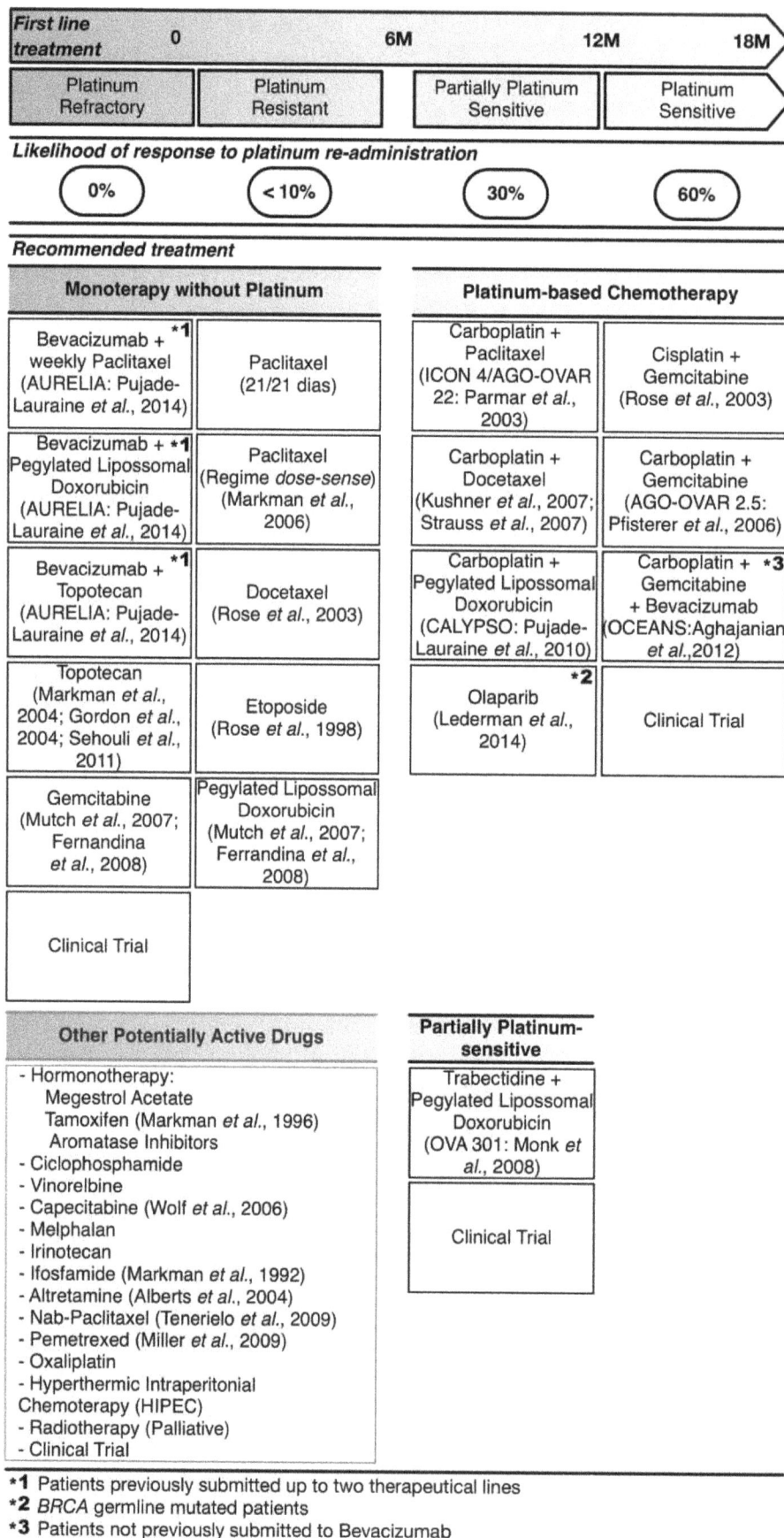

Figure 2. EOC recurrence treatment algorithm based on platinum-free interval, according to the clinical trial that determines its approval.

The administration of bevacizumab in combination with carboplatin/gemcitabine, followed by maintenance until progression or toxicity, was approved by EMA as the first-line treatment for platinum-sensitive relapse (for bevacizumab-naïve patients), being associated with an improvement in PFS despite no impact on OAS [8, 63]. In December 2016, US Food and Drug Administration (FDA) also approved bevacizumab administration to platinum-sensitive recurrent patients, either in combination with carboplatin/paclitaxel or carboplatin/gemcitabine, followed by bevacizumab alone.

Patients with PFI between 6 and 12 months, considered as partially sensitive, also benefit from platinum-based second-line therapy, although with a lower therapeutic effect (**Figure 2**). For these patients, the administration of trabectedin associated with PLD might also be an option, according to the results of the OVA301 trial, probably by restoring platinum sensitivity due to the artificial prolongation of the platinum-free interval [8, 64].

For relapses linked to a disease-free interval less than 6 months, the tumor is defined as platinum resistant and another treatment strategy should be instituted, with monotherapy regimens being recommended [8, 40, 65]. The treatment of platinum-resistant/refractory patients is mostly directed toward improvement in the quality of life and symptom control, as these patients are usually associated with a reduced prognosis with a reduced OAS (generally less than 12 months) [8]. Surgery as a therapeutic alternative in these cases might be considered only in need of symptom palliation. Monotherapy regimens with paclitaxel (preferably weekly), PLD, gemcitabine, and topotecan, among others, have shown similar response rates (not exceeding 15%) and PFS between 3 and 4 months [8, 66–73]. Thus, the choice for one of these agents should be based on previously performed therapies, toxicity profiles, administration convenience, cost, and patient opinion. Combination therapy regimens did not significantly improve response rates or survival for platinum-resistant disease, when compared to monotherapy regimens, even when considering toxicity [8, 40].

Recently, promising results have been achieved with biological maintenance treatments, in particular with anti-angiogenic agents (bevacizumab, pazopanib, and trebananib) and PARP (poly(ADP-ribose) polymerase) inhibitors (olaparib, niraparib, and rucaparib) [74]. Bevacizumab was the first antiangiogenic agent to demonstrate clinical benefit in platinum sensitive and resistant relapse, concomitantly with chemotherapy and as maintenance therapy. As previously mentioned, according to the results published in the OCEANS trial, EMA approved the combination of bevacizumab with carboplatin/gemcitabine for patients with platinum-sensitive OC relapse, if there was no previous exposure to this antiangiogenic drug [63]. According to the AURELIA results, the addition of bevacizumab to the chemotherapy (weekly paclitaxel, PLD or topotecan) in patients with platinum-resistant OC (previously treated with up to two therapeutic lines) has been shown to be associated with an improvement in PFS, response rates, and quality of life, although without impact on OAS [75]. Therefore, this regimen could be an alternative in this subgroup until the development of toxicity or progression (**Figure 2**).

In addition to bevacizumab, olaparib is also considered as a target therapy option in OC recurrence. This drug was the first PARP inhibitor to be authorized by EMA as maintenance treatment of BRCA-mutated patients, with partial or complete responses to platinum-based chemotherapy. The results have shown almost a 7-month extension in PFS for patients with

BRCA mutations exposed to Olaparib (11.2 versus 4.3 months; HR, 0.18), although the impact on OAS was not observed [76]. Response rates to this drug correlate with the platinum-free interval, being 69.2, 45.8 and 23.1% for the sensitive, resistant, and platinum-refractory disease, respectively [77]. Furthermore, olaparib administration allows for a time extension for a subsequent therapy which suggests that its administration did not adversely affect the treatment recurrence.

With the existence of several treatment alternatives that allow for sequential approaches and the emergence of new targeted therapies, most of which are well tolerated, it is possible to administrate extended therapeutic regimens concomitantly with significant symptomatic control and a positive impact in the quality of life.

6.3. Emergent therapeutic approaches

The duplet platinum/taxane is considered the standard first-line therapy for advanced OC treatment. Nevertheless, chemotherapy response rates remain disappointing, and the introduction of newer treatment strategies at recurrence is essential to increase the long-term survival. The recent adoption of molecular therapies targeting the inhibition of angiogenesis and DNA repair is a step forward in the OC medical treatment, aiming to delay disease progression and the re-treatment with chemotherapy [33]. The encouraging study results with bevacizumab, in first-line treatment and both platinum sensitive and resistant recurrence, illustrate the importance of angiogenesis inhibition in the success of OC treatment [46, 63, 75].

PARP is an enzyme involved in the response to DNA single-strand breaks, and so it was initially suggested that its inhibition could be used to enhance the effects of chemotherapy [78]. However, the finding that the survival of tumor cells carrying *BRCA* homozygous deletions is significantly lower with the administration of PARP inhibitors prompted the development of a new therapeutic strategy for OC [79, 80]. The molecular rationale for this association is based on the fact that cells with BRCA defective proteins are not able to repair DNA double-strand breaks by homologous recombination (HR), depending on other pathways to repair the damage, namely the base excision repair (BER) pathway, in which PARP is involved. In the BER pathway, PARP is responsible to detect single-strand breaks and to activate effector proteins to repair the damage. Thus, homologous recombination deficiencies (HRD), as in the presence of *BRCA* mutations, in concomitance with PARP inhibition lead to cell death due to the excessive accumulation of unrepaired damage. This phenomenon is designated as synthetic lethality and occurs when two nonlethal defects are combined to culminate in cell death. This strategy is also of benefit in that toxicity is reduced for normal tissues, as nontumor cells can repair DNA by the HR pathway [80, 81].

As molecular and genetic knowledge of OC is increasing, studies with PARP inhibitors are indicating that more patients with OC may benefit. According to data published by the TCGA project, the presence of *BRCA* mutations is identified in about 20% of high-grade serous ovarian cancer (HGSOC), and about 50% of these tumors have a positive HRD phenotype, even in the absence of a familial history of breast/ovarian cancer [34, 78]. In addition to the excellent results obtained with olaparib for the subgroup of patients with *BRCA* mutations, the study published by Ledermann et al. also demonstrated that PARP inhibition is also useful for *BRCA* wild-type patients, although to a less extent [76].

The promising results achieved with olaparib encouraged the development of new PARP inhibitors, including niraparib and rucaparib [82, 83]. Maintenance clinical trials ongoing with both agents include *BRCA* wild-type patients to test the effect of PARP inhibitors in this major group, incorporating additional molecular tests for HDR. Namely, for patients with platinum-sensitive recurrence, the PFS mean duration is significantly higher for patients receiving niraparib when compared to placebo, regardless of the presence/absence of *BRCA* germline mutations or HRD status [83]. Thus, clinical trials are being developed to evaluate not only the impact of PARP inhibitors on limiting recurrence, as in the SOLO2 trial [84], but also as a maintenance strategy for first-line treatment, as in SOLO1 [85]. In addition, the GOG3005 trial evaluates the addition of the PARP inhibitor veliparib to first-line therapy (carboplatin/paclitaxel), as well as its role in subsequent maintenance [78].

A possible synergy between PARP inhibitors and other pathways inhibitors, such as anti-angiogenic, has also been hypothesized. In fact, preclinical studies have demonstrated an additive effect on the association of inhibitors of these two pathways, since hypoxia leads to a decreased expression of DNA repair proteins, thereby increasing the sensitivity for PARP inhibitors [86, 87]. Thus, a recent phase I clinical trial, which combined a tyrosine kinase inhibitor of VEGF receptor, cediranib, with olaparib, achieved an objective response rate of 44% in recurrent disease [88]. The results of this study prompted the development of a randomized phase II trial, demonstrating an improvement in PFS and in the objective response rate for the cediranib/olaparib combination when compared to olaparib alone (17.7 versus 9.0 months; HR, 0.42; 95% CI, 0.23–0.76; $P = 0.005$ and 79.6% versus 47.8%; OR, 4.24; 95% CI, 1.53–12.22; $P = 0.002$) in patients with platinum-sensitive recurrence [89]. Although the results must be interpreted carefully, due to the low number of recruited patients, they are of high interest as it suggests a synergistic action for the combined use of angiogenesis/DNA repair inhibitors. Thus, numerous clinical trials exploring these pathways are under development, either isolated or in combination, for first-line therapy or maintenance, with the prospect of increasing the treatment opportunities for OC patients.

6.4. Monitoring treatment response

The treatment response evaluation in OC is based on CT, following RECIST criteria, complemented by the CA125 serum measurement following Gynecologic Cancer InterGroup (GCIG) criteria [90]. In fact, despite the limitations as a diagnostic biomarker, CA125 is a good predictor of relapse as it proved to be a useful biomarker for monitoring treatment response in more than 80% of OC patients [91]. Normalization of CA125 serum levels following first-line therapy does have clinical implications, especially when considering maintenance treatment in OC. However, even the systemic therapy in early recurrence stages had the potential to improve survival, studies have demonstrated that the premature treatment in asymptomatic patients with single elevation of CA125 levels (without clinical or radiological evidence) had no positive impact [92].

In Medical Oncology clinical practice, high heterogeneity in the response and toxicity to cytotoxic agents are observed. There are subgroups of patients who, despite being at an early disease stage, have a higher risk of tumor progression. In these cases, surgery and classic prognostic factors do not allow to predict the biological behavior of these tumors correctly. In the current era of individualized therapy, and according to the OC heterogeneity, biomarkers need to be developed to identify patients at an early disease stage but with the potential to progress and disseminate [93].

6.5. Predictive factors

Several biomarkers are considered to have prognostic relevance, independent of the therapeutic approach. In OC, as previously mentioned, FIGO staging, histological subtype, or the extent of residual disease are considered as key prognostic factors. The identification and characterization of predictive biomarkers for OC have proven to be a challenge, and none of the molecular determinants that underlie platinum-sensitivity/resistant phenotypes have reached the clinical setting [91].

Additionally, the inability to select those patients that will benefit from bevacizumab to maximize survival and minimize toxicity and costs complicates treatment planning. Several studies have been performed to unravel the role of the VEGF signaling pathway and the key drivers of response to antiangiogenic agents in OC. VEGF serum levels are thought to be representative of the VEGF-mediated OC angiogenesis, but the results were not systematically concordant [94]. Also, VEGFR-2 plasma levels were not predictive for patients treated with bevacizumab in the GOG-218 trial [95]. Translational research conducted within the ICON7 trial identified three candidate biomarkers (mesothelin, VEGFR-3, and alpha-1-acid glycoprotein) for patients treated concomitantly with this antiangiogenic agent and first-line chemotherapy. Each of these biomarkers was considered as an independent factor and, in combination with CA125 measurement, was included in a predictive nomogram for bevacizumab [96]. However, though several promising candidate angiogenesis biomarkers for OC were identified, it was neither possible to achieve meaningful results for their use in routine clinical practice nor possible to select patients for this targeted therapy [97, 98].

Failure to improve the therapeutic strategies in OC has resulted in studies focusing on genomic features, such as the TCGA project. This project aims to determine the impact of OC genomic and epigenomic changes and, thus, to identify molecular markers influencing clinical outcome and possible therapeutic targets for OC. One of the most interesting findings obtained from this study is the presence of HRD in about 50% of HGSOC, which could represent a patient subgroup which could benefit from PARP inhibitor treatment [34]. In fact, the presence of BRCA mutations and an HRD positive phenotype is both positive predictive factors for PARP inhibition, thus indicating personalized OC therapy defined by a genetic biomarker [76, 83]. The impact of BRCA mutations as predictive biomarkers has been published for other agents such as PLD and trabectedin [99, 100]. The implications of these advances are still being investigated, and as a result, genetic testing for BRCA mutations should be offered for all patients with nonmucinous tumors, regardless of age or familial history. The test should be performed at diagnosis, as it provides information on the likelihood of response to chemotherapy and can then be systematically incorporated into clinical practice to promote an individualized therapeutic strategy [33]. The TCGA project also provided the opportunity to identify four OC subtypes based on the expression of marker genes (differentiated, immunoreactive, mesenchymal, and proliferative), and several retrospective subanalyses have already demonstrated that is possible to correlate distinct outcomes between the subgroups [101, 102].

Based on the TCGA data, other studies have also proposed molecular signatures, namely the prognostic model "Classification of Ovarian Cancer" (CLOVAR), for which 23 genes involved in the platinum-induced DNA damage repair are predictive of treatment response among HGSOC patients [103]. Recently, the ARIEL2 clinical trial showed that the combination of *BRCA* mutational status with the degree of genome-wide loss of heterozygosity (LOH) in the tumor could predict the rucaparib treatment response. *BRCA*-mutated patients (germline or somatic) or *BRCA* wild-type with high LOH had longer PFS and clinical response to rucaparib, when compared with *BRCA* wild-type and low LOH patients [104].

The concept of *BRCA*ness must be promptly clarified, as the associated phenotypes define a clinical subpopulation of EOC patients with common characteristics. These include high response rates to both first-line platinum-based treatment and to relapse therapies (including platinum based), long treatment-free intervals (even in recurrent disease), and improved OAS and include mainly serous tumors. The HRD phenotype (somatic or germline) might be complemented with other molecular defects, beyond *BRCA* deficiencies, which lead to an analogous clinical profile and be targeted for PARP inhibition [34, 105]. Commercial tests are already available, and multiple clinical trials (as ARIEL3 and NOVA) are ongoing to investigate PARP inhibition in *BRCA* wild-type patients and to identify a putative predictive signature.

7. Pharmacogenomics for future predictive marker definition

Although *BRCA*ness signature definition can provide valuable information regarding the magnitude of the benefit of targeted therapy, these biomarkers may not be unique for the determination of the likelihood of treatment sensitivity/resistance. To date, besides *BRCA* mutations and HRD status, platinum sensitivity remains the best biomarker of PARP inhibitor response. Platinum sensitivity correlates with HRD, and platinum-sensitive tumors are more responsive to PARP inhibitors than platinum-resistant tumors, whatever the genetic background [33, 78]. Therefore, perhaps the PARP inhibitors administration should be offered to all OC patients that respond to platinum-based treatment.

Platinum-based compounds are among the most active and used cytotoxic agents in the clinical practice. They exert their biological effect by acting as alkylating agents by the ability to covalently bind to DNA, leading to the formation of intrastrand and interstrand DNA adducts that promote cell-cycle arrest and tumor cell apoptosis. The mechanisms underlying the development of chemoresistant phenotypes in OC are not fully recognized. Interindividual variation in platinum-drug response might be a major determinant for OC. This is suggested from the wide variability in the PFI and its direct association with a platinum response, as well as the finding that intrinsic resistance to these compounds, occur in up to a fifth of OC patients [106–109]. Mechanisms involved in platinum resistance are likely to be multifactorial although seems to be greatly determined by the platinum detoxification pathway and DNA damage repair ability [54, 108, 110–113].

While platinum therapy is prescribed to achieve a target exposure based on renal function, the dose of taxanes is based on body surface area. Taxanes are microtubule-stabilizing drugs, inducing cell cycle arrest and activating proapoptotic signaling. The cellular toxicity to taxanes is controlled by the action of multiple mediators, namely those involved in transport (i.e., ABCB1, ABCC1, and ABCC2), metabolism, and metabolism-associated proteins (cytochrome P450s and nuclear receptors), as well as pharmacodynamics (i.e., TP53 and CDKN1A), which appear to play a role in taxane efficacy [54, 108, 114–116]. However, to date, no reliable biomarker or signature exists to predict the sensitivity or resistance to paclitaxel. Although the duplet platinum/taxane is associated with better outcome, rather than platinum alone, the results of the GOG132 trial showed that only 42% of patients are likely to benefit from paclitaxel administration [117], and thus, further study into the mechanisms of resistance is needed.

8. Conclusion

Achieving an individualized therapeutic strategy will only be possible through the identification of feasible, validated, and reproducible biomarkers in the clinical practice that will allow the prediction of the likelihood of response to a given treatment. Biomarker validation is crucial, both in respect of predictive ability and sensitivity/specificity, and should be stated previously in the definition of treatment subgroups [106, 107, 118, 119].

Research in OC treatment evolution and improvement needs to focus on the identification of interindividual determinants, which is often associated with genetic polymorphisms to identify potential biomarkers and/or treatment targets. Circulating tumor cells or tumor nanovesicles (as exosomes) may help to identify the molecular targets. Consequently, the incorporation of molecular and genetic information into integrated clinical models may be a potential approach in order to define predictive nomograms. Pharmacogenomics will be important in clinical practice to improve efficacy, reduce toxicity, and predict nonresponders to several therapies, thus allowing for individualized treatment strategies.

Author details

Joana Assis[1,2], Deolinda Pereira[3,4], Augusto Nogueira[1,2] and Rui Medeiros[1,5,6*]

*Address all correspondence to: ruimedei@ipoporto.min-saude.pt

1 Molecular Oncology and Viral Pathology Group-Research Center, Portuguese Institute of Oncology, Porto, Portugal

2 FMUP, Faculty of Medicine, Porto University, Porto, Portugal

3 Oncology Department, Portuguese Institute of Oncology, Porto, Portugal

4 ICBAS, Abel Salazar Institute for the Biomedical Sciences, Porto, Portugal

5 Research Department, Portuguese League Against Cancer (NRNorte), Porto, Portugal

6 CEBIMED, Faculty of Health Sciences, Fernando Pessoa University, Porto, Portugal

References

[1] Ferlay J, Soerjomataram I, Dikshit R, Eser S, et al. Cancer incidence and mortality worldwide: Sources, methods and major patterns in GLOBOCAN 2012. International Journal of Cancer. 2015;**136**(5):E359-E386. DOI: 10.1002/ijc.29210

[2] Kurman R, Carcangiu M, Herrington C, Young R. WHO Classification of Tumors of Female Reproductive Organs, WHO Classification of Tumors. 4th ed. Vol. 6. Lyon (France): World Health Organization; 2014

[3] Ferlay J, Steliarova-Foucher E, Lortet-Tieulent J, Rosso S, et al. Cancer incidence and mortality patterns in Europe: Estimates for 40 countries in 2012. European Journal of Cancer. 2013;**49**(6):1374-1403. DOI: 10.1016/j.ejca.2012.12.027

[4] Ferlay J, Soerjomataram I, Ervik M, Dikshit R. et al. GLOBOCAN 2012 v1.0, Cancer Incidence and Mortality Worldwide: IARC CancerBase No.11 [Internet]. 2013. Available from: http://globocan.iarc.fr

[5] Jelovac D, Armstrong DK. Recent progress in the diagnosis and treatment of ovarian cancer. CA: A Cancer Journal for Clinicians. 2011;**61**(3):183-203. DOI: 10.3322/caac.20113

[6] Hennessy BT, Coleman RL, Markman M. Ovarian cancer. Lancet. 2009;**374**(9698):1371-1382. DOI: 10.1016/S0140-6736(09)61338-6

[7] Bast RC Jr, Hennessy B, Mills GB. The biology of ovarian cancer: New opportunities for translation. Nature Reviews. Cancer. 2009;**9**(6):415-428. DOI: 10.1038/nrc2644

[8] Ledermann JA, Raja FA, Fotopoulou C, Gonzalez-Martin A, et al. Newly diagnosed and relapsed epithelial ovarian carcinoma: ESMO Clinical Practice Guidelines for diagnosis, treatment and follow-up. Annals of Oncology. 2013;**24**(Suppl 6):vi24-vi32. DOI: 10.1093/annonc/mdt333

[9] Folkins AK, Longacre TA. Hereditary gynaecological malignancies: Advances in screening and treatment. Histopathology. 2013;**62**(1):2-30. DOI: 10.1111/his.12028

[10] Romero I, López-Guerrero J, Poveda A. Molecular genetics in epithelial ovarian cancer. In: Poveda A, editor. 100 Key Questions on Ovarian Cancer. Permanyer; 2015

[11] Schuler S, Ponnath M, Engel J, Ortmann O. Ovarian epithelial tumors and reproductive factors: A systematic review. Archives of Gynecology and Obstetrics. 2013;**287**(6):1187-1204. DOI: 10.1007/s00404-013-2784-1

[12] Temkin S, Minassian L, Kohn E. Early diagnosis. In: Poveda A, editor. 100 Key Questions on Ovarian Cancer. Barcelona (Spain): Permanyer; 2015

[13] Fleming G, Seidman J, Lengyel E. Epithelial Ovarian Cancer. In: Barakat R, Berchuck A, Markman M, editors. Principles and Practice of Gynecologic Oncology. Philadelphia: Lippincott Williams & Wilkins; 2013. pp. 757-847

[14] Morch LS, Lokkegaard E, Andreasen AH, Kruger-Kjaer S, et al. Hormone therapy and ovarian cancer. JAMA. 2009;**302**(3):298-305. DOI: 10.1001/jama.2009.1052

[15] Forstner R, Sala E, Kinkel K, Spencer JA, et al. ESUR guidelines: Ovarian cancer staging and follow-up. European Radiology. 2010;**20**(12):2773-2780. DOI: 10.1007/s00330-010-1886-4

[16] Deffieux X, Castaigne D, Pomel C. Role of laparoscopy to evaluate candidates for complete cytoreduction in advanced stages of epithelial ovarian cancer. International Journal of Gynecological Cancer. 2006;**16**(Suppl 1):35-40. DOI: 10.1111/j.1525-1438.2006.00323.x

[17] Cannistra SA. Cancer of the ovary. The New England Journal of Medicine. 2004;**351**(24): 2519-2529. DOI: 10.1056/NEJMra041842

[18] Jemal A, Siegel R, Ward E, Hao Y, et al. Cancer statistics, 2009. CA: A Cancer Journal for Clinicians. 2009;**59**(4):225-249. DOI: 10.3322/caac.20006

[19] Levanon K, Crum C, Drapkin R. New insights into the pathogenesis of serous ovarian cancer and its clinical impact. Journal of Clinical Oncology. 2008;**26**(32):5284-5293. DOI: 10.1200/JCO.2008.18.1107

[20] Jayson GC, Kohn EC, Kitchener HC, Ledermann JA. Ovarian cancer. Lancet. 2014; **384**(9951):1376-1388. DOI: 10.1016/S0140-6736(13)62146-7

[21] Romero I, Bast RC Jr. Minireview: Human ovarian cancer: Biology, current management, and paths to personalizing therapy. Endocrinology. 2012;**153**(4):1593-1602. DOI: 10.1210/en.2011-2123

[22] Prat J, FCoG. Oncology: Staging classification for cancer of the ovary, fallopian tube, and peritoneum. International Journal of Gynaecology and Obstetrics. 2014;**124**(1):1-5. DOI: 10.1016/j.ijgo.2013.10.001

[23] Halkia E, Spiliotis J, Sugarbaker P. Diagnosis and management of peritoneal metastases from ovarian cancer. Gastroenterology Research and Practice. 2012;**2012**:541842. DOI: 10.1155/2012/541842

[24] Lengyel E. Ovarian cancer development and metastasis. The American Journal of Pathology. 2010;**177**(3):1053-1064. DOI: 10.2353/ajpath.2010.100105

[25] Naora H, Montell DJ. Ovarian cancer metastasis: Integrating insights from disparate model organisms. Nature Reviews. Cancer. 2005;**5**(5):355-366. DOI: 10.1038/nrc1611

[26] Kleppe M, Wang T, Van Gorp T, Slangen BF, et al. Lymph node metastasis in stages I and II ovarian cancer: A review. Gynecologic Oncology. 2011;**123**(3):610-614. DOI: 10.1016/j. ygyno.2011.09.013

[27] McLachlan J, Gore M. Prognostic factors in epithelial ovarian cancer. In: Poveda A, editor. 100 Key Questions on Ovarian Cancer. Barcelona (Spain): Permanyer; 2015

[28] Chan JK, Munro EG, Cheung MK, Husain A, et al. Association of lymphadenectomy and survival in stage I ovarian cancer patients. Obstetrics and Gynecology. 2007;**109**(1):12-19. DOI: 10.1097/01.AOG.0000249610.95885.ef

[29] Bristow RE, Tomacruz RS, Armstrong DK, Trimble EL, et al. Survival effect of maximal cytoreductive surgery for advanced ovarian carcinoma during the platinum era: A meta-analysis. Journal of Clinical Oncology. 2002;**20**(5):1248-1259. DOI: 10.1200/JCO. 2002.20.5.1248

[30] Vergote I, Trope CG, Amant F, Kristensen GB, et al. Neoadjuvant chemotherapy or primary surgery in stage IIIC or IV ovarian cancer. The New England Journal of Medicine. 2010;**363**(10):943-953. DOI: 10.1056/NEJMoa0908806

[31] du Bois A, Reuss A, Pujade-Lauraine E, Harter P, et al. Role of surgical outcome as prognostic factor in advanced epithelial ovarian cancer: A combined exploratory analysis of 3 prospectively randomized phase 3 multicenter trials: By the Arbeitsgemeinschaft Gynaekologische Onkologie Studiengruppe Ovarialkarzinom (AGO-OVAR) and the Groupe d'Investigateurs Nationaux Pour les Etudes des Cancers de l'Ovaire (GINECO). Cancer. 2009;**115**(6):1234-1244. DOI: 10.1002/cncr.24149

[32] van der Burg ME, van Lent M, Buyse M, Kobierska A, et al. The effect of debulking surgery after induction chemotherapy on the prognosis in advanced epithelial ovarian cancer. Gynecological Cancer Cooperative Group of the European Organization for Research and Treatment of Cancer. The New England Journal of Medicine. 1995;**332**(10):629-634. DOI: 10.1056/NEJM199503093321002

[33] Poveda A, Romero I. Advanced ovarian cancer: 20 years of ovarian cancer treatment. Annals of Oncology. 2016;**27**(Suppl 1):i72-i73. DOI: 10.1093/annonc/mdw081

[34] Cancer Genome Atlas Research, N. Integrated genomic wild of ovarian carcinoma. Nature. 2011;**474**(7353):609-615. DOI: 10.1038/nature10166

[35] Swart A, oboI Collaborators.Long-term follow-up of women enrolled in a randomized trial of adjuvant chemotherapy for early stage ovarian cancer (ICON1). In: American Society of Clinical Oncology Annual Meeting. 2007

[36] Colombo N, Guthrie D, Chiari S, Parmar M, et al. International collaborative ovarian neoplasm trial 1: A randomized trial of adjuvant chemotherapy in women with early-stage ovarian cancer. Journal of the National Cancer Institute. 2003;**95**(2):125-132

[37] Trimbos JB, Vergote I, Bolis G, Vermorken JB, et al. Impact of adjuvant chemotherapy and surgical staging in early-stage ovarian carcinoma: European Organisation for Research and Treatment of Cancer-adjuvant ChemoTherapy in Ovarian Neoplasm trial. Journal of the National Cancer Institute. 2003;**95**(2):113-125

[38] McGuire WP, Hoskins WJ, Brady MF, Kucera PR, et al. Cyclophosphamide and cisplatin compared with paclitaxel and cisplatin in patients with stage III and stage IV ovarian cancer. The New England Journal of Medicine. 1996;**334**(1):1-6. DOI: 10.1056/ NEJM199601043340101

[39] Piccart MJ, Bertelsen K, James K, Cassidy J, et al. Randomized intergroup trial of cisplatin-paclitaxel versus cisplatin-cyclophosphamide in women with advanced epithelial ovarian cancer: Three-year results. Journal of the National Cancer Institute. 2000;92(9): 699-708

[40] Pignata S, Cecere S, Pujade-Lauraine E. Treatment of advanced disease. In: Poveda A, editor. 100 Key Questions on Ovarian Cancer. Barcelona (Spain): Permanyer; 2015

[41] Ozols RF, Bundy BN, Greer BE, Fowler JM, et al. Phase III trial of carboplatin and paclitaxel compared with cisplatin and paclitaxel in patients with optimally resected stage III ovarian cancer: A Gynecologic Oncology Group study. Journal of Clinical Oncology. 2003;21(17):3194-3200. DOI: 10.1200/JCO.2003.02.153

[42] Vasey PA, Jayson GC, Gordon A, Gabra H, et al. Phase III randomized trial of docetaxel-carboplatin versus paclitaxel-carboplatin as first-line chemotherapy for ovarian carcinoma. Journal of the National Cancer Institute. 2004;96(22):1682-1691. DOI: 10.1093/jnci/djh323

[43] Neijt JP, Engelholm SA, Tuxen MK, Sorensen PG, et al. Exploratory phase III study of paclitaxel and cisplatin versus paclitaxel and carboplatin in advanced ovarian cancer. Journal of Clinical Oncology. 2000;18(17):3084-3092. DOI: 10.1200/JCO.2000.18.17.3084

[44] Bookman MA, Brady MF, McGuire WP, Harper PG, et al. Evaluation of new platinum-based treatment regimens in advanced-stage ovarian cancer: A Phase III Trial of the Gynecologic Cancer Intergroup. Journal of Clinical Oncology. 2009;27(9):1419-1425. DOI: 10.1200/JCO.2008.19.1684

[45] Pignata S, Scambia G, Ferrandina G, Savarese A, et al. Carboplatin plus paclitaxel versus carboplatin plus pegylated liposomal doxorubicin as first-line treatment for patients with ovarian cancer: The MITO-2 randomized phase III trial. Journal of Clinical Oncology. 2011;29(27):3628-3635. DOI: 10.1200/JCO.2010.33.8566

[46] Burger RA, Brady MF, Bookman MA, Fleming GF, et al. Incorporation of bevacizumab in the primary treatment of ovarian cancer. The New England Journal of Medicine. 2011;365(26):2473-2483. DOI: 10.1056/NEJMoa1104390

[47] Perren TJ, Swart AM, Pfisterer J, Ledermann JA, et al. A phase 3 trial of bevacizumab in ovarian cancer. The New England Journal of Medicine. 2011;365(26):2484-2496. DOI: 10.1056/NEJMoa1103799

[48] van der Burg ME, Onstenk W, Boere IA, Look M, et al. Long-term results of a randomised phase III trial of weekly versus three-weekly paclitaxel/platinum induction therapy followed by standard or extended three-weekly paclitaxel/platinum in European patients with advanced epithelial ovarian cancer. European Journal of Cancer. 2014;50(15):2592-2601. DOI: 10.1016/j.ejca.2014.07.015

[49] Armstrong DK, Bundy B, Wenzel L, Huang HQ, et al. Intraperitoneal cisplatin and paclitaxel in ovarian cancer. The New England Journal of Medicine. 2006;354(1):34-43. DOI: 10.1056/NEJMoa052985

[50] Hess LM, Benham-Hutchins M, Herzog TJ, Hsu CH, et al. A meta-analysis of the efficacy of intraperitoneal cisplatin for the front-line treatment of ovarian cancer. International Journal of Gynecological Cancer. 2007;**17**(3):561-570. DOI: 10.1111/j.1525-1438.2006.00846.x

[51] Chiva LM, Gonzalez-Martin A. A critical appraisal of hyperthermic intraperitoneal chemotherapy (HIPEC) in the treatment of advanced and recurrent ovarian cancer. Gynecologic Oncology. 2015;**136**(1):130-135. DOI: 10.1016/j.ygyno.2014.11.072

[52] Kehoe S, Hook J, Nankivell M, Jayson GC, et al. Primary chemotherapy versus primary surgery for newly diagnosed advanced ovarian cancer (CHORUS): An open-label, randomised, controlled, non-inferiority trial. Lancet. 2015;**386**(9990):249-257. DOI: 10.1016/S0140-6736(14)62223-6

[53] Rose PG, Nerenstone S, Brady MF, Clarke-Pearson D, et al. Secondary surgical cytoreduction for advanced ovarian carcinoma. The New England Journal of Medicine. 2004;**351**(24):2489-2497. DOI: 10.1056/NEJMoa041125

[54] Agarwal R, Kaye SB. Ovarian cancer: Strategies for overcoming resistance to chemotherapy. Nature Reviews. Cancer. 2003;**3**(7):502-516. DOI: 10.1038/nrc1123

[55] Sandercock J, Parmar MK, Torri V, Qian W. First-line treatment for advanced ovarian cancer: Paclitaxel, platinum and the evidence. British Journal of Cancer. 2002;**87**(8):815-824. DOI: 10.1038/sj.bjc.6600567

[56] Greenlee RT, Hill-Harmon MB, Murray T, Thun M. Cancer statistics, 2001. CA: A Cancer Journal for Clinicians. 2001;**51**(1):15-36

[57] Friedlander M, Trimble E, Tinker A, Alberts D, et al. Clinical trials in recurrent ovarian cancer. International Journal of Gynecological Cancer. 2011;**21**(4):771-775. DOI: 10.1097/IGC.0b013e31821bb8aa

[58] Gonzalez-Martin AJ, Calvo E, Bover I, Rubio MJ, et al. Randomized phase II trial of carboplatin versus paclitaxel and carboplatin in platinum-sensitive recurrent advanced ovarian carcinoma: A GEICO (Grupo Espanol de Investigacion en Cancer de Ovario) study. Annals of Oncology. 2005;**16**(5):749-755. DOI: 10.1093/annonc/mdi147

[59] Parmar MK, Ledermann JA, Colombo N, du Bois A, et al. Paclitaxel plus platinum-based chemotherapy versus conventional platinum-based chemotherapy in women with relapsed ovarian cancer: The ICON4/AGO-OVAR-2.2 trial. Lancet. 2003;**361**(9375):2099-2106

[60] Pfisterer J, Plante M, Vergote I, du Bois A, et al. Gemcitabine plus carboplatin compared with carboplatin in patients with platinum-sensitive recurrent ovarian cancer: An intergroup trial of the AGO-OVAR, the NCIC CTG, and the EORTC GCG. Journal of Clinical Oncology. 2006;**24**(29):4699-4707. DOI: 10.1200/JCO.2006.06.0913

[61] Pujade-Lauraine E, Wagner U, Aavall-Lundqvist E, Gebski V, et al. Pegylated liposomal doxorubicin and carboplatin compared with paclitaxel and carboplatin for patients with platinum-sensitive ovarian cancer in late relapse. Journal of Clinical Oncology. 2010;**28**(20):3323-3329. DOI: 10.1200/JCO.2009.25.7519

[62] Bast RC Jr, Markman M. Chemotherapy: A new standard combination for recurrent ovarian cancer? Nature Reviews. Clinical Oncology. 2010;**7**(10):559-560. DOI: 10.1038/ nrclinonc.2010.152

[63] Aghajanian C, Blank SV, Goff BA, Judson PL, et al. OCEANS: A randomized, double-blind, placebo-controlled phase III trial of chemotherapy with or without bevacizumab in patients with platinum-sensitive recurrent epithelial ovarian, primary peritoneal, or fallopian tube cancer. Journal of Clinical Oncology. 2012;**30**(17):2039-2045. DOI: 10.1200/ JCO.2012.42.0505

[64] Monk BJ, Herzog TJ, Kaye SB, Krasner CN, et al. Trabectedin plus pegylated liposomal doxorubicin in recurrent ovarian cancer. Journal of Clinical Oncology. 2010;**28**(19):3107-3114. DOI: 10.1200/JCO.2009.25.4037

[65] Fung-Kee-Fung M, Oliver T, Elit L, Oza A, et al. Optimal chemotherapy treatment for women with recurrent ovarian cancer. Current Oncology. 2007;**14**(5):195-208

[66] Gordon AN, Tonda M, Sun S, Rackoff W, et al. Long-term survival advantage for women treated with pegylated liposomal doxorubicin compared with topotecan in a phase 3 randomized study of recurrent and refractory epithelial ovarian cancer. Gynecologic Oncology. 2004;**95**(1):1-8. DOI: 10.1016/j.ygyno.2004.07.011

[67] Gynecologic Oncology G, Markman M, Blessing J, Rubin SC, et al. Phase II trial of weekly paclitaxel (80 mg/m^2) in platinum and paclitaxel-resistant ovarian and primary peritoneal cancers: A Gynecologic Oncology Group study. Gynecologic Oncology. 2006; **101**(3):436-440. DOI: 10.1016/j.ygyno.2005.10.036

[68] ten Bokkel Huinink W, Gore M, Carmichael J, Gordon A, et al. Topotecan versus paclitaxel for the treatment of recurrent epithelial ovarian cancer. Journal of Clinical Oncology. 1997;**15**(6):2183-2193. DOI: 10.1200/JCO.1997.15.6.2183

[69] Friedlander M, Millward MJ, Bell D, Bugat R, et al. A phase II study of gemcitabine in platinum pre-treated patients with advanced epithelial ovarian cancer. Annals of Oncology. 1998;**9**(12):1343-1345

[70] Burger RA, Sill MW, Monk BJ, Greer BE, et al. Phase II trial of bevacizumab in persistent or recurrent epithelial ovarian cancer or primary peritoneal cancer: A Gynecologic Oncology Group Study. Journal of Clinical Oncology. 2007;**25**(33):5165-5171. DOI: 10. 1200/JCO.2007.11.5345

[71] Cannistra SA, Matulonis UA, Penson RT, Hambleton J, et al. Phase II study of bevacizumab in patients with platinum-resistant ovarian cancer or peritoneal serous cancer. Journal of Clinical Oncology. 2007;**25**(33):5180-5186. DOI: 10.1200/JCO.2007.12.0782

[72] Berkenblit A, Seiden MV, Matulonis UA, Penson RT, et al. A phase II trial of weekly docetaxel in patients with platinum-resistant epithelial ovarian, primary peritoneal serous cancer, or fallopian tube cancer. Gynecologic Oncology. 2004;**95**(3):624-631. DOI: 10.1016/j.ygyno.2004.08.028

[73] Rose PG, Blessing JA, Mayer AR, Homesley HD. Prolonged oral etoposide as second-line therapy for platinum-resistant and platinum-sensitive ovarian carcinoma: A

Gynecologic Oncology Group study. Journal of Clinical Oncology. 1998;**16**(2):405-410. DOI: 10.1200/JCO.1998.16.2.405

[74] Ray-Coquard I, Oaknin A, Linossi C, Kandalaft L. New targeted therapies and development. In: Poveda A, editor. 100 Key Questions on Ovarian Cancer. Barcelona (Spain): Permanyer; 2015

[75] Pujade-Lauraine E, Hilpert F, Weber B, Reuss A, et al. Bevacizumab combined with chemotherapy for platinum-resistant recurrent ovarian cancer: The AURELIA open-label randomized phase III trial. Journal of Clinical Oncology. 2014;**32**(13):1302-1308. DOI: 10.1200/JCO.2013.51.4489

[76] Ledermann J, Harter P, Gourley C, Friedlander M, et al. Olaparib maintenance therapy in patients with platinum-sensitive relapsed serous ovarian cancer: A preplanned retrospective analysis of outcomes by BRCA status in a randomised phase 2 trial. The Lancet Oncology. 2014;**15**(8):852-861. DOI: 10.1016/S1470-2045(14)70228-1

[77] Fong PC, Yap TA, Boss DS, Carden CP, et al. Poly(ADP)-ribose polymerase inhibition: Frequent durable responses in BRCA carrier ovarian cancer correlating with platinum-free interval. Journal of Clinical Oncology. 2010;**28**(15):2512-2519. DOI: 10.1200/JCO.2009.26.9589

[78] Ledermann JA. PARP inhibitors in ovarian cancer. Annals of Oncology. 2016;**27**(Suppl 1): i40-i44. DOI: 10.1093/annonc/mdw094

[79] Farmer H, McCabe N, Lord CJ, Tutt AN, et al. Targeting the DNA repair defect in BRCA mutant cells as a therapeutic strategy. Nature. 2005;**434**(7035):917-921. DOI: 10.1038/nature03445

[80] Helleday T, Petermann E, Lundin C, Hodgson B, et al. DNA repair pathways as targets for cancer therapy. Nature Reviews. Cancer. 2008;**8**(3):193-204. DOI: 10.1038/nrc2342

[81] Brunen D, Bernards R. Drug therapy: Exploiting synthetic lethality to improve cancer therapy. Nature Reviews. Clinical Oncology. 2017;**14**(6):331-332. DOI: 10.1038/nrclinonc.2017.46

[82] Drew Y, Ledermann J, Hall G, Rea D, et al. Phase 2 multicentre trial investigating intermittent and continuous dosing schedules of the poly(ADP-ribose) polymerase inhibitor rucaparib in germline BRCA mutation carriers with advanced ovarian and breast cancer. British Journal of Cancer. 2016;**114**(12):e21. DOI: 10.1038/bjc.2016.133

[83] Mirza MR, Monk BJ, Herrstedt J, Oza AM, et al. Niraparib maintenance therapy in platinum-sensitive, recurrent ovarian cancer. The New England Journal of Medicine. 2016;**375**(22):2154-2164. DOI: 10.1056/NEJMoa1611310

[84] US National Library of Medicine. 2017. Available from: https://www.clinicaltrials.gov/ct2/show/NCT01874353

[85] US National Library of Medicine. 2017. Available from: http://www.clinicaltrials.gov/ct2/show/NCT01844986

[86] Bindra RS, Gibson SL, Meng A, Westermark U, et al. Hypoxia-induced down-regulation of BRCA1 expression by E2Fs. Cancer Research. 2005;**65**(24):11597-11604. DOI: 10.1158/0008-5472.CAN-05-2119

[87] Chan N, Pires IM, Bencokova Z, Coackley C, et al. Contextual synthetic lethality of cancer cell kill based on the tumor microenvironment. Cancer Research. 2010;**70**(20):8045-8054. DOI: 10.1158/0008-5472.CAN-10-2352

[88] Liu JF, Tolaney SM, Birrer M, Fleming GF, et al. A phase 1 trial of the poly(ADP-ribose) polymerase inhibitor olaparib (AZD2281) in combination with the anti-angiogenic cediranib (AZD2171) in recurrent epithelial ovarian or triple-negative breast cancer. European Journal of Cancer. 2013;**49**(14):2972-2978. DOI: 10.1016/j.ejca.2013.05.020

[89] Liu JF, Barry WT, Birrer M, Lee JM, et al. Combination cediranib and olaparib versus olaparib alone for women with recurrent platinum-sensitive ovarian cancer: A randomised phase 2 study. The Lancet Oncology. 2014;**15**(11):1207-1214. DOI: 10.1016/S1470-2045(14)70391-2

[90] Rustin GJ, Vergote I, Eisenhauer E, Pujade-Lauraine E, et al. Definitions for response and progression in ovarian cancer clinical trials incorporating RECIST 1.1 and CA 125 agreed by the Gynecological Cancer Intergroup (GCIG). International Journal of Gynecological Cancer. 2011;**21**(2):419-423. DOI: 10.1097/IGC.0b013e3182070f17

[91] Yang WL, Lu Z, Bast RC Jr. The role of biomarkers in the management of epithelial ovarian cancer. Expert Review of Molecular Diagnostics. 2017;**17**(6):577-591. DOI: 10.1080/14737159.2017.1326820

[92] Rustin GJ, van der Burg ME, Griffin CL, Guthrie D, et al. Early versus delayed treatment of relapsed ovarian cancer (MRC OV05/EORTC 55955): A randomised trial. Lancet. 2010;**376**(9747):1155-1163. DOI: 10.1016/S0140-6736(10)61268-8

[93] Colombo PE, Fabbro M, Theillet C, Bibeau F, et al. Sensitivity and resistance to treatment in the primary management of epithelial ovarian cancer. Critical Reviews in Oncology/Hematology. 2014;**89**(2):207-216. DOI: 10.1016/j.critrevonc.2013.08.017

[94] Yu L, Deng L, Li J, Zhang Y, et al. The prognostic value of vascular endothelial growth factor in ovarian cancer: A systematic review and meta-analysis. Gynecologic Oncology. 2013;**128**(2):391-396. DOI: 10.1016/j.ygyno.2012.11.002

[95] Birrer MJ, Choi YJ, Brady MF, Mannel RS, et al. Retrospective analysis of candidate predictive tumor biomarkers (BMs) for efficacy in the GOG-0218 trial evaluating frontline carboplatin-paclitaxel (CP) +/− bevacizumab (BEV) for epithelial ovarian cancer (EOC). Journal of Clinical Oncology. 2015;**33**(15 suppl; abstr 5505):5505. DOI: 10.1200/jco.2015.33.15_suppl.5505

[96] Collinson F, Hutchinson M, Craven RA, Cairns DA, et al. Predicting response to bevacizumab in ovarian cancer: A panel of potential biomarkers informing treatment selection. Clinical Cancer Research. 2013;**19**(18):5227-5239. DOI: 10.1158/1078-0432.CCR-13-0489

[97]   Lambrechts D, Lenz HJ, de Haas S, Carmeliet P, et al. Markers of response for the anti-angiogenic agent bevacizumab. Journal of Clinical Oncology. 2013;31(9):1219-1230. DOI: 10.1200/JCO.2012.46.2762

[98]   Secord AA, Nixon AB, Hurwitz HI. The search for biomarkers to direct antiangiogenic treatment in epithelial ovarian cancer. Gynecologic Oncology. 2014;135(2):349-358. DOI: 10.1016/j.ygyno.2014.08.033

[99]   Kaye SB, Lubinski J, Matulonis U, Ang JE, et al. Phase II, open-label, randomized, multicenter study comparing the efficacy and safety of olaparib, a poly (ADP-ribose) polymerase inhibitor, and pegylated liposomal doxorubicin in patients with BRCA1 or BRCA2 mutations and recurrent ovarian cancer. Journal of Clinical Oncology. 2012; 30(4):372-379. DOI: 10.1200/JCO.2011.36.9215

[100] Monk BJ, Ghatage P, Parekh T, Henitz E, et al. Effect of BRCA1 and XPG mutations on treatment response to trabectedin and pegylated liposomal doxorubicin in patients with advanced ovarian cancer: Exploratory analysis of the phase 3 OVA-301 study. Annals of Oncology. 2015;26(5):914-920. DOI: 10.1093/annonc/mdv071

[101] Konecny GE, Wang C, Hamidi H, Winterhoff B, et al. Prognostic and therapeutic relevance of molecular subtypes in high-grade serous ovarian cancer. Journal of the National Cancer Institute. 2014;106(10). DOI: 10.1093/jnci/dju249

[102] Winterhoff B, Hamidi H, Wang C, Kalli KR, et al. Molecular classification of high grade endometrioid and clear cell ovarian cancer using TCGA gene expression signatures. Gynecologic Oncology. 2016;141(1):95-100. DOI: 10.1016/j.ygyno.2016.02.023

[103] Verhaak RG, Tamayo P, Yang JY, Hubbard D, et al. Prognostically relevant gene signatures of high-grade serous ovarian carcinoma. The Journal of Clinical Investigation. 2013;123(1):517-525. DOI: 10.1172/JCI65833

[104] Swisher EM, Lin KK, Oza AM, Scott CL, et al. Rucaparib in relapsed, platinum-sensitive high-grade ovarian carcinoma (ARIEL2 Part 1): An international, multicentre, open-label, phase 2 trial. The Lancet Oncology. 2017;18(1):75-87. DOI: 10.1016/S1470-2045(16)30559-9

[105] Muggia F, Safra T. 'BRCAness' and its implications for platinum action in gynecologic cancer. Anticancer Research. 2014;34(2):551-556

[106] Lambrechts S, Lambrechts D, Despierre E, Van Nieuwenhuysen E, et al. Genetic variability in drug transport, metabolism or DNA repair affecting toxicity of chemotherapy in ovarian cancer. BMC Pharmacology and Toxicology. 2015;16:2. DOI: 10.1186/s40360-015-0001-5

[107] Paige AJ, Brown R. Pharmaco(epi)genomics in ovarian cancer. Pharmacogenomics. 2008;9(12):1825-1834. DOI: 10.2217/14622416.9.12.1825

[108] Assis J, Pereira C, Nogueira A, Pereira D, et al. Genetic variants as ovarian cancer first-line treatment hallmarks: A systematic review and meta-analysis. Cancer Treatment Reviews. 2017;61:35-52. DOI: 10.1016/j.ctrv.2017.10.001

[109] Pinto R, Assis J, Nogueira A, Pereira C, et al. Rethinking ovarian cancer genomics: Where genome-wide association studies stand? Pharmacogenomics. 2017;**18**(17):1611-1625. DOI: 10.2217/pgs-2017-0108

[110] Siddik ZH. Cisplatin: Mode of cytotoxic action and molecular basis of resistance. Oncogene. 2003;**22**(47):7265-7279. DOI: 10.1038/sj.onc.1206933

[111] Pereira D, Assis J, Gomes M, Nogueira A, et al. Improvement of a predictive model in ovarian cancer patients submitted to platinum-based chemotherapy: Implications of a GST activity profile. European Journal of Clinical Pharmacology. 2016;**72**(5):545-553. DOI: 10.1007/s00228-016-2015-3

[112] Medeiros R, Pereira D, Afonso N, Palmeira C, et al. Platinum/paclitaxel-based chemotherapy in advanced ovarian carcinoma: Glutathione S-transferase genetic polymorphisms as predictive biomarkers of disease outcome. International Journal of Clinical Oncology. 2003;**8**(3):156-161. DOI: 10.1007/s10147-003-0318-8

[113] Assis J, Pereira D, Medeiros R. Ovarian cancer and DNA repair: DNA ligase IV as a potential key. World Journal of Clinical Oncology. 2013;**4**(1):14-24. DOI: 10.5306/wjco.v4.i1.14

[114] Assis J, Pereira D, Gomes M, Marques D, et al. Influence of CYP3A4 genotypes in the outcome of serous ovarian cancer patients treated with first-line chemotherapy: Implication of a CYP3A4 activity profile. International Journal of Clinical and Experimental Medicine. 2013;**6**(7):552-561

[115] Santos AM, Sousa H, Portela C, Pereira D, et al. TP53 and P21 polymorphisms: Response to cisplatinum/paclitaxel-based chemotherapy in ovarian cancer. Biochemical and Biophysical Research Communications. 2006;**340**(1):256-262. DOI: 10.1016/j.bbrc.2005.11.176

[116] Pinto D, Pereira D, Portela C, da Silva JL, et al. The influence of HER2 genotypes as molecular markers in ovarian cancer outcome. Biochemical and Biophysical Research Communications. 2005;**335**(4):1173-1178. DOI: 10.1016/j.bbrc.2005.08.012

[117] Muggia FM, Braly PS, Brady MF, Sutton G, et al. Phase III randomized study of cisplatin versus paclitaxel versus cisplatin and paclitaxel in patients with suboptimal stage III or IV ovarian cancer: A gynecologic oncology group study. Journal of Clinical Oncology. 2000;**18**(1):106-115. DOI: 10.1200/JCO.2000.18.1.106

[118] Caiola E, Porcu L, Fruscio R, Giuliani D, et al. DNA-damage response gene polymorphisms and therapeutic outcomes in ovarian cancer. The Pharmacogenomics Journal. 2013;**13**(2):159-172. DOI: 10.1038/tpj.2011.50

[119] Gurwitz D, Pirmohamed M. Pharmacogenomics: The importance of accurate phenotypes. Pharmacogenomics. 2010;**11**(4):469-470. DOI: 10.2217/pgs.10.41

9

Chemotherapy for Primary and Recurrent Epithelial Ovarian Cancer

Nora Naqos

Abstract

Epithelial ovarian cancer is the second most common gynecological cancer. It causes more deaths despite advances in treatment over the last few decades. Following explorative surgery and after histological assessment, the tumor can be formally "staged" according to the size, extent and location of the cancer. Staging during surgery determines the appropriate treatment regimen and the long-term outcome (prognosis). Recommendations for treatment after surgery are dependent on the stage of the cancer. Chemotherapy is recommended after surgery for stage III or IV ovarian cancer; certain tumor factors determine its use in stage I or II disease.

Keywords: chemotherapy, ovarian cancer, recurrence

1. Introduction

Epithelial ovarian cancer is the second most common gynecological cancer. It causes more deaths despite advances in treatment over the last few decades.

Epithelial ovarian cancer is the most common histological subtype diagnosed, accounting for 80% of cases [1]. It arises from the coelomic epithelium, 75% are serous cystadenocarcinoma, other types are less frequent and include endometrioid, mucinous, Brenner transitional cell, clear cell and unclassified carcinomas. Germ cell and sex cord-stromal tumors represent the other 20% [1].

2. Staging

Following explorative surgery and after histological assessment, the tumor can be formally "staged" according to the size, extent and location of the cancer. Staging during surgery determines the appropriate treatment regimen and the long-term outcome (prognosis).

Recommendations for treatment after surgery are dependent on the stage of the cancer. Chemotherapy is recommended after surgery for stage III or IV ovarian cancer; certain tumor factors determine its use in stage I or II disease.

3. Chemotherapy in advanced and metastatic ovarian cancer

3.1. History of chemotherapy

Twenty years ago, patients with advanced ovarian cancer were treated most commonly with the alkylating agents such as cyclophosphamide, chlorambucil, thiotepa and melphalan, all as monotherapy. These drugs have resulted in overall objective response rates between 33 and 65% and complete clinical responses in nearly 20% of patients [2].

In 1970, cisplatin was established by Wiltshaw and Kroner [3] as one of the most active agents for ovarian cancer, with a reported overall response rate of 26.5% in 34 patients who were resistant to alkylating agents. Moreover, Young et al. [2] obtained objective responses (one was complete) in 29% of 25 patients refractory to alkylating agents.

The North Thames Cooperative Group reported in 1985 the results of the first randomized comparison of first-line cisplatin and an alkylating agent cyclophosphamide in women with advanced ovarian cancer, it demonstrated significantly longer survival and response duration rates in patients receiving platinum therapy [4].

3.2. Which platinum: carboplatin or cisplatin?

The meta-analysis of the advanced ovarian cancer trialists group and two trials comparing cisplatinum with cyclophosphamide and carboplatin + cyclophosphamide showed that cisplatin and carboplatin have the same activity in ovarian cancer [1].

3.3. What is the effective dose of platinum?

A retrospective review reported a significant correlation between the dose intensity of cisplatin and response rates and survival [4]. Data from 10 trials focusing on platinum agents in approximately 2000 patients showed improvements in outcomes with doses up to 25 mg/m^2/week [5]. When the dose is increased above this there is increasing toxicity but without any clinical benefit observed [5]. In respect to carboplatin, clinicians use AUC from 5 to 7.5 [1].

3.4. What drug should be combined with platinum (the role of taxane)?

3.4.1. Anthracycline

Five meta-analyses from 10 trials in 1702 patients compared cyclophosphamide plus cisplatin with cyclophosphamide, cisplatin and doxorubicine (C A P), a modest but significant improvement in survival was seen for the regimen using doxorubicine (overall hazard ratio 0.85, P 1/4 0.003) [5] . Most investigators in the United States abandoned the use of anthracycline in 1986 due to cardiotoxicity that may outweigh the clinical benefit [5].

3.4.2. Paclitaxel

A significant development in the treatment of ovarian cancer was the discovery of the taxane class of cytotoxics. Two randomized controlled trials of first-line cisplatin based dual therapy showed additional clinical benefit when cyclophosphamide was replaced by paclitaxel [6, 7].

The Gynecological Oncology Group (GOG) 111 trial studied 386 women with stage III suboptimally debulked or stage IV disease [6]. Whereas the intergroup OV10 trial had wider selection criteria and assessed 675 women with FIGO stage IIb, IIc, III or IV disease with or without successful debulking surgery [7].

In GOG 111, patients received paclitaxel at 135 mg/m^2 over 24 h with cisplatin at 75 mg/m^2 or cyclophosphamide at 750 mg/m^2 every 3 weeks for a total of 6 courses. The same drugs were studied in OV10 and paclitaxel was given at 175 mg/m^2 over 3 h. The median follow-up intervals were 38.5 and 37 months in the OV10 and GOG 111 studies, respectively; the combination of platinum and paclitaxel is more effective with respect to OS and PFS. Hence the chemotherapy regimen is based on this combination.

3.5. Carboplatin as a substitute for cisplatin

Regimens containing carboplatin and paclitaxel were generally better tolerated than cisplatin plus paclitaxel in three major studies in which the two doublets showed similar efficacity.

The Dutch/Danish study [8], treated 208 patients and Arbeitsgemeinschaft Gyneco-oncology (AGO) study [9] examined 798 patients (3 weekly paclitaxel at 175 or 185 mg/m^2 given over 3 h plus cisplatin at 75 mg/m^2 with carboplatin AUC 5 or 6 plus the same dose of paclitaxel). Patients in both studies had stage IIb, IV and were followed up for a median of 37 months [8]. The GOG 158 trial compared 792 eligible patients with optimal stage III disease given paclitaxel 135 mg/m^2 over 24 h added to cisplatin at 75 mg/m^2 with paclitaxel 175 mg/m^2 over 3 hrs added to carboplatin AUC 7.5 [10].

The final results from AGO, GOG 158 and Dutch/Danish study noted little difference between treatments in the median PFS (the median overall survival was similar between treatment arms in each study), toxicities were mainly as expected, paclitaxel plus carboplatin were better tolerated [8–10].

4. Neoadjuvant chemotherapy

Neoadjuvant chemotherapy (NAC) followed by interval debulking surgery (IDS) has been pro-posed in the management of advanced Epithelial ovarian cancer in order to increase the rate of complete optimal surgery with less surgical morbidity [11–13]. Reserved initially for unresect-able disease or for patients in bad and poor general condition, the use of NAC and IDS has increased over the past two decades and frequently the first debulking is now realized only after several cycles of chemotherapy [11, 13]. Vergote et al. [11] in a large phase III randomized trial including patients with advanced stages IIIc-IV reported the non-inferiority of interval surgery after 3 cycles of NAC compared to upfront surgery [11] s The hazard ratio for death (intention-to-treat analysis) in the group assigned to neoadjuvant chemotherapy followed by interval debulking was 0.98 (90% confidence interval [CI], 0.84–1.13; P = 0.01 for non-inferiority) [11].

However, in clinical practice, optimal surgical timing and selection criteria for neoadjuvant chemotherapy and interval surgery remain controversial. Retrospective studies and meta-analyses observed a large survival advantage for patients receiving initial and complete removal of all macroscopic tumors prior to chemotherapy [14]. Moreover, the quality of sur-gery was heterogeneous in the EORTC trial among participating centres with variations in surgical aggressiveness and rates of complete resection, residual tumor of 1 cm or less was achieved in 42% of patients in the primary cytoreduction arm and in 81% of patients in the NACT arm. In the intent to treat analysis, the NACT arm was non inferior to the primary surgery arm with respect to the primary outcome of overall survival [14]. This argument explains the comparatively low survival observed for those treated with upfront surgery in this study. Furthermore, retrospective data have also suggested that NAC and IDS compared to primary surgery may increase the risk of developing platinum-resistant disease and less sensitive recurrent disease [15]. A minimum of 6 cycles of treatment is recommended includ-ing at least 3 cycles of adjuvant therapy after interval debulking surgery [16].

5. Targeted therapy

The addition of bevacizumab (a humanized monoclonal antibody to VEGF) to first-line che-motherapy based on platinum-taxane in advanced ovarian cancer demonstrated a significant improvement of PFS. This was evaluated in GOG-218 [17] a phase 3 trial in which they ran-domly assigned patients with newly diagnosed stage III (incompletely resectable) or stage IV epithelial ovarian cancer who had debulking surgery to receive one of these three treatments:

1. Cycles 1–6: carboplatin, AUC 6 Paclitaxel, 175 mg/m^2 Placebo (starting in cycle 2) every 3 wk. Cycles 7–22: placebo every 3 weeks.

2. Cycles 1–6: carboplatin, AUC 6 Paclitaxel, 175 mg/m^2 Bevacizumab, 15 mg/kg (starting in cycle 2) every 3 weeks the Cycles from 7 to 22 patients received Placebo every 3 weeks.

3. Cycles 1–6: carboplatin, AUC 6 Paclitaxel, 175 mg/m^2 Bevacizumab, 15 mg/kg (starting in cycle 2) every 3 weeks the Cycles from 7 to 22 patients received Bevacizumab at 15 mg/kg every 3 weeks.

The median progression-free survival was 10.3 months in the control group, 11.2 in the bevacizumab-initiation group, and 14.1 in the bevacizumab-throughout group [18].

The administration of bevacizumab during and up to 10 months after paclitaxel and carboplatin chemotherapy prolongs the median progression-free survival by about 4 months in patients with advanced epithelial ovarian cancer [18].

Similar results were obtained in the ICON-7 trial [19] where a total of 1528 women from 11 countries were studied, 70% had stage IIIC or IV ovarian cancer. In this study patients were randomly assigned to carboplatin and paclitaxel (175 mg/m^2) every 3 weeks for 6 cycles, or to this regimen plus bevacizumab (7.5 mg/Kg), given every 3 weeks for 5 or 6 cycles and continued for 12 more cycles or until disease progression. The PFS at 36 months was 20.3 months with chemotherapy alone, as compared with 21.8 months with chemotherapy plus bevacizumab. In the updated analyses, PFS at 42 months was 22.4 months without bevacizumab versus 24.1 months with bevacizumab (P = 0.04); in patients at high risk for disease progression, the benefit was greater with bevacizumab than without it, with PFS at 42 months of 18.1 months with bevacizumab, versus 14.5 months with standard chemotherapy, with median overall survival of 36.6 and 28.8 months, respectively [19].

These observations suggest that effectiveness of anti-angiogenic therapy may be greater in more advanced disease. However this was not supported by other studies testing the impact of different anti-angiogenesis factors added to chemotherapy in advanced ovarian cancer [18]. Both pazopanib [20] and nindetanib [18] showed a significant increase in PFS in patients with small tumors. The PFS benefit of the addition of nindetanib to first-line chemotherapy resulted in a more pronounced effect in the non-high-risk subgroup (stage II or stage III and residual ≤1 c m) with 27.1 vs. 20.8 months. In contrast, there was no significant benefit noted for high risk patients (FIGO IV or stage III with residual tumors). Pazopanib as maintenance therapy after first line chemotherapy showed a significant advantage with respect to PFS compared to the control group 17.9 vs. 12.3 months, HR 0,77, P = 0.0021) [18].

6. Intraperitoneal chemotherapy

The peritoneal cavity is the most common route of ovarian cancer spread.

The rational for giving chemotherapy directly into the peritoneal cavity is supported by preclinical, pharmacodynamics and pharmacocinetic data [21]. Compared with intravenous (IV) treatment, intraperitoneal (IP) administration allows an increase in drug concentration inside the abdominal cavity.

In the majority of patients, epithelial ovarian cancer is confined to the peritoneal cavity at initial diagnosis and in recurrence [22]. As a result ovarian cancer is a good target for intraperitoneal therapy.

The hypothesis of improved effectiveness is explained by the increasing concentration of the cytotoxic agent in the tumor microenvironment. Analysis of intratumoral drug concentrations demonstrates that higher drug exposure is observed for lesions 2–3 mm or smaller when intraperitoneal administration is performed compared with intravenous infusion [23]. Moreover, avascular tumors are more exposed to higher drug concentrations with intraperitoneal rather than intravenous administration [24].

A meta-analysis of five clinical trials confirmed a benefit in OS for intraperitoneal chemotherapy [25]. This led to a National Cancer Institute alert in 1996 recommending that intraperitoneal chemotherapy should be considered in patients with small volume (<1 cm) or no residual disease after surgery [16]. However, this has not been adopted as a standard care of in the majority of institutions and countries due to its great toxicity [16].

7. Adjuvant chemotherapy in early stage disease

After surgery, there is still a risk that cancer cells remain and may return or spread to other organs of the body. Adjuvant chemotherapy is administered after surgery to destroy these cells and improve the chance of curing ovarian cancer and to decrease the risk of the death due to ovarian cancer.

A recent Cochrane meta-analyses of five prospective clinical trials (4 of 10 with platinum-based chemotherapy) demonstrated that chemotherapy is more beneficial than observation in patients with adequately staged early-stage ovarian cancer [26]. Patients who received adjuvant chemotherapy had better OS [hazard ratio (HR) 0.71; 95% confidence interval (CI) 0.53–0.93] and PFS (HR 0.67; 95% CI 0.53–0.84) than patients who did not receive adjuvant treatment [26].

Two-thirds of the patients included in the two major studies were suboptimally staged, in optimally staged patients, benefit for chemotherapy cannot be excluded, Long-term follow-up of the ICON 1 trial confirms the benefit of adjuvant chemotherapy, particularly in those patients at higher risk of recurrence (stage 1B/C grade 2/3, any grade 3 or clear-cell histology) [26].

Therefore, adjuvant chemotherapy should be recommended not only to suboptimally staged patients but also to those optimally staged at higher risk of recurrence [16].

8. Recurrent ovarian cancer

Recurrent ovarian cancer can be diagnosed by the appearance of new symptoms, radiologic evidence of recurrent disease or a rising CA-125 level in an asymptomatic patient.

In the past, treatment for recurrent ovarian cancer was given based on rising levels of tumor markers alone even without symptoms. However, a phase III randomized study (OV05-EORTC 55955) demonstrated no survival benefit of starting chemotherapy based on the increasing level of CA-125 alone and that quality of life may be improved by awaiting the appearance of symptoms or signs of ovarian cancer recurrence.

In this study treatment was delayed by a median of 4.8 months with no benefice on OS (HR 1.01; 95% CI 0.82–1.25; P = 0.91) [27]. Similarly, third-line treatment was started 4.6 months earlier in the patients who had regular CA 125 monitoring. Quality of life was lower in the early treatment group [27].

The choice of chemotherapy agents in recurrent disease is based on the response to first line treatment, the current symptoms; the time elapsed from last chemotherapy and the side effects of previous drugs administered.

The prognosis and the response to second-line therapy and subsequent lines depends in great part on the progression-free interval after the last dose of the preceding line of chemotherapy.

We define:

- Platinum-refractory disease when the progression occurs during treatment or within 4 weeks after the last dose.

- Platinum-resistant disease as a progression within 6 months of platinum-based therapy;

- Partially platinum-sensitive disease when the progression occurs between 6 and 12 months;

- Platinum-sensitive patients progressing with an interval of more than 12 months (GCIG Consensus) [28].

- For patients with platinum-sensitive recurrent ovarian cancer: carboplatin-doublet should be the treatment of choice [16].

A meta-analysis including four randomized trials confirmed an improvement in PFS with a HR of 0, 68 (95% CI 0.57–0.81) and OS with a HR of 0.8 (95% CI 0.64–1.0) [29].The phase III Calypso [30] trial compared two doublets, taxol and carboplatin vs. carboplatin with pegylated lipososmal doxorubicin (PLD). The PFS with the second regimen (11.3 months) was not inferior to the taxane-carboplatin (9.4 months, P < 0.001, HR = 0.82) [3]. However the PLD regimen was better tolerated because of the minimal incidence of neuropathy, alopecia, and arthralgia and with less hypersensitivity reactions [3].

Again, the selection between the different options of platinum-based doublets should be based on the previous toxicity profile and convenience of administration [16].

Bevacizumab (Avastin) has also been studied as a treatment option in patients with recurrent ovarian cancer. The phase III OCEANS [31], study performed in women with platinum-sensitive recurrent ovarian cancer compared gemcitabine plus carboplatin with or without bevacizumab for 10 cycles followed by bevacizumab alone until disease progression or toxicity as compared to placebo. Chemotherapy with bevacizumab improved PFS, 12 months with bevacizumab vs. 8 months in the placebo group, as well as the response rate (79 vs. 57%, P < 0.001) [31].

Regimens based on non-platinum combinations are another option for patients with platinum-sensitive disease. In a phase III randomized trial OVA 301 [32], PLD alone was compared with PLD combined with the Mariane-derived alkaloid trabectidin (Yondelis), this combination regimen improved the PFS [32], Median PFS was 7.3 months with trabectedin/PLD v 5.8 months with PLD (hazard ratio, 0.79; 95% CI, 0.65–0.96; P = 0.0190). Overall response rate (ORR) was 27.6% for trabectedin/PLD vs. 18.8% for PLD (P = 0.0080) [32].

It has been hypothesized that this benefit is due to the restoration of 'platinum-sensitivity' by prolonging the platinum- free interval. This is now being explored in two prospective randomized trials [16].

8.1. Maintenance therapy in platinum-sensitive recurrent ovarian cancer

Many clinical trials have evaluated the role of drugs aimed at prolonging the second remission. One of these is the OCEANS trial that demonstrated the role of bevacizumab as noted above in combination with chemotherapy and as maintenance therapy [31]. Chemotherapy with bevacizumab improved PFS, 12 months with bevacizumab vs. 8 months in the placebo group, as well as the response rate (79 vs. 57%, P < 0.001) [31].

In women with the BRCA mutation, the Poly-ADP ribose polymerase (PARP) inhibitor: rucaparib, olaparib is an active drug; a trial assessed olaparib in women with recurrent advanced ovarian cancer; the overall response rate was 34% (complete response, 2% and partial response, 32%) [33].

The FDA approved olaparib for patients with advanced ovarian cancer who have received treatment with 3 or more lines of chemotherapy and have germline BRCA mutation [34].

8.2. Platinum-resistant recurrent ovarian cancer

8.2.1. Treatment selection

In platinum-resistant recurrent cancer, patients should be treated with non-platinum based chemotherapy. The treatment aims to palliate symptoms, optimizing quality of life and prolonging life. In general in this case, response rates are low and the prognosis is poor.

We should use non cross-resistant agents and avoid toxicities based on side effects that have developed from previous therapies, in general higher response rates and PFS rates longer than 2–3 months are obtained with the use of combination regimens. But combination drugs is associated with higher toxicity without any improvement in OS compared with the use of single agent therapy [16]. In fact, for the platinum-resistant cancer, a treatment based on single agent is preferable since it may offer a balance between efficacy and toxicity.

8.2.1.1. Taxane

Many drugs have documented activity in platinum-resistant disease. In phase II and III trials, the use of single agent paclitaxel has permitted objective responses in 22–30% of patients [35].

8.2.1.2. Pegylated liposomal doxorubicin

A phase III trial compared PLD with topotecan [36] in women with recurrent ovarian cancer, patients were stratified prior to being randomized according to the platinum sensitivity of their tumor. Similar results were obtained for each of these regimens with respect to the overall RR (20 vs. 17%), time to progression (22 vs. 20 weeks) and median OS (60 vs. 56.7 weeks) [36]. PLD has resulted in a significant OS benefit with longer follow up, mainly for patients with platinum-sensitive disease, and PLD was found to be significantly superior to topotecan (P = 0.0.08) [36].

Compared with topotecan, PLD caused lower rates of neutropenia, thrombocytopenia and was associated with higher rates of hand foot syndrome and stomatitis [36].

8.2.1.3. Topotecan

Topotecan has similar efficacy to paclitaxel and PLD in the treatment of platinum-resistant recurrent ovarian cancer [36, 37]. Its use is usually associated with some degree of myelosuppression especially neutropenia.

Monochemotherapy is therefore the standard of early "platinum-resistant" relapse of ovarian cancers [16].

The use of bevacizumab was demonstrated in the AURELIA trial that showed an improved PFS in patients with platinum-resistant ovarian cancer treated with bevacizumab in combination with single agent chemotherapy when compared to treatment with chemotherapy alone (5.7 vs. 4 months) [38].

9. Summary

Chemotherapy is the first systemic treatment of epithelial ovarian cancer at all disease stages. It is based on platinum with paclitaxel in the adjuvant and neoadjuvant setting. In advanced stage cases chemotherapy with bevacizumab improved the response.

Most cases of newly diagnosed ovarian cancer will respond to initial therapy, but 80% or more will ultimately relapse and further chemotherapy may be indicated. Newer strategies involving gene testing such as BRCA has proven to be an important addition to the treatment strategy. The choice of treatment for recurrent disease is based on the duration of response to prior therapy, previous treatment toxicity and quality of life.

Author details

Nora Naqos

Address all correspondence to: noura.naqos@gmail.com

Department of Medical Oncology, Mohammed VI University Hospital of Marrakech, Morocco

References

[1] McGuire WP et al. Primary ovarian cancer chemotherapy: Current standards of care. British Journal of Cancer. 2003;**89**:S3-S8

[2] Young RC, Von Hoff DD, Gormley P, Makuch R, Cassidy J, Howser D, et al. Cis-dichlorodiammine platinum (II) for the treatment of advanced ovarian cancer. Cancer Treatment Reports. 1979;**63**:1539-1544

[3] Wiltshaw E, Kroner T. Phase II study of cis-dichlorodiammine platinum in advanced adenocarcinoma of the ovary. Cancer Treatment Reports. 1976;**60**(55):60

[4] Lambert HE, Berry RJ. High dose cisplatin compared with high dose cyclophosphamide in the management of advanced epithelial ovarian cancer (FIGO stages III and IV): Report from the North Thames Cooperative Group. BMJ (Clin Res Ed). 1985;**290**:889-893

[5] Ahern RP, Gore ME. Impact of doxorubicin on survival in advanced ovarian cancer. Journal of Clinical Oncology. 1995;**13**:726-732

[6] McGuire WP, Hoskins WJ, Brady MF, Kucera PR, Partridge EE, Look KY, et al. Cyclophosphamide and cisplatin compared with paclitaxel and cisplatin in patients with stage III and stage IV ovarian cancer. The New England Journal of Medicine. 1996;**334**:16

[7] Piccart MJ, Bertelsen K, James K, Cassidy J, Mangioni C, Simonsen E, et al. Ranomized intergroup trial of cisplatin paclitaxel vs cisplatin cyclophosphamide in women with advanced epithelial ovarian cancer: Three-year results. Journal of the National Cancer Institute. **92**:699-708

[8] Neijt JP, Engelholm SA, Tuxen MK, Sorensen PG. Exploratory phase III study of paclitaxel and cisplatin vs paclitaxel and carboplatin i n advanced ovarian cancer. Journal of Clinical Oncology. **18**:3084-3092

[9] Du Bois A, LuCK H, Meier W, Adams H-P, Mobus V, Costa S, et al. A randomized clinical trial of cisplatin/paclitaxel vs carboplatin/paclitaxel as first-line treatment of ovarian cancer. Journal of the National Cancer Institute. 2003;**95**:1320-1329

[10] Ozols RF, Bundy BN, Greer BE, et al. Phase III trial of carboplatin and paclitaxel compared with cisplatin and paclitaxel in patients with optimally resected stage III ovarian cancer: A gynecologic oncology group study. Journal of Clinical Oncology. **21**:3194-3200

[11] Vergote I, Trope CG, Amant F, Kristensen GB, Ehlen T, Johnson N, et al. Neoadjuvant chemotherapy or primary surgery in stage IIIC or IV ovarian cancer. The New England Journal of Medicine. 2010;**363**:94353

[12] Du Bois A, Reuss A, Pujade-Lauraine E, et al. Role of surgical outcome as prognostic factor in advanced epithelial ovarian cancer: A combined exploratory analysis of 3 prospectively randomized phase 3 multicenter trials: By the Arbeitsemeinschaft Gynaekologische Onkologie Studiengruppe Ovarialkarzinom (AGO-OVAR) and the Groupe d'Investigateurs Nationaux pour les etudes des cancers de l'Ovaire (GINECO). Cancer. 2009;**115**:123444

[13] Morice P, Dubernard G, Rey A, Atallah D, Pautier P, Pomel C, et al. Results of interv al debulking surgery compared with primary debulking surgery in advanced stage ovarian cancer. Journal of the American College of Surgeons. 2003;**197**:95563

[14] Chi DS, Musa F, Dao F, Zivanovic O, Sonoda Y, Leitao MM, et al. An analysis of patients with bulky advanced stage ovarian, tubal, and peritoneal carcinoma treated with primary debulking surgery (PDS) during an identical time period as the randomized EORTC NCIC trial of PDS vs neoadjuvant chemotherapy (NACT). Gynecologic Oncology. 2012; **124**:104

[15] Rauh-Hain JA, Nitschmann CC, Worley MJ Jr, BradFord LS, BerkOwitz RS, Schorge JO, et al. Platinum resistance after neoadjuvant chemotherapy compared to primary surgery in patients with advanced epithelial ovarian carcinoma. Gynecologic Oncology. 2013;**129**:638

[16] Ledermann JA et al. Newly diagnosed and relapsed epithelial ovarian carcinoma: ESMO clinical practice guidelines for diagnosis, treatment and follow-up. Annals of Oncology. 2013;**24**(Supplement 6):vi24-vi32

[17] Burger RA, Brady MF, Bookman MA, et al. Incorporation of bevacizumab in the primary treatment of ovarian cancer. The New England Journal of Medicine. 2011;**365**:24732483

[18] Perren TJ, Swart AM, Pfisterer J, et al. A phase 3 trial of bevacizumab in ovarian cancer. The New England Journal of Medicine. 2011;**365**:24842496

[19] Ataseven B et al. FIGO stage IV epithelial ovarian, fallopian tube and peritoneal cancer revisited. Gynecologic Oncology. 2016

[20] du Bois A, Floquet A, Kim JW, et al. Incorporation of pazopanib in maintenance therapy of ovarian cancer. Journal of Clinical Oncology. 2014;**32**:33743382

[21] Wagner U, Marth C, Largillier R, Kaern J, et al. Final overall survival results of phase III GCIG CALYPSO trial of pegylated liposomal doxorubicin and carboplatin vs paclitaxel and carboplatin in platinum-sensitive ovarian canc er patients. British Journal of Cancer. 2012;**107**(4):588-591

[22] Markman M. Intraperitoneal chemotherapy in the management of malignant disease. Expert Review of Anticancer Therapy. 2001;**1**(1):142-148

[23] Helm CW. The role of hyperthermic intraperitoneal chemotherapy (HIPEC) in ovarian cancer. The Oncologist. 2009;**14**(7):683-694. Epub 2009 Jul 16

[24] Los G, Mutsaers PH, Lenglet WJ, Baldew GS, McVie JG. Platinum distribution in intraperitoneal tumors after intraperitoneal cisplatin treatment. Cancer Chemotherapy and Pharmacology. 1990;**25**(6):389-394

[25] Dedrick RL, Myers CE, Bungay PM, DeVita VT Jr. Pharmacokinetic rationale for peritoneal drug administration in the treatment of ovarian cancer. Cancer Treatment Reports. 1978;**62**(1):1

[26] Winter-Roach BA, Kitchener HC, Dickinson HO. Adjuvant (post-surgery) chemotherapy for early stage epithelial ovarian cancer. Cochrane Database of Systematic Reviews. 2009:CD004706

[27] Swart AC, On behalf of ICON collaborators. Long-term follow-up of women enrolled in a randomized trial of adjuvant chemotherapy for early stage ovarian cancer (ICON1). Journal of Clinical Oncology (Meeting Abstracts). 2007;**25**(18 suppl):Abstr 5509

[28] Rustin GJ, van der Burg ME, On behalf of MRC and EORTC collaborators. A randomized trial in ovarian cancer (OC) of early treatment of relapse based on CA125 level alone versus delayed treatment based on conventional clinical indicators (MRC OV05/EORTC 55955 trials). Journal of Clinical Oncology (Meeting Abstracts). 2009;**27**(18s):1

[29] Friedlander M, Trimble E, Tinker A, et al. Clinical trials in recurrent ovarian cancer. International Journal of Gynecological Cancer. 2011;**21**:771-775

[30] Raja FA, Counsell N, Colombo N, et al. Platinum combination chemotherapy versus platinum monotherapy in platinum-sensitive recurrent ovarian cancer: A metaanalysis of randomised trials using individual patients data (IPD). Annals of Oncology. 2012; **23**:abstr 982P

[31] Aghajanian C, Blank SV, Goff BA, Judson PL, et al. OCEANS: A randomied, double-blind, placebo-controlled phase III trial of chemotherapy with or without bevacizumab in patients with platinum-sensitive recurrent epithelial ovarian, primary peritoneal, or fallopian tube cancer. Journal of Clinical Oncology. 2012;**30**(17):2039-2045. DOI: 10.1200/ JCO.2012.42.0505. Epub 2012 Apr 23

[32] Monck BJ, Herzog TJ, Kaye SB, et al. Trabectedin plus pegyla - ted li posomal doxorubicin in recurrent ovarian cancer. Journal of Clinical Oncology. 2010;**28**:3107-3114

[33] Kaufman B, Shapira-Frommer R, et al. Olaparib monotherapy in patients with advanced cancer and germline BRCA 1/2 mutation. Journal of Clinical Oncology. 2015;**33**:244-250

[34] Butler T, Maravent S, et al. A review of 2014 cancer drug approvals with a look at 2015 and beyond. Pharmacy and Therapeutics. 2015;**40**:191-205

[35] Markman M, Hall J, Spitz D, et al. Phase II trial of weekly single-agent paclitaxel in platinum/paclitaxel-refractory ovarian cancer. Journal of Clinical Oncology. 2002;**20**(9): 2365-2369

[36] Gordon AN et al. Recurrent epithelial ovarian carcinoma: A randomized phase III study of pegylated liposomal doxorubicin versus topotecan. Journal of Clinical Oncology. 2001; **19**(14):3312-3322

[37] ten Bokkel Huinink W, Gore M, et al. Topotecan versus paclitaxel for the treatment of recurrent epithelial ovarian cancer. Journal of Clinical Oncology. 1997;**15**(6):2183-2193

[38] Pujade-Lauraine E, Hilpert F, Weber B, On behalf of the EnGOT- GCIG Investigators, et al. AURELIA: A randomized phase III trial evaluating bevacizumab combined with chemotherapy for platinum- resistant recurrent ovarian cancer. Journal of Clinical Oncology. 2012;**30**, Abst 5002ASCO

10

The Role of Circulating Biomarkers in the Early Diagnosis of Ovarian Cancer

Ece Gumusoglu and Tuba Gunel

Abstract

Ovarian cancer is the leading cause of gynecologic-related cancer death and epithelial ovarian cancer (EOC) is the most lethal sub-type. EOC is usually asymptomatic, and few screening tests are available. Diagnosis of ovarian cancer can be difficult because of the nonspecific symptoms. Despite the various diagnostic methods used, there is no reliable early diagnostic test and it needs to be developed. Specific biomarkers may have potential with the least possible invasive procedure. Biomarkers with a high sensitivity to ovarian cancer should be identified. Circulating biomarkers that are significant tools for non-invasive early diagnosis can be analyzed using circulating tumor cells, exosomes, and circulating nucleic acids. Protein, gene, metabolite, and miRNA-based biomarkers can be used for ovarian cancer diagnosis. As non-coding RNAs, MiRNAs may have an important role in ovarian cancer diagnosis due to their effects on mRNA expression levels. The most recent developments regarding the potential of circulating biomarkers to detect early ovarian cancer is presented in this chapter.

Keywords: ovarian cancer, biomarker, cell-free nucleic acids, early diagnosis, miRNA

1. Introduction

Ovarian cancer is a heterogeneous disease and the most important cause of gynecological cancer-induced deaths [1]. It is the fifth most important cause of cancer-related deaths among women in the world [2]. Different types of tumors may develop from each cell type. These tumors are epithelial tumors, germ cell tumors (originating from the ovary cell and follicular), and stromal tumors [3].

Molecular and cellular analyses of these tumor types may lead to earlier diagnosis of ovarian cancer and it is hoped better survival rates. Many factors play a role in the development of cancer, while genomic mutations and epigenetic changes are very important. For this reason, studies on mutations and epigenetic alterations may provide information about features such as early diagnosis, surveillance, and response to treatment.

2. Biomarkers used in the diagnosis of ovarian cancer

Tumor biomarkers are molecules that are produced by cancer cells or cells around them, which can be measured in body fluids or in the blood during the diagnosis, screening or treatment of cancer. Molecules that can be used as tumor biomarkers can be counted as cytoplasmic proteins, enzymes, hormones, surface antigens, receptors, oncofetal antigens (re-emerging proteins in cancer that is normally lost after birth), oncogenes or their products. An ideal tumor biomarker should be sensitive enough for early detection of small tumors while retaining the specificity of the identified cancer type. Unfortunately, however, today there is no known tumor biomarker carrying these features [4].

The features that should be found in an ideal tumor biomarker are given below [5]:

- It should have high specificity; it should be specific to only one type of tumor.

- Must have high sensitivity, should not be detected in cases of physiological or benign tumors.

- Levels should be proportional to tumor characteristics and size.

- The predictive and prognostic benefit of tumor biomarkers should be known.

- Half-life should be short, frequent and serial monitoring is possible.

- It should be cheap and easy to apply.

- Can be used as a screening test.

- Sample taking should be easy.

Potential biomarkers used in ovarian cancer are grouped as gene, protein, metabolite, and miRNA-based biomarkers according to their type [5].

The vast majority of ovarian tumors arise from the accumulation of genetic damage, but the specific genetic pathways that are involved in the development of epithelial, borderline, and malignant tumors are largely unknown. Considering the important relationship between genetic alterations and ovarian tumors, potential ovarian-cancer biomarkers can be found at gene-level (hereditary gene mutations, epigenetic changes, and gene expression) studies. The most common genes associated with epithelial ovarian cancer are shown in **Table 1** [6].

BRCA1, BRCA2, and Lynch syndrome genes show high penetrance and offer lifetime risks of 7–40% for ovarian cancer. Nowadays, the multigene panels used for clinical genetic testing

Gene	Gene full name	Protein class	Score[a]	No. of PMIDs[b]	No. of SNPs[c]
TP53	Tumor protein p53	Transcription factor	0.245958	144	2
CLDN7	Claudin 7	Cell junction protein	0.201099	5	0
ABO	ABO, alpha 1–3-N-acetylgalactosaminyltransferase and alpha 1–3-galactosyltransferase	Transferase	0.200549	3	0
SYNPO2	Synaptopodin 2	Cytoskeletal protein	0.200275	1	0
GPX6	Glutathione peroxidase 6	Oxidoreductase	0.200275	1	0
RSPO1	R-spondin 1		0.200275	1	0
WNT4	Wnt family member 4	Signaling molecule	0.200275	1	0
ATAD5	ATPase family, AAA domain containing 5	Nucleic acid binding	0.200275	1	0
EHMT2	Euchromatic histone lysine methyltransferase 2	Transferase; nucleic acid binding	0.2	1	0
MIR376C	MicroRNA 376c		0.2	1	0
BRCA1	BRCA1, DNA repair associated		0.02933	99	5
ERBB2	erb-b2 receptor tyrosine kinase 2		0.017792	57	0
BRCA2	BRCA2, DNA repair associated	Nucleic acid binding	0.01422	44	4
VEGFA	Vascular endothelial growth factor A	Signaling molecule	0.012847	39	0
MUC16	Mucin 16, cell-surface associated		0.009	25	0
EGFR	Epidermal growth factor receptor		0.008176	22	0
PIK3CA	Phosphatidylinositol-4,5-bisphosphate 3-kinase catalytic subunit alpha	Transferase; kinase	0.007627	20	3
PGR	Progesterone receptor	Transcription factor; receptor; nucleic acid binding	0.007287	10	0
ERCC1	ERCC excision repair 1, endonuclease non-catalytic subunit	Nucleic acid binding	0.007077	18	0
EGF	Epidermal growth factor	Extracellular matrix protein; receptor	0.006528	16	0
ESR1	Estrogen receptor 1	Transcription factor; receptor; nucleic acid binding	0.006528	16	0
IGF2	Insulin like growth factor 2		0.006253	15	1
NBR1	NBR1, autophagy cargo receptor		0.006044	22	0
CDKN1A	Cyclin dependent kinase inhibitor 1A	Enzyme modulator	0.005704	13	0
TNF	Tumor necrosis factor	Signaling molecule	0.005704	13	0
ABCB1	ATP binding cassette subfamily B member 1		0.005495	20	3

Gene	Gene full name	Protein class	Score[a]	No. of PMIDs[b]	No. of SNPs[c]
MLH1	mutL homolog 1	Nucleic acid binding	0.005154	11	0
PTGS2	Prostaglandin-endoperoxide synthase 2	Oxidoreductase	0.005154	11	1
BRAF	B-Raf proto-oncogene, serine/threonine kinase	Transferase; kinase	0.00488	10	1
CDKN2A	Cyclin dependent kinase inhibitor 2A	Enzyme modulator	0.004605	9	0

[a]Gene-Disease Score.

[b]Total Number of PubMed ID (PMIDs) Supporting the Association.

[c]The Number of Associated Single Nucleotide Polymorphism (SNPs).

Table 1. The most common genes associated with epithelial ovarian cancer.

include the mild-penetrance genes (lifetime risks of 6–13%) such as BRIP1, RAD51C, and RAD51D. The common low-penetrance susceptibility genes make up the rest of the genetic risk. Besides, SNPs have approximately 1% risk which is shown by population-based genome-wide association studies (GWASs) [7]. Expression analyses of quantitative or semi-quantitatively specific genes in serum or tumor tissue can potentially contribute to tumor recognition. In the last decade, analysis of gene expression has gained momentum due to improvements in microarray technology. This is because microarray technology enables analysis of tens or hundreds of gene expressions in a single piece of tissue. Gene expression profiling has focused on three main topics: the separation of tumor tissue by normal ovarian tissue, the identification of different subtypes of ovarian cancer, and the determination of cancer according to possible responses to treatment.

DNA methylation and histone modification are epigenetic mechanisms that play important roles in gene regulation, tumor formation, and progression. Measuring the rate of methylation in specific genes in the promoter region helps early detection of cancer, detection of disease progression, and prediction of therapeutic response. Identification of specific genes that change with epigenetic regulation is one of the areas that are actively studied in ovarian cancer. In this chapter, we want to focus on circulating biomarkers and other types of biomarkers will not be discussed.

3. Tumor materials in circulation: liquid biopsy and their biomarker potentials

Non-invasive tumor diagnosis and screening has become an important area of study. Contrary to tissue biopsy, through detection of circulating tumor cells (CTCs), tumor nucleic acids ("circulating tumor DNA/RNA"), and exosomes, predictive and prognostic markers may potentially be developed which is far less invasive. Hence early and multiple evaluations of the disease can be made, including retrospective follow-up, identification of treatment effects and investigation of clonal development. Isolation and characterization of CTCs, exosomes, and circulating tumor DNA (ctDNA) will improve cancer diagnosis, treatment, and imaging. Liquid biopsy can be performed "real-time" and at every stage of cancer. Although, it has some potential disadvantages such as; still is not certain to use in cancer diagnosis, difficulties in analysis of data obtaining from high-throughput screening and lack of data verification through clinical trials; it has significant potential for clinical cancer diagnosis in future [8].

3.1. Circulating tumor cells (CTCs)

Some cancer derived cells are detected in peripheral blood, and appear as solid tumor cells that have broken away into the circulation [9]. There are two main types of CTCs to explain this phenomenon. The majority are "Accidental CTCs", and these are CTCs that are passively pushed by external forces, such as tumor growth, mechanical forces during surgical operation or friction. The rest are CTCs which gain more plasticity and metastatic potential via the epithelial-mesenchymal transition (EMT) process [8]. These CTCs can stay in the non-divided form in the vein, can spread together, or settle into a new tissue to compose the metastatic deposit. Regardless of the CTC pathway, these cells carry important information about tumor composition, metastasis, drug sensitivity, and treatment.

CTCs have been demonstrated to have prognostic value among patients with breast, colorectal, gastric, lung, and pancreatic cancers in previous meta-analyses. However, the value of CTCs in ovarian cancer still remains controversial. Some studies did not observe any correlation between CTC status and prognosis. In contrast, other studies demonstrated an association Zhou et al. has shown that the prognostic value of CTCs was not associated with disease stage but with an elevated CA-125, both of which are known to correlate with prognosis either directly or indirectly. It has also been known that the CTC status was significant in respect to the overall survival (OS), progression-free survival (PFS), and disease-free survival (DFS) in ovarian cancer [10].

CTCs can be detected in both metastatic patients and patients with early, localized tumors. There is a significant potential for CTCs in the clinical management of cancers such as ovarian cancer. CTCs may enable real-time monitoring of treatment efficacy, identification of new therapy targets, and detecting and understanding drug resistance mechanisms [11]. CTC imaging and separation from leukocytes is dependent on reliable cell-surface markers. Based on the precipitation of CTCs in the low-speed centrifuge, the leukocyte fractions can be distinguished via physical features as well. Lee et al. used a nanoroughened microfluidic platform and detected CTCs in the sera of nearly all female participants (53/54, 98.1%) with ovarian cancer [12]. They also showed that although there is no relationship between CTC count and PFS in patients with newly diagnosed epithelial ovarian cancer (EOC), in patients with recurrent disease and chemoresistance; a relationship was found between CTC-cluster positivity and diminished OS [12]. It has been postulated that CTCs could result in metastatic progression and recurrence by way of epithelial-mesenchymal-transition (EMT) or development of stem-like features and hence a reduced OS. Therefore, researchers have tried to identify therapy-resistant tumor cells and to overcome treatment failure by analyzing CTCs transcriptional profiles [13]. In this study, the authors analyzed 15 single CTCs from 3 ovarian cancer patients and found them to be positive for stem cell (CD44, ALDH1A1, Nanog, Oct4) and EMT markers (N-cadherin, vimentin, Snai2, CD117, CD146) [13].

3.2. Circulating cell-free tumor DNA

Chang et al. were the first to examine the amount of cell-free DNA (cfDNA) in a patient's serum as a marker of disease presence in gynecologic malignancies [14, 15]. Cell free tumor DNAs (ctDNAs) circulate in the bloodstream and are derived from tumor cells. The presence of ctDNAs has been proven by detection of tumor-specific anomalies such as the presence of mutation in circulating tumor DNA (ctDNA), loss of heterozygosity of microsatellite, and methylation of CpG islands [16–18]. Similar to CTCs source; ctDNAs are released into the bloodstream in two ways: passively whereby ctDNAs from dead tumor cells and actively whereby ctDNAs are derived from live tumor cells spontaneously [8, 19]. ctDNA and apoptotic cell levels are lower in healthy individuals compared to cancer patients because chronic inflammation and excessive cell death cause accumulation of cell residues. cfDNA (cell-free DNA) is believed to originate from apoptotic cells content and found in elevated levels in cancer patients and related to higher tumor stage [20, 21].

The level of ctDNA is higher in the bloodstream of patients with solid tumors and metastatic disease compared to those without metastases [20, 21]. In patients with metastatic disease, the serum ctDNA level is higher (prevalence 86–100%) when compared to early-staged cancer types and patients with no radiographic evidence of disease (prevalence 49–78%) [20, 22]. Olsen et al. showed that in 86% of patients, ctDNA can be detected approximately 1 year before metastases while they are not observed in those clear of recurrence [23, 24] The anticipated short half-life of ctDNA of around 2 hours allows for an almost continuous analysis of tumor features including development, metastatic progression, and treatment efficacy. Thus, the identification of ctDNA has extraordinary potential as a potential biomarker for observing tumor load in the patient both prior and during treatment and in follow up [23].

Earlier studies in gynecological malignancies evaluated the presence of ctDNA at one time point using pelvic washings, ascites, serum, and plasma. Pereira et al. has demonstrated that serial estimation of ctDNA is a surveillance biomarker in gynecologic malignancies that is as sensitive and specific as the FDA-approved serum biomarker CA-125 [25]. Additionally, disease recurrence can be detected months earlier with ctDNA than CT checking [25]. Furthermore, the survival profiles of patients can be predicted with ctDNA level during the start of primary treatment, debulking surgery, and combined platinum/taxane doublet chemotherapy [25]. Both improved progression free and overall survival appear to be associated with undetectable levels of ctDNA [25] Additionally, ctDNA level maybe a stronger predictor than CA-125 of tumor size because of the longer half-life of CA-125 (9–44 days). It is also shown that in some patients, relapse of disease can be detected with ctDNA approximately 7 months before any CT scan changes [25]. Pereira et al. detected occult ovarian cancer cases by continuously monitoring the ctDNA even during apparent clinical remission [25]. These studies demonstrate that ctDNA could be used in early detection, it can act as a marker of disease stage as well as disease progression for gynecological cancers especially ovarian cancer.

Early diagnosis seems to be the best solution to reduce rates of ovarian cancer deaths unless highly effective drugs are developed with fewer side effects. Bettegowda et al. showed that for ctDNA detection in solid tumors, patients are treated at an earlier stage resulting in improved survival [21]. Moreover, even in stage I patients (usually curable with surgery alone), detection of ctDNA level can be observed in around 47% of all patients [21]. Using ctDNA-level analysis, ovarian cancer can be detected in around 70% of all stage III patients [21].

3.3. Circulating cell-free tumor RNA (ctRNA)

Cancer cells have a very specific gene expression profile which differs from normal tissues. These tumor-specific gene transcripts can be detected in the circulation of cancer patients [26]. Despite the high amount of RNase present in the blood, circulating RNAs have been found to be surprisingly stable. This can be explained by the possibility that RNA is destructively protected by exosomes (such as microparticles, microvesicles, multivesiculas) that pass through the cell membrane into the bloodstream [26]. In addition, these mRNAs that are present in blood can be used as prognostic and predictive biomarkers [27]. Similar to ctDNA, ctRNA requires further study to assess the exact value as a biomarker in ovarian cancer.

3.3.1. Circulating microRNAs

MicroRNAs (miRNAs) are RNAs that do not encode proteins, at about 22 nucleotides in length, but they are involved with translation suppression, mRNA degradation, or sequencing specific gene regulation. Thus these molecules regulate various biological processes such as development, cell proliferation, differentiation, and apoptosis [28]. Approximately 3% of human genes encode miRNAs, while about 30% of genes encoding protein are regulated by miRNAs. These miRNAs vary according to the type of each cell, the stage of development, and differentiation of the cell. The release and biological functions of extracellular miRNAs are still not fully understood [29].

It has been shown that blood miRNAs in cancer patients have the similar importance as the miRNAs in tissues, and the relationship between solid tumors and miRNA expression profiles in the blood have been investigated [30, 31]. Circulating miRNAs are not bonded to the cell but are protected against endogenous RNase breakdown by binding to microvesicles, exosomes, microparticles, apoptotic bodies, and protein-miRNA complexes [32]. MiRNAs are resistant to severe conditions such as high temperature, low/high pH, long-term storage, and over-applied freezing/thawing [29]. Measurement of circulating miRNA level is difficult because it can be contaminated with cellular miRNAs of different hematopoietic origin [29]. The isolation and stabilization protocols of circulating miRNAs should be standardized and the cancer patient's plasma should be selectively distinguishable at the single molecule level [33]. MiRNA expression varies in tumor tissue with respect to normal tissue, and these changes can be detected in serum/plasma samples of cancer patients when compared to healthy individuals [34]. Further work is needed because of the low level of difference detected [29]; however miRNA has been shown to play an important role in cancer development as a new oncogene or tumor-suppressor gene class that varies according to the target gene [35].

In eukaryotic cells, there are several stages in miRNA biogenesis stages (transcription, pri-miRNA clipping, pre-miRNA transport, and pre-miRNA cloning) [36, 37]. MiRNA expression levels vary from normal to ovarian cancer, with epigenetic changes, genetic changes (such as copy number changes), or differentiated expression of transcriptional factors, targeting miRNA genes. Transcriptional gene silencing in cancer cells is often associated with epigenetic defects [38, 39]. Studies have suggested that dysfunction or irregularity may occur in key proteins that are effective in miRNA biogenesis and may lead to tumor formation [39].

In recent years, many studies have been performed on the miRNA expression profile in EOC and it has been shown that there are significant differences in the miRNA expression profile compared to normal [35]. Iorio et al. compared 59 EOC operation samples with 15 normal ovarian species using a "custom" microarray and found 29 differently expressed miRNAs [35]. In EOC patients, miRNA expression profiles obtained from circulating tumor exosomes were compared with benign tumors and normal individuals and separated by different expression profiles. In this study, exosomes were separated by magnetic beads and anti-EPCAM antibodies, and miRNAs were analyzed by isolated microarray. As a result, there are several differentially expressed miRNAs in ovarian cancer samples [40]. In a study by Resnick et al., real-time PCR analysis of miRNA expression was performed on the serum collected from ovarian cancer patients and normal subjects, with different miRNAs expression found [41]. Patients with the three up-regulated miRNAs (miR-21, miR-92, and miR-93) were found to have a normal level of CA-125. Therefore, miRNA analysis may be complementary to other diagnostic methods [41].

It is clear that miRNAs play a crucial role in both normal and pathological processes due to their ability to regulate the expression of specific genes. However, no consensus has been reached as to the exact role/potential in diagnosis, metastasis, and prediction of response to treatment in EOC [28]. In addition, ovarian cancer is a heterogeneous disease, treatment and diagnostic options may vary from individual to individual; in this context, the tissue and origin specificity of miRNAs may be exploited and individualized treatment methods may be applied [42].

3.3.2. Circulating long non-coding RNAs

The Long Non-Coding RNAs (lncRNAs) are defined as >200 nucleotides in length and divided into five subclasses, which are intergenic, intronic, sense overlapping, anti-sense, and bidirectional lncRNAs [43]. LncRNAs are involved in various regulation processes which include protein-coding genes, functions at the level of splicing, chromatin remodeling, transcriptional control, and post-transcriptional processing after binding to DNA, RNA, or proteins [44]. These differ from tissue to tissue [45, 46] and lncRNAs play a role in growth, metabolism, and cancer metastasis [20, 47]. In several human cancer types, differentially expressed lncRNAs have been identified [48] which can be related to cancer metastasis and prognosis [49–51]. In addition, lncRNAs are specific for certain tumor origins such as the lymphatics, the cardiovascular or nervous system, circulating peripheral blood cells, or hematologic stem cells. Therefore, circulating lncRNAs may be informative about the tumor microenvironment [20, 52].

In ovarian cancer, lncRNAs have been shown to regulate several cancer processes such as development, metastasis, and relapse. Gao et al. [53] showed that a lncRNA named *HOST1* (human ovarian cancer-specific transcript 1) plays a role in key biological pathways of EOC through the stimulation of tumor cell migration, invasion, and proliferation by inhibiting let-7b which is one of the most important miRNA involved in EOC [54]. In another study, Tong et al. showed that a lncRNA named RP11-190D6.2 regulates the WW domain-containing oxidoreductase (*WWOX*) expression by acting like an antisense transcript of this gene [55]. WWOX is linked with poor prognosis in several cancers, including EOC [56]. In addition, RP11-190D6.2 appears to play a role in the regulation of tumor metastasis, thus it can be counted as a potential biomarker and therapeutic target for EOC [55]. Zhou et al. compared several lncRNA expression profiles in a large number of OvCa patients from TCGA and found an eight-lncRNA signature predictive of overall survival [57]. Moreover, using lncRNA expression profiles, they could separate similarly aged patient into high-risk and low-risk groups, identify good or poor survival potential of patients, the eight-lncRNA signature maintained independent prognostic value, and was significantly correlated with the response to chemotherapy [57]. In a separate study [51], examining the expression profiles of lncRNAs and mRNAs in the high-throughput molecular profiles of OV patients; they found a correlation between lncRNA and malignant OV progression. Therefore; they suggest that two specific lncRNAs (RP11-284 N8.3.1 and AC104699.1.1) as may be candidate biomarkers for prognosis [51]. Clearly further study is required to understand their clinical application as a biomarker in EOC.

3.3.3. Circulating Piwi RNAs(piRNA)

Piwi RNAs (PiRNAs) are single-stranded, 26–31 nucleotide long RNAs which may inhibit transposons and target mRNAs through the formation of the miRNA silencer complex (RISC). Post-transcriptional regulation of piRNA (piRISC) happens in the cytoplasm [58]. The piRISC protects the integrity of the genome from alterations made by transposable elements (TE)—by silencing them; mRNA and lncRNA are other targets of piRNA complexes [58, 59]. piRNAs pathways play an important role to regulate some cancer-related pathways such as DNA hypomethylation and transposable element (TE) derepression. *L1* is a piRNA pathway gene that regulates these pathways, also overexpression of these genes (PIWIL1 and 2), have been shown in several tumor tissues [60]. Lim et al. showed that overexpression piRNA pathway genes and L1 elements may have a role in EOC [60]. They compared the EOC tissues and cell lines to benign and normal ovaries and found overexpression of PIWIL1 and MAEL, known as a cancer/testis gene [61] which are two genes of piRNA pathway which is a germ-line-specific RNA silencing mechanism. In situ analysis indicated that L1, PIWIL1, PIWIL2, and MAEL are up-regulated in cancerous cells, while MAEL and PIWIL2 genes are expressed in the stromal cells lining tumor tissues as well. PIWI, MAEL genes are essential for Drosophila and other vertebrates' germ-line stem-cell differentiation [60, 62]. These gene changes may promote a change in cell composition or identity in the tissue surrounding the cancer cells [60]. Also cancer stem cells may have potential as a biomarker for stem-cell definition [60, 63].

In addition, synthetic piRNAs may offer a new therapeutic approach through their use in silencing the expression of cancer-related genes. This approach has an advantage over other miRNA-based blocking methods because it does not require extra components for processing such as Dicer [59].

3.4. Exosomes and circulating microvesicles

Exosomes are multivesicular endosomal-derived extracellular vesicles (EVs) which are 30–120 nm size [64–67]. Exosomes can be distinguished from microvesicles which are heterogeneous in size (50–1500 nm) and result from the plasma membrane directly via a budding mechanism [68, 69]. Exosomes include several molecules such as proteins, metabolites, RNAs (mRNA, miRNA, long non-coding RNA), DNAs (mtDNA, ssDNA, dsDNA), and lipids and are used in cell communication [64, 70, 71]. Similar to circulating microvesicles, exosomes have also been shown to have specific functions and play an important role in coagulation, intercellular signaling, and the management of debris. Both circulating parts of the cell are found in different body and interstitial fluids [72, 73].

Tumor-derived exosomes are different from circulating healthy exosomes in terms of number of exosomes, content, and also cell-surface proteins [74]. Exosomes can be detected and isolated with several markers especially cell-surface proteins including those found only in the primary tissue. TGF β1, MAGE 3/6 proteins have a cell-surface biomarker feature special for ovarian cancer. These markers can be detected by filtration and ultracentrifugation methods in ovarian cancer plasma samples and can be used for prognosis/therapy monitoring of disease [74, 77]. Exosome contents are variable for cancer types as well. Taylor et al. indicated that several ovarian cancer specific exosomal miRNAs, (miR-21, miR-141, miR-200a, miR-200c, miR-200b, miR-203, miR-205, miR-214), have been differentiated in serum samples by magnetic-activated cell-sorting (MACs) using anti-EpCAM array for diagnosis and screening of stage [40]. Exosomes are informative about tumor-specific features such as metastatic or benign form, stage, response to chemotherapies, and other drugs at that point in time via a possible blood sample [64].

Microvesicles have several common features with the primary cell such as membrane lipids, receptors, and diverse types of nucleic acids and proteins [75]. As in exosomes, microvesicles also have a potential to be biomarkers in several malignancies. Galindo-Hernandez et al. demonstrated that there were an increased number of microvesicles in breast cancer serum compared to healthy control samples [76]. It is also revealed that microvesicles derived from renal cancer stem cells include different miRNAs and mRNAs and these appear to play a function in tumor vascularization [75, 77, 78]. Microvesicles originated from tumor cells have been found in biological fluids in ovarian cancer. It has been shown that the number of microvesicles in malignant ovarian tumors is higher when compared to benign and nonmalignant pathologies (e.g., ovarian serous cysts, mucinous cystoadenomas, and fibromas) [79]. Ovarian cancer-induced ascites contains high levels of proteolytic enzymes such as matrix metalloproteinase (MMP-2, MMP-9) and urokinase-type plasminogen activator (uPA), which are the enzymes carried inside microvesicles [80–82]. Microvesicles may represent an ideal biomarker for ovarian cancer diagnosis and prognosis.

4. Biomarker detection technologies for ovarian cancer

High-throughput techniques of cellular transcriptome analysis mean that gene expression can be correlated with various aspects of disease in a variety of cancer types. This technology used today in ovarian cancer research, such as expression microarrays and CGH, Real-time PCR, and Next-Generation Sequencing (NGS) allow genome-wide scanning and the discovery of altered genes involved in cancer.

4.1. Real-time PCR

Cell-free nucleic acids reflect both normal and tumor-derived nucleic acids released into the circulation through cellular necrosis and apoptosis. Stroun et al. have demonstrated with Reverse Transcription Quantitative PCR (RT-qPCR) that there is a consistent correlation between tumor load and quantity of cell-free DNA detected in a wide range of malignancies including ovarian cancer [83]. Several studies in OC with free DNA have also shown that miRNAs are abnormally expressed. Initial studies identifying tumor-derived miRNAs in the circulation of OC patients was published by Taylor et al. [40]. Zou et al. identified nine differentially expressed microRNAs (microRNA199a-5p, microRNA199a-3p, microRNA199-b3p, microRNA-645, microRNA-335, microR-NA-18b, and microRNA-141) through qRT-PCR expression analysis in SKOV3/DDP and A2780/DDP cells and these agreed with microRNA chip results [84].

4.2. Microarray

Microarrays together with clustering analysis have allowed genome-wide expression patterns in a lot of cancer types to be deciphered and compared. Wong et al. studied a group of genes (CLDN7, EPHA1, FOXM1, and FGF7), for the validation of the microarray findings; these were selected as these genes were associated with the alteration of crucial pathways involved in the regulation of cell cycle and cell proliferation [85]. Liu et al. [86] using the bioinformatics analyses of mRNA expression profiles retrieved from the Oncomine and Gene Expression Omnibus (GEO) Profiles online databases, they enriched two biological processes (cell cycle- and microtubule-related) and identified six genes (ALDH1A2, ADH1B, NELL2, HBB, ABCA8, and HBA1) that all were associated with ovarian cancer progression.

4.3. Next-generation sequencing

Clinical cancer next-generation sequencing (NGS) assays are dependent on many software subsystems and databases to deliver their results. The building of software systems for clinical use is a mandatory requirement of reliability and reproducibility imposed by diagnostic laboratory accreditation bodies such as Clinical Laboratory Improvement Amendments (CLIA), National Association of Testing Authorities (NATA), and the International Organization for Standardization (ISO 15189).

Pinto et al. [87] validated the use of next-generation sequencing (NGS) for the detection of BRCA1/BRCA2 point mutations in a diagnostic setting and also investigated the role of other genes associated with hereditary breast and ovarian cancer in Portuguese families. They obtained 100% sensitivity and specificity (total of 506 variants) for the detection of BRCA1/BRCA2 point mutations with their bioinformatics pipeline using a targeted enrichment approach when compared to the gold standard Sanger sequencing.

5. Conclusion

Ovarian cancer is one of the most significant and fatal gynecological cancer types worldwide. The earlier this disease can be detected, the better the success of treating it. There are several detection methods for ovarian cancer, but molecular diagnosis methods are more accurate, faster, and suitable for early detection. Recent developments have focused on identifying biological material with newer technological devices and these have become more precise, reliable, and more widely available over a short period of time. Although molecular markers, which are specific for ovarian cancer, have been extensively studied, they are still not used in a clinical setting. Clearly a greater understanding of their mechanisms and specificities are needed before they can be applied to early detection of OC.

Liquid biopsy using body fluids (e.g. blood, urine, saliva, and ascites) to isolate and characterize CTCs, exosomes, circulating tumor DNA, RNAs, and circulating free small RNAs is a new technique used in the detection and treatment of several diseases. Clearly further investigation is required but it is hoped that this may become a very important tool for early detection of ovarian cancer. In addition, these biomarkers may become an important part of the clinical strategies used in cancer diagnosis, treatment, and imaging. In this chapter, their roles in the early detection and management of ovarian cancer have been discussed. It is hoped that as our understanding of these markers increases, we will see an improvement in the rate of early cancer detection and ultimately increased survival.

Author details

Ece Gumusoglu[1]* and Tuba Gunel[1,2]

*Address all correspondence to: ece.gumusoglu@istanbul.edu.tr

1 Faculty of Science, Molecular Biology and Genetics, Istanbul University, Istanbul, Turkey

2 Center for Research and Practice in Bio-technology and Genetic Engineering, Istanbul, Turkey

References

[1] Chu CS, Rubin SC. Screening for ovarian cancer in the general population. Best Practice & Research. Clinical Obstetrics & Gynaecology. 2006;**20**(2):307-320

[2] Allain DC. Genetic counseling and testing for common hereditary breast cancer syndromes: A paper from the 2007 William Beaumont hospital symposium on molecular pathology. The Journal of Molecular Diagnostics. 2008;**10**(5):383-395

[3] Berek JS, Crum C, Friedlander M. Cancer of the ovary, fallopian tube, and peritoneum. International Journal of Gynaecology and Obstetrics. 2015;**131**(Suppl 2):S111-S122

[4]   Burtis CA, Ashwood E, Bruns DE, Sawyer BG. Tietz Fundamentals of Clinical Chemistry; 2008

[5]   Sharma S. Tumor markers in clinical practice: General principles and guidelines. Indian Journal of Medical and Paediatric Oncology. 2009;**30**(1):1-8

[6]   Zhang S, Lin H, Kong S, Wang S, Wang H, Wang H, et al. Physiological and molecular determinants of embryo implantation. Molecular Aspects of Medicine. 2013;**34**(5):939-980

[7]   Rahman B, Side L, Gibbon S, Meisel SF, Fraser L, Gessler S, et al. Moving towards population-based genetic risk prediction for ovarian cancer. BJOG: An International Journal of Obstetrics and Gynaecology. 2017;**124**(6):855-858

[8]   Zhang W, Xia W, Lv Z, Ni C, Xin Y, Yang L. Liquid biopsy for cancer: Circulating tumor cells, circulating free DNA or exosomes? Cellular Physiology and Biochemistry. 2017; **41**(2):755-768

[9]   Joosse SA, Pantel K. Biologic challenges in the detection of circulating tumor cells. Cancer Research. 2013;**73**(1):8-11

[10]   Zhou Y, Bian B, Yuan X, Xie G, Ma Y, Shen L. Prognostic value of circulating tumor cells in ovarian cancer: A meta-analysis. PLoS One. 2015;**10**(6):e0130873

[11]   Kolostova K, Pinkas M, Cegan M, Matkowski R, Jakabova A, Pospisilova E, Svobodova P, Spicka J, Bobek V. Molecular characterization of circulating tumor cells in ovarian cancer. American Journal of Cancer Research. 2016;**6**(5):973-980

[12]   Lee M, Kim EJ, Cho Y, Kim S, Chung HH, Park NH, et al. Predictive value of circulating tumor cells (CTCs) captured by microfluidic device in patients with epithelial ovarian cancer. Gynecologic Oncology. 2017;**145**(2):361-365

[13]   Blassl C, Kuhlmann JD, Webers A, Wimberger P, Fehm T, Neubauer H. Single cell gene expression analysis of circulating tumor cells in ovarian cancer reveals CTCs co-expressing stem cell and mesenchymal markers. Geburtshilfe und Frauenheilkunde. 2016; **76**(10):P005

[14]   Chang H-W, Lee SM, Goodman SN, Singer G, Cho SKR, Sokoll LJ, et al. Assessment of plasma DNA levels, allelic imbalance, and CA 125 as diagnostic tests for cancer. JNCI: Journal of the National Cancer Institute. 2002;**94**(22):1697-1703

[15]   Kamat AA, Sood AK, Dang D, Gershenson DM, Simpson JL, Bischoff FZ. Quantification of total plasma cell-free DNA in ovarian cancer using real-time PCR. Annals of the New York Academy of Sciences. 2006;**1075**(1):230-234

[16]   Silva JM, Dominguez G, Villanueva MJ, Gonzalez R, Garcia JM, Corbacho C, et al. Aberrant DNA methylation of the p16INK4a gene in plasma DNA of breast cancer patients. British Journal of Cancer. 1999;**80**:1262

[17]   Esteller M, Sanchez-Cespedes M, Rosell R, Sidransky D, Baylin SB, Herman JG. Detection of aberrant promoter hypermethylation of tumor suppressor genes in serum DNA from non-small cell lung cancer patients. Cancer Research. 1999;**59**(1):67-70

[18] Nawroz H, Koch W, Anker P, Stroun M, Sidransky D. Microsatellite alterations in serum DNA of head and neck cancer patients. Nature Medicine. 1996;**2**(9):1035-1037

[19] Crowley E, Di Nicolantonio F, Loupakis F, Bardelli A. Liquid biopsy: Monitoring cancergenetics in the blood. Nature Reviews Clinical Oncology. 2013;**10**:472

[20] Rapisuwon S, Vietsch EE, Wellstein A. Circulating biomarkers to monitor cancer progression and treatment. Computational and Structural Biotechnology Journal. 2016;**14**:211-222

[21] Bettegowda C, Sausen M, Leary RJ, Kinde I, Wang Y, Agrawal N, et al. Detection of circulating tumor DNA in early- and late-stage human malignancies. Science Translational Medicine. 2014;**6**(224):224ra24

[22] Speicher MR, Pantel K. Tumor signatures in the blood. Nature Biotechnology. 2014;**32**(5):441-443

[23] Harris FR, Kovtun IV, Smadbeck J, Multinu F, Jatoi A, Kosari F, et al. Quantification of somatic chromosomal rearrangements in circulating cell-free DNA from ovarian cancers. Scientific Reports. 2016;**6**:29831

[24] Olsson E, Winter C, George A, Chen Y, Howlin J, Tang MH, et al. Serial monitoring of circulating tumor DNA in patients with primary breast cancer for detection of occult metastatic disease. EMBO Molecular Medicine. 2015;**7**(8):1034-1047

[25] Pereira E, Camacho-Vanegas O, Anand S, Sebra R, Catalina Camacho S, Garnar-Wortzel L, et al. Personalized circulating tumor DNA biomarkers dynamically predict treatment response and survival in gynecologic cancers. PLoS One. 2015;**10**(12):e0145754

[26] Zhou J, Shi YH, Fan J. Circulating cell-free nucleic acids: Promising biomarkers of hepatocellular carcinoma. Seminars in Oncology. 2012;**39**(4):440-448

[27] Pucciarelli S, Rampazzo E, Briarava M, Maretto I, Agostini M, Digito M, et al. Telomerespecific reverse transcriptase (hTERT) and cell-free RNA in plasma as predictors of pathologic tumor response in rectal cancer patients receiving neoadjuvant chemoradiotherapy. Annals of Surgical Oncology. 2012;**19**(9):3089-3096

[28] Zhang B, Cai FF, Zhong XY. An overview of biomarkers for the ovarian cancer diagnosis. European Journal of Obstetrics, Gynecology, and Reproductive Biology. 2011;**158**(2):119-123

[29] Gold B, Cankovic M, Furtado LV, Meier F, Gocke CD. Do circulating tumor cells, exosomes, and circulating tumor nucleic acids have clinical utility? The Journal of Molecular Diagnostics. 2015;**17**(3):209-224

[30] van Schooneveld E, Wouters MC, Van der Auwera I, Peeters DJ, Wildiers H, Van Dam PA, et al. Expression profiling of cancerous and normal breast tissues identifies microRNAs that are differentially expressed in serum from patients with (metastatic) breast cancer and healthy volunteers. Breast Cancer Research. 2012;**14**(1):R34

[31] Mitchell PS, Parkin RK, Kroh EM, Frits BR, Wyman SK, Pogosova-Agadjanyan EL, et al. Circulating microRNAs as stable blood-based markers for cancer detection. Proceedings of the National Academy of Sciences of the United States of America. 2008:105

[32] Vickers KC, Palmisano BT, Shoucri BM, Shamburek RD, Remaley AT. MicroRNAs are transported in plasma and delivered to recipient cells by high-density lipoproteins. Nature Cell Biology. 2011;**13**(4):423-433

[33] Hastings ML, Palma J, Duelli DM. Sensitive PCR-based quantitation of cell-free circulating microRNAs. Methods. 2012;**58**(2):144-150

[34] Godfrey AC, Xu Z, Weinberg CR, Getts RC, Wade PA, LA DR, et al. Serum microRNA expression as an early marker for breast cancer risk in prospectively collected samples from the Sister Study cohort. Breast Cancer Research : BCR. 2013;**15**(3):R42-R4R

[35] Iorio MV, Visone R, Di Leva G, Donati V, Petrocca F, Casalini P, et al. MicroRNA signatures in human ovarian cancer. Cancer Research. 2007;**67**(18):8699-8707

[36] Lee YS, Dutta A. MicroRNAs in cancer. Annual Review of Pathology. 2009;**4**:199-227

[37] Ozsolak F, Poling LL, Wang Z, Liu H, Liu XS, Roeder RG, et al. Chromatin structure analyses identify miRNA promoters. Genes & Development. 2008;**22**(22):3172-3183

[38] Soto-Reyes E, González-Barrios R, Cisneros-Soberanis F, Herrera-Goepfert R, Pérez V, Cantú D, et al. Disruption of CTCF at the miR-125b1 locus in gynecological cancers. BMC Cancer. 2012;**12**(1):40

[39] Zhang L, Volinia S, Bonome T, Calin GA, Greshock J, Yang N, et al. Genomic and epigenetic alterations deregulate microRNA expression in human epithelial ovarian cancer. Proceedings of the National Academy of Sciences. 2008;**105**(19):7004-7009

[40] Taylor DD, Gercel-Taylor C. MicroRNA signatures of tumor-derived exosomes as diagnostic biomarkers of ovarian cancer. Gynecologic Oncology. 2008;**110**(1):13-21

[41] Resnick KE, Alder H, Hagan JP, Richardson DL, Croce CM, Cohn DE. The detection of differentially expressed microRNAs from the serum of ovarian cancer patients using a novel real-time PCR platform. Gynecologic Oncology. 2009;**112**(1):55-59

[42] Hausler SF, Keller A, Chandran PA, Ziegler K, Zipp K, Heuer S, et al. Whole blood-derived miRNA profiles as potential new tools for ovarian cancer screening. British Journal of Cancer. 2010;**103**(5):693-700

[43] Archer K, Broskova Z, Bayoumi AS, Teoh JP, Davila A, Tang Y, et al. Long non-coding RNAs as master regulators in cardiovascular diseases. International Journal of Molecular Sciences. 2015;**16**(10):23651-23667

[44] Mercer TR, Dinger ME, Mattick JS. Long non-coding RNAs: Insights into functions. Nature Reviews Genetics. 2009;**10**:155

[45] Harrow J, Frankish A, Gonzalez JM, Tapanari E, Diekhans M, Kokocinski F, et al. GENCODE: The reference human genome annotation for the ENCODE project. Genome Research. 2012;**22**(9):1760-1774

[46] Derrien T, Johnson R, Bussotti G, Tanzer A, Djebali S, Tilgner H, et al. The GENCODE v7 catalog of human long noncoding RNAs: Analysis of their gene structure, evolution, and expression. Genome Research. 2012;**22**(9):1775-1789

[47] Silva A, Bullock M, Calin G. The clinical relevance of long non-coding RNAs in cancer. Cancers (Basel). 2015;**7**(4):2169-2182

[48] Yang TY. A simple rank product approach for analyzing two classes. Bioinformatics and Biology Insights. 2015;**9**:119-123

[49] Han L, Zhang EB, Yin DD, Kong R, Xu TP, Chen WM, et al. Low expression of long noncoding RNA PANDAR predicts a poor prognosis of non-small cell lung cancer and affects cell apoptosis by regulating Bcl-2. Cell Death & Disease. 2015;**6**:e1665

[50] Liz J, Esteller M. lncRNAs and microRNAs with a role in cancer development. Biochimica et Biophysica Acta. 2016;**1859**(1):169-176

[51] Guo Q, Cheng Y, Liang T, He Y, Ren C, Sun L, et al. Comprehensive analysis of lncRNA-mRNA co-expression patterns identifies immune-associated lncRNA biomarkers in ovarian cancer malignant progression. Scientific Reports. 2015;**5**:17683

[52] Arita T, Ichikawa D, Konishi H, Komatsu S, Shiozaki A, Shoda K, et al. Circulating long non-coding RNAs in plasma of patients with gastric cancer. Anticancer Research. 2013;**33**(8):3185-3193

[53] Gao Y, Meng H, Liu S, Hu J, Zhang Y, Jiao T, et al. LncRNA-HOST2 regulates cell biological behaviors in epithelial ovarian cancer through a mechanism involving microRNA let-7b. Human Molecular Genetics. 2015;**24**(3):841-852

[54] Yun J, Frankenberger CA, Kuo WL, Boelens MC, Eves EM, Cheng N, et al. Signalling pathway for RKIP and Let-7 regulates and predicts metastatic breast cancer. The EMBO Journal. 2011;**30**(21):4500-4514

[55] Tong W, Yang L, Yu Q, Yao J, He A. A new tumor suppressor lncRNA RP11-190D6.2 inhibits the proliferation, migration, and invasion of epithelial ovarian cancer cells. Onco Targets and Therapy. 2017;**10**:1227-1235

[56] Yan H, Tong J, Lin X, Han Q, Huang H. Effect of the WWOX gene on the regulation of the cell cycle and apoptosis in human ovarian cancer stem cells. Molecular Medicine Reports. 2015;**12**(2):1783-1788

[57] Zhou M, Sun Y, Sun Y, Xu W, Zhang Z, Zhao H, et al. Comprehensive analysis of lncRNA expression profiles reveals a novel lncRNA signature to discriminate nonequivalent outcomes in patients with ovarian cancer. Oncotarget. 2016;**7**(22):32433-32448

[58] Siomi MC, Sato K, Pezic D, Aravin AA. PIWI-interacting small RNAs: The vanguard of genome defence. Nature Reviews Molecular Cell Biology. 2011;**12**:246

[59] Assumpção CB, Calcagno DQ, Araújo TMT, Batista dos Santos SE, Ribeiro dos Santos ÂKC, Riggins GJ, et al. The role of piRNA and its potential clinical implications in cancer. Epigenomics. 2015;**7**(6):975-984

[60] Lim SL, Ricciardelli C, Oehler MK, Tan IM, Russell D, Grutzner F. Overexpression of piRNA pathway genes in epithelial ovarian cancer. PLoS One. 2014;9(6):e99687

[61] Xiao L, Wang Y, Zhou Y, Sun Y, Sun W, Wang L, et al. Identification of a novel human cancer/testis gene MAEL that is regulated by DNA methylation. Molecular Biology Reports. 2010;37(5):2355-2360

[62] Pek JW, Lim AK, Kai T. Drosophila maelstrom ensures proper germline stem cell lineage differentiation by repressing microRNA-7. Developmental Cell. 2009;17(3):417-424

[63] Foster R, Buckanovich RJ, Rueda BR. Ovarian cancer stem cells: Working towards the root of stemness. Cancer Letters. 2013;338(1):147-157

[64] Soung YH, Ford S, Zhang V, Chung J. Exosomes in cancer diagnostics. Cancers (Basel). 2017;9(1):1-11

[65] Tkach M, Thery C. Communication by extracellular vesicles: Where we are and where we need to go. Cell. 2016;164(6):1226-1232

[66] Théry C, Zitvogel L, Amigorena S. Exosomes: Composition, biogenesis and function. Nature Reviews Immunology. 2002;2:569

[67] Keller S, Sanderson MP, Stoeck A, Altevogt P. Exosomes: From biogenesis and secretion to biological function. Immunology Letters. 2006;107(2):102-108

[68] Colombo M, Raposo G, Thery C. Biogenesis, secretion, and intercellular interactions of exosomes and other extracellular vesicles. Annual Review of Cell and Developmental Biology. 2014;30:255-289

[69] Raposo G, Stoorvogel W. Extracellular vesicles: Exosomes, microvesicles, and friends. The Journal of Cell Biology. 2013;200(4):373-383

[70] El Andaloussi S, Mäger I, Breakefield XO, Wood MJA. Extracellular vesicles: Biology and emerging therapeutic opportunities. Nature Reviews Drug Discovery. 2013;12:347

[71] De Toro J, Herschlik L, Waldner C, Mongini C. Emerging roles of exosomes in normal and pathological conditions: New insights for diagnosis and therapeutic applications. Frontiers in Immunology. 2015;6:203

[72] Muralidharan-Chari V, Clancy JW, Sedgwick A, D'Souza-Schorey C. Microvesicles: Mediators of extracellular communication during cancer progression. Journal of Cell Science. 2010;123(10):1603-1611

[73] Camussi G, Deregibus MC, Bruno S, Cantaluppi V, Biancone L. Exosomes/microvesicles as a mechanism of cell-to-cell communication. Kidney International. 2010;78(9):838-848

[74] Szajnik M, Derbis M, Lach M, Patalas P, Michalak M, Drzewiecka H, et al. Exosomes in plasma of patients with ovarian carcinoma: Potential biomarkers of tumor progression and response to therapy. Gynecology & Obstetrics (Sunnyvale). 2013;(Suppl 4):3

[75] Verma M, Lam TK, Hebert E, Divi RL. Extracellular vesicles: Potential applications in cancer diagnosis, prognosis, and epidemiology. BMC Clinical Pathology. 2015;15:6

[76] Galindo-Hernandez O, Villegas-Comonfort S, Candanedo F, Gonzalez-Vazquez MC, Chavez-Ocana S, Jimenez-Villanueva X, et al. Elevated concentration of microvesicles isolated from peripheral blood in breast cancer patients. Archives of Medical Research. 2013;**44**(3):208-214

[77] Atala A. Re: Microvesicles released from human renal cancer stem cells stimulate angiogenesis and formation of lung premetastatic niche. The Journal of Urology. 2012; **187**(4):1506-1507

[78] Grange C, Tapparo M, Collino F, Vitillo L, Damasco C, Deregibus MC, et al. Microvesicles released from human renal cancer stem cells stimulate angiogenesis and formation of lung premetastatic niche. Cancer Research. 2011;**71**(15):5346-5356

[79] Ginestra A, Miceli D, Dolo V, Romano FM, Vittorelli ML. Membrane vesicles in ovarian cancer fluids: A new potential marker. Anticancer Research. 1999;**19**(4C):3439-3445

[80] Young TN, Rodriguez GC, Rinehart AR, Bast JRC, Pizzo SV, Stack MS. Characterization of gelatinases linked to extracellular matrix invasion in ovarian adenocarcinoma: Purification of matrix metalloproteinase 2. Gynecologic Oncology. 1996;**62**(1):89-99

[81] Dolo V, D'Ascenzo S, Violini S, Pompucci L, Festuccia C, Ginestra A, Vittorelli ML, Canevari S, Pavan A. Matrix-degrading proteinases are shed in membrane vesicles by ovarian cancer cells *in vivo* and *in vitro*. Clinical & Experimental Metastasis. 1999;**17**: 131-140

[82] Graves LE, Ariztia EV, Navari JR, Matzel HJ, Stack MS, Fishman DA. Proinvasive properties of ovarian cancer ascites-derived membrane vesicles. Cancer Research. 2004; **64**(19):7045-7049

[83] Stroun M, Maurice P, Vasioukhin V, Lyautey J, Lederrey C, Lefort F, et al. The origin and mechanism of circulating DNA. Annals of the New York Academy of Sciences. 2000;**906**(1):161-168

[84] Zou J, Yin F, Wang Q, Zhang W, Li L. Analysis of microarray-identified genes and microRNAs associated with drug resistance in ovarian cancer. International Journal of Clinical and Experimental Pathology. 2015;**8**(6):6847-6858

[85] Wong YL, Dali AZ, Mohamed Rose I, Jamal R, Mokhtar NM. Potential molecular signatures in epithelial ovarian cancer by genome wide expression profiling. Asia-Pacific Journal of Clinical Oncology. 2016;**12**(2):e259-e268

[86] Liu S, Goldstein RH, Scepansky EM, Rosenblatt M. Inhibition of rho-associated kinase signaling prevents breast cancer metastasis to human bone. Cancer Research. 2009;**69**(22): 8742-8751

[87] Pinto P, Paulo P, Santos C, Rocha P, Pinto C, Veiga I, et al. Implementation of next-generation sequencing for molecular diagnosis of hereditary breast and ovarian cancer highlights its genetic heterogeneity. Breast Cancer Research and Treatment. 2016;**159**(2): 245-256

Permissions

List of Contributors

Hans Nagar
Northern Ireland Cancer Centre, Belfast Trust, UK

Seiya Sato and Hiroaki Itamochi
Department of Obstetrics and Gynecology, Iwate Medical University School of Medicine, Iwate, Morioka, Japan

Joe R. Delaney and Dwayne G. Stupack
Division of Gynecologic Oncology, UCSD Department of Reproductive Medicine, UCSD Moores Cancer Center, USA

Olga Kurmyshkina
Laboratory of Molecular Genetics of Innate Immunity, Institute of High-Tech Biomedicine, Petrozavodsk State University, Petrozavodsk, Russian Federation

Pavel Kovchur
Department of Hospital Surgery, ENT Diseases, Ophthalmology, Dentistry, Oncology, Urology, Institute of Medicine, Petrozavodsk State University, Petrozavodsk, Russian Federation

Ludmila Schegoleva
Department of Applied Mathematics and Cybernetics, Institute of Mathematics and Information Technologies, Petrozavodsk State University, Petrozavodsk, Russian Federation

Tatyana Volkova
Department of Biomedical Chemistry, Immunology and Laboratory Diagnostics, Institute of Medicine, Petrozavodsk State University, Petrozavodsk, Russian Federation
Institute of High-Tech Biomedicine, Petrozavodsk State University, Petrozavodsk, Russia

Poonam Jani and Rema Iyer
Department of Gynaecological Oncology, Women's Health Directorate, East Kent Hospitals University NHS Foundation Trust, Kent, England, United Kingdom

Alda Pereira da Silva
Genetics Laboratory and Environmental Health of Faculty of Medicine of University of Lisbon, Lisbon, Portugal

Andreia Matos and Manuel Bicho
Genetics Laboratory and Environmental Health of Faculty of Medicine of University of Lisbon, Lisbon, Portugal
Instituto de Investigação Científica Bento da Rocha Cabral, Lisbon, Portugal

Maria Clara Bicho
Genetics Laboratory and Environmental Health of Faculty of Medicine of University of Lisbon, Lisbon, Portugal
Instituto de Investigação Científica Bento da Rocha Cabral, Lisbon, Portugal
Dermatology Research Unit, Instituto de Medicina Molecular, Lisboa, Portugal

Rui Medeiros
Faculty of Medicine, University of Porto, Portugal
Research Department, Portuguese League Against Cancer, CEBIMED, Portugal
Faculty of Health Sciences of the Fernando Pessoa University, Porto, Portugal

Andrey Khrunin and Svetlana Limborska
Department of Molecular Bases of Human Genetics, Institute of Molecular Genetics, Russian Academy of Sciences, Moscow, Russia

Alexey Moisseev
Institute of Modern Information Technologies in Medicine, Russian Academy of Sciences, Moscow, Russia

Vera Gorbunova
Department of Chemotherapy, N.N.Blokhin Cancer Research Centre, Ministry of Healthcare of the Russian Federation, Moscow, Russia

Joana Assis and Augusto Nogueira
Molecular Oncology and Viral Pathology Group-Research Center, Portuguese Institute of Oncology, Porto, Portugal
FMUP, Faculty of Medicine, Porto University, Porto, Portugal

Rui Medeiros
Molecular Oncology and Viral Pathology Group-Research Center, Portuguese Institute of Oncology, Porto, Portugal
Research Department, Portuguese League Against Cancer (NRNorte), Porto, Portugal
CEBIMED, Faculty of Health Sciences, Fernando Pessoa University, Porto, Portugal

Deolinda Pereira
Oncology Department, Portuguese Institute of Oncology, Porto, Portugal
ICBAS, Abel Salazar Institute for the Biomedical Sciences, Porto, Portugal

Nora Naqos
Department of Medical Oncology, Mohammed VI University Hospital of Marrakech, Morocco

Ece Gumusoglu
Faculty of Science, Molecular Biology and Genetics, Istanbul University, Istanbul, Turkey

Tuba Gunel
Faculty of Science, Molecular Biology and Genetics, Istanbul University, Istanbul, Turkey
Center for Research and Practice in Bio-technology and Genetic Engineering, Istanbul, Turkey

Index

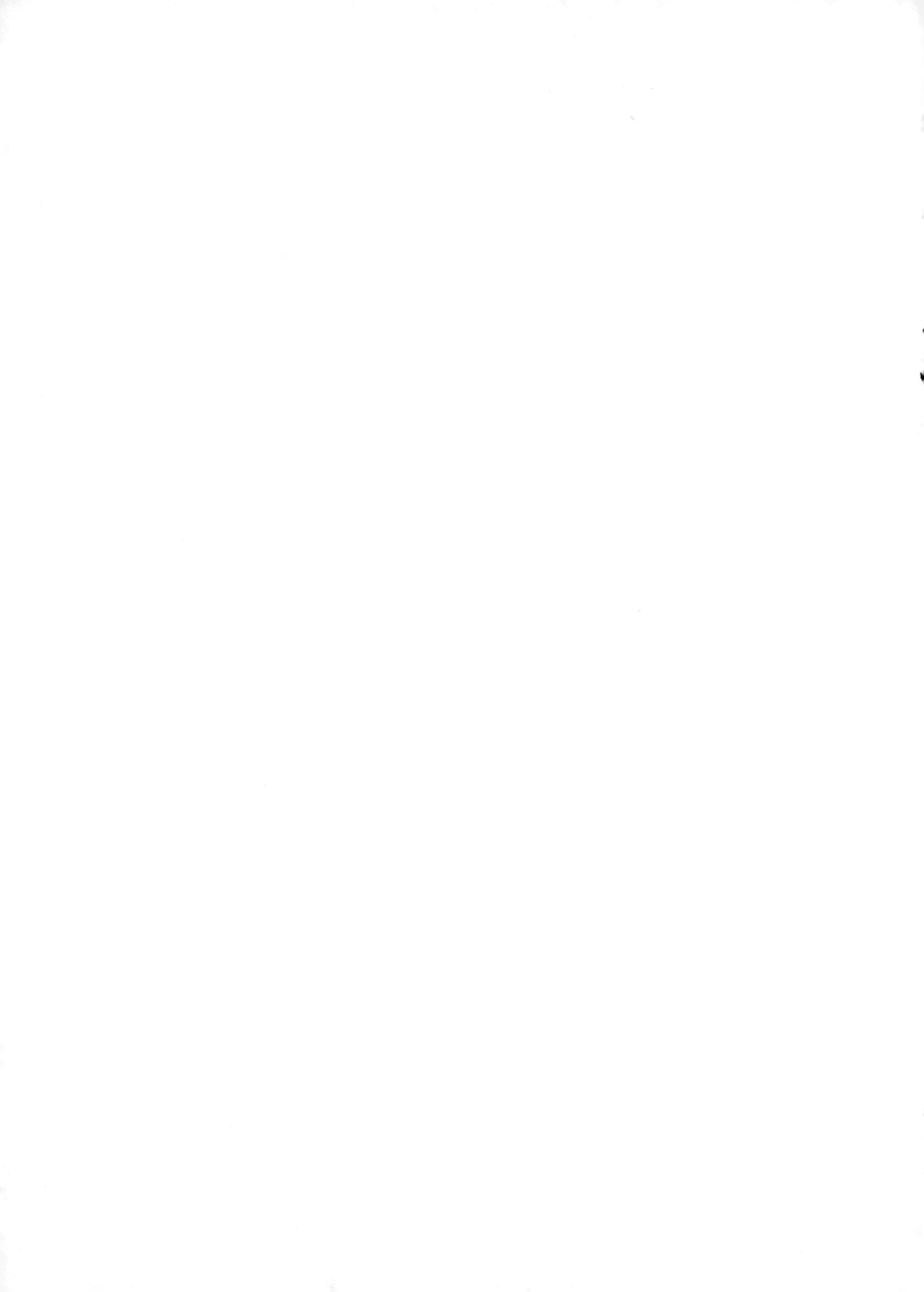

www.ingramcontent.com/pod-product-compliance
Lightning Source LLC
Chambersburg PA
CBHW080259230326
41458CB00097B/5178